Schizophrenia: An Issue of Psychiatric Clinics

Schizophrenia: An Issue of Psychiatric Clinics

Edited by **Willey Campbell**

FOSTER ACADEMICS
New Jersey

Published by Foster Academics,
61 Van Reypen Street,
Jersey City, NJ 07306, USA
www.fosteracademics.com

Schizophrenia: An Issue of Psychiatric Clinics
Edited by Willey Campbell

International Standard Book Number: 978-1-63242-451-8 (Hardback)

Printed in China.

Contents

	Preface	**IX**
Chapter 1	**Prolactin and Psychopathology in Schizophrenia: A Literature Review and Reappraisal** Ravi Philip Rajkumar	**1**
Chapter 2	**A Comparative Study between Olanzapine and Risperidone in the Management of Schizophrenia** Saeed Shoja Shafti and Mahsa Gilanipoor	**13**
Chapter 3	**Gender Identity Disorder and Schizophrenia: Neurodevelopmental Disorders with Common Causal Mechanisms?** Ravi Philip Rajkumar	**18**
Chapter 4	**Dimensional Information-Theoretic Measurement of Facial Emotion Expressions in Schizophrenia** Jihun Hamm, Amy Pinkham, Ruben C. Gur, Ragini Verma and Christian G. Kohler	**26**
Chapter 5	**Pomaglumetad Methionil (LY2140023 Monohydrate) and Aripiprazole in Patients with Schizophrenia: A Phase 3, Multicenter, Double-Blind Comparison** David H. Adams, Lu Zhang, Brian A. Millen, Bruce J. Kinon and Juan-Carlos Gomez	**36**
Chapter 6	**Vascular Endothelial Growth Factor and Brain-Derived Neurotrophic Factor in Quetiapine Treated First-Episode Psychosis** Brendan P. Murphy, Terence Y. Pang, Anthony J. Hannan, Tina-Marie Proffitt, Mirabel McConchie, Melissa Kerr, Connie Markulev, Colin O'Donnell, Patrick D. McGorry and Gregor E. Berger	**47**
Chapter 7	**The Impact of Childhood Adversity on the Clinical Features of Schizophrenia** Ravi Philip Rajkumar	**57**
Chapter 8	**Twenty Years of Schizophrenia Research in the Northern Finland Birth Cohort 1966: A Systematic Review** Erika Jääskeläinen, Marianne Haapea, Nina Rautio, Pauliina Juola, Matti Penttilä, Tanja Nordström, Ina Rissanen, Anja Husa, Emmi Keskinen, Riikka Marttila, Svetlana Filatova, Tiina-Mari Paaso, Jenni Koivukangas, Kristiina Moilanen, Matti Isohanni and Jouko Miettunen	**64**
Chapter 9	**Residual Negative Symptoms Differentiate Cognitive Performance in Clinically Stable Patients with Schizophrenia and Bipolar Disorder** Rajeev Krishnadas, Seethalakshmi Ramanathan, Eugene Wong, Ajita Nayak and Brian Moore	**76**

Chapter 10 **Arousal Predisposition as a Vulnerability Indicator for Psychosis: A General Population Online Stress Induction Study** 82
Annika Clamor, A. Malika Warmuth and Tania M. Lincoln

Chapter 11 **Long-Term Risperidone Treatment Induces Visceral Adiposity Associated with Hepatic Steatosis in Mice: A Magnetic Resonance Approach** 90
Florent Auger, Patrick Duriez, Françoise Martin-Nizard, Nicolas Durieux, Régis Bordet and Olivier Pétrault

Chapter 12 **Schizophrenia and Suicide Attempts: Findings from a Representative Community-Based Canadian Sample** 101
Esme Fuller-Thomson and Bailey Hollister

Chapter 13 **Delusional Disorder over the Reproductive Life Span: The Potential Influence of Menopause on the Clinical Course** 112
Alexandre González-Rodríguez, Oriol Molina-Andreu, Rafael Penadés, Marina Garriga, Alexandre Pons, Rosa Catalán and Miguel Bernardo

Chapter 14 **Irony and Proverb Comprehension in Schizophrenia: Do Female Patients "Dislike" Ironic Remarks?** 120
Alexander M. Rapp, Karin Langohr, Dorothee E. Mutschler and Barbara Wild

Chapter 15 **Parents' Experiences of Caring Responsibility for their Adult Child with Schizophrenia** 130
Ann Blomgren Mannerheim, Ulla Hellström Muhli and Eleni Siouta

Chapter 16 **Investigation of Anti-*Toxocara* and Anti-*Toxoplasma* Antibodies in Patients with Schizophrenia Disorder** 142
Shahram Khademvatan, Niloufar Khajeddin, Sakineh Izadi and Elham Yousefi

Chapter 17 **Not All Distraction is Bad: Working Memory Vulnerability to Implicit Socioemotional Distraction Correlates with Negative Symptoms and Functional Impairment in Psychosis** 149
Quintino R. Mano, Gregory G. Brown, Heline Mirzakhanian, Khalima Bolden, Kristen S. Cadenhead and Gregory A. Light

Chapter 18 **"Sometimes It's Difficult to Have a Normal Life": Results from a Qualitative Study Exploring Caregiver Burden in Schizophrenia** 155
Adam Gater, Diana Rofail, Chloe Tolley, Chris Marshall, Linda Abetz-Webb, Steven H. Zarit and Carmen Galani Berardo

Chapter 19 **Polyphenols from Berries of *Aronia melanocarpa* Reduce the Plasma Lipid Peroxidation Induced by Ziprasidone** 168
Anna Dietrich-Muszalska, Justyna Kopka and Bogdan Kontek

Chapter 20 **Explaining Attitudes and Adherence to Antipsychotic Medication: The Development of a Process Model** 175
Martin Wiesjahn, Esther Jung, Fabian Lamster, Winfried Rief and Tania M. Lincoln

Chapter 21 **Eating Disorders in Schizophrenia: Implications for Research and Management** 186
Youssef Kouidrat, Ali Amad, Jean-Daniel Lalau and Gwenole Loas

Chapter 22 **Effect of a System-Oriented Intervention on Compliance Problems in Schizophrenia: A Pragmatic Controlled Trial** 193
Hanne Skarsholm, Henrik Stoevring and Bent Nielsen

Chapter 23 **Traditional Knowledge and Formulations of Medicinal Plants used by the Traditional Medical Practitioners of Bangladesh to Treat Schizophrenia like Psychosis** **201**
Md. Nasir Ahmed and Md. Nur Kabidul Azam

Permissions

List of Contributors

Preface

Schizophrenia is the mental disorder caused by environmental and genetic factors. A schizophrenic person shows abnormal behavior and finds it difficult to conform to social norms. Symptoms include confused thinking, hallucinations, thought disorders, delusions and lack of motivation. Antipsychotics, coordinated special care and psychosocial treatments are some of the curative measures. This book discusses the fundamental as well as modern approaches towards schizophrenia. It collates contributions made by international experts which explore innovative aspects revolving around causes, diagnosis and treatment of this disorder. This book strives to provide a fair idea about this discipline and to help develop a better understanding of the latest advances within this field. Students, researchers, psychiatrists, experts and all associated with this area of study will benefit alike from this book.

This book is a result of research of several months to collate the most relevant data in the field.

When I was approached with the idea of this book and the proposal to edit it, I was overwhelmed. It gave me an opportunity to reach out to all those who share a common interest with me in this field. I had 3 main parameters for editing this text:

1. Accuracy – The data and information provided in this book should be up-to-date and valuable to the readers.
2. Structure – The data must be presented in a structured format for easy understanding and better grasping of the readers.
3. Universal Approach – This book not only targets students but also experts and innovators in the field, thus my aim was to present topics which are of use to all.

Thus, it took me a couple of months to finish the editing of this book.

I would like to make a special mention of my publisher who considered me worthy of this opportunity and also supported me throughout the editing process. I would also like to thank the editing team at the back-end who extended their help whenever required.

Editor

1

Prolactin and Psychopathology in Schizophrenia: A Literature Review and Reappraisal

Ravi Philip Rajkumar

Department of Psychiatry, Jawaharlal Institute of Postgraduate Medical Education and Research (JIPMER), Dhanvantari Nagar, 605 006 Pondicherry, India

Correspondence should be addressed to Ravi Philip Rajkumar; ravi.psych@gmail.com

Academic Editor: Brian Kirkpatrick

Secretion of the anterior pituitary hormone prolactin can be significantly increased by antipsychotic drugs, leading to a range of adverse effects in patients with schizophrenia. However, there is evidence from a variety of studies that prolactin may also be related to symptom profile and treatment response in these patients, and recent work has identified variations in prolactin secretion even in drug-free patients. In this paper, a selective review of all relevant studies pertaining to prolactin and schizophrenia, including challenge and provocation studies, is presented. The implications of this work are discussed critically. A tentative model, which synthesizes these findings and argues for a significant role for prolactin in the development of schizophrenia, is outlined.

1. Introduction

Prolactin is a polypeptide hormone secreted by the anterior pituitary gland. Prolactin has multiple functions, including lactation and maternal-infant bonding, in mammals. Recent work has found it to be relevant to parental and sexual behaviour in humans [1, 2] as well. Various factors, including gender, sexual activity, childbirth, stress, smoking, and drugs, can affect the release of prolactin [3, 4].

The production of prolactin is inhibited by dopamine release in the hypothalamo-pituitary circuit and can be increased by blocking type 2 (D_2) dopamine receptors. Most available antipsychotic drugs can therefore cause elevations in prolactin secretion. This increase is associated with a variety of adverse effects: lack of libido and erectile dysfunction in men [5], amenorrhoea and galactorrhoea in women [6], acceleration of osteoporosis in women [7], weight gain [8], and—potentially—an increased risk of cancer, particularly breast cancer in women [9]. The association of prolactin with male sexual dysfunction is complex and has been challenged by some authors [10] but is supported by research showing that antipsychotics which cause greater elevations in prolactin also have more marked sexual adverse effects [11]. Besides this, a variety of studies over the past four decades have examined other facets of the relationship between prolactin and schizophrenia and call for a reappraisal of this relationship. In this paper, the author highlights the important findings pertaining to prolactin and schizophrenia, excluding the literature on drug-induced hyperprolactinemia which has been extensively reviewed elsewhere. The author also proposes a model that may explain these findings. In the discussion that follows, the term "prolactin levels" refers to plasma prolactin, unless otherwise specified.

2. Studies of Prolactin Levels in Drug-Naïve Patients

As antipsychotic treatment generally causes hyperprolactinemia, measuring prolactin levels in drug-naïve patients is a useful method of assessing their relationship with schizophrenia itself. These studies are summarized in Table 1.

As seen from Table 1, the results of these studies are equivocal and are confounded by various methodological issues, including sampling time, gender, the use of medications, and the form of prolactin being assayed (total plasma, bioactive, or CSF). The two most recent studies to be published both

Table 1: Studies measuring prolactin levels in schizophrenia.

Study and authors	Patient sample	Results
Garcia-Rizo et al., 2012 [61]	Newly diagnosed patients with first-episode, nonaffective psychosis; comparison group of matched healthy controls	Significant elevation in prolactin even after controlling for confounders; more marked in women
Riecher-Rössler et al., 2013 [54]	74 antipsychotic-naïve patients with first-episode psychosis	39% of the study subjects had hyperprolactinemia
Warner et al., 2001 [62]	7 drug-free male patients with schizophrenia; 7 male controls	Lower levels of bioactive prolactin in the patient group
Rao et al., 1984 [63]	10 acutely ill patients with schizophrenia; 10 healthy controls	Lower levels of prolactin in patients; the authors also found lower levels of TSH and L-thyroxine
Kuruvilla et al., 1993 [64]	116 patients with schizophrenia; 120 healthy controls	No difference in prolactin levels between the two groups
Muck-Seler et al., 2004 [65]	20 women with schizophrenia drug-free for 7 days, compared with 25 depressed and 25 normal women	No difference in prolactin levels across the three groups
Rimon et al., 1981 [66] *(CSF prolactin)*	28 lobotomized and 28 nonlobotomized patients with "chronic schizophrenia"	Higher CSF prolactin levels in women and in nonlobotomized patients
Hyyppä et al., 1980 [67] *(CSF prolactin)*	Lobotomized and nonlobotomized patients with "chronic schizophrenia"	Higher CSF prolactin levels in nonlobotomized patients

found elevated plasma prolactin in drug-naïve patients with first-episode psychosis, while older studies found lower or equivalent levels.

3. Studies Reporting Relationships between Prolactin and Symptom Profile

The next question to be considered is whether elevated prolactin is related to specific symptoms or dimensions of schizophrenia, which is a multidimensional entity. Results of these studies are described in Table 2.

Examining the above studies yields a clearer, though not unequivocal, picture: there is a fairly consistent and negative association between plasma prolactin and surrogate measures of positive symptoms—such as specific delusions or the paranoid subtype of schizophrenia. Segal et al. [12] have interpreted these results in terms of increased dopaminergic tone in patients with paranoid symptoms, which is consistent with the dopamine hypothesis of schizophrenia. However, our interpretation remains confounded by the presence of studies with negative findings and by the variations in methodology adopted by different authors—particularly in terms of patient gender and the measures used to assess symptom dimensions.

4. Challenge and Provocative Test-Based Studies

Given the inconsistent results of studies measuring basal plasma prolactin, another fruitful line of enquiry would be assessing the prolactin response to various external stimuli in patients with schizophrenia, as these would give us a clearer notion of the physiological processes implicated in the altered levels. A variety of drugs—hormones, adrenergic agonists, serotonergic agonists, and dopamine antagonists—have been used to study prolactin release in patients with schizophrenia. The results of these studies are outlined in Table 3.

Some consistent findings emerge across these studies. A blunted prolactin response to pharmacological challenge in schizophrenia is documented across various classes of agents—adrenergic [13], serotonergic [14, 15], and dopaminergic [16–20]. However, these results are confounded by variables such as the dose of the pharmacological challenge, the effects of treatment, age and gender, and the duration of psychosis, and negative or inverse results have also been reported. With reference to drugs that inhibit prolactin release, results are more consistent, with many studies reporting a reduced suppression in patients [21–23]. Only one study has examined the effects of stress in this patient population and found a significantly greater increase in stress-stimulated prolactin in schizophrenia [24].

Relations with specific symptom dimensions have not been found consistently across studies. Positive correlations have been reported between the prolactin response to a serotonergic challenge and negative symptoms [25] as well as affective symptoms [26] and between prolactin release after TRH administration and thought disorder [27]. Negative correlations have been reported between prolactin response and inattention [28] as well as the severity of delusions [29]. Blunted prolactin responses have been associated with a "Kraepelinian" diagnosis of schizophrenia [17] and with schizophreniform disorder [20] in particular. A greater prolactin response to fenfluramine was associated with treatment resistance in one study [30]. Incidentally, one study found an association between a lower basal prolactin and positive symptoms [31], which is consistent with the results of Segal's studies [12, 32].

The interpretation of these findings is complicated by the wide range of potential mechanisms involved. The blunting of the prolactin response to dopamine antagonists [16–18] may indicate dopamine receptor supersensitivity,

TABLE 2: Studies examining the relationship between symptom profile and prolactin in schizophrenia.

Study and authors	Patient sample	Results
Segal et al., 2007 [12]	57 unmedicated male patients with schizophrenia (off medication for at least 3 months); 32 controls	Significantly lower prolactin levels in patients with the paranoid subtype of schizophrenia
Segal et al., 2004 [32]	48 first-episode and 38 recurrent patients with schizophrenia	Significantly lower prolactin levels in paranoid schizophrenia compared to schizoaffective and disorganized subtypes; no effect of illness duration on levels
Segal et al., 2007 [68]	45 male patients with schizophrenia, receiving risperidone	Significantly greater elevation of prolactin in patients with the paranoid subtype of schizophrenia
Otani et al., 1996 [69]	56 unmedicated patients with schizophrenia (28 male, 28 female)	Weak negative correlation between prolactin and hostility scores; no relation with other measures of psychopathology on the Brief Psychiatric Rating Scale
Newcomer et al., 1992 [70]	24 patients with schizophrenia on maintenance treatment with haloperidol	Significant positive correlation between prolactin levels and negative symptoms
Akhondzadeh et al., 2006 [71]	54 male patients with schizophrenia on maintenance treatment with haloperidol or risperidone; 25 healthy male controls	Significant positive correlation between prolactin levels and negative symptoms
Rinieris et al., 1985 [72]	Male patients with paranoid schizophrenia with or without "homosexual delusions"; healthy heterosexual controls	Lower prolactin levels associated with delusions having a homosexual content
Johnstone et al., 1977 [73]	16 unmedicated male patients with "chronic schizophrenia"	Serum prolactin was negatively correlated with both speech incoherence and total positive symptoms
Kleinman et al., 1982 [74]	17 drug-free patients with "chronic schizophrenia"	Inverse relationship between prolactin and total psychotic symptoms but only in those patients who did not show ventricular enlargement on computed tomography
Csernansky et al., 1986 [75]	33 male patients with schizophrenia on treatment; 8 off treatment; 18 normal male controls	"Prolactin index" (plasma prolactin divided by plasma neuroleptic activity) was negatively correlated with paranoid symptoms in younger patients receiving treatment
Prasad, 1986 [76]	13 patients off medication for 12 months: 4 with positive symptoms, 9 with negative symptoms	Higher prolactin levels in the group with positive symptoms
Luchins et al., 1984 [77]	23 patients with schizophrenia	No relationship between prolactin levels and psychopathology

while the worsening of positive symptoms [15] associated with a blunted response to serotonergic challenge may implicate reduced serotonin receptor sensitivity in these symptoms. In contrast, the exaggerated prolactin response to serotonin in resistant schizophrenia is indicative of serotonergic hyperfunction; this is consistent with the fact that clozapine, an antagonist at multiple serotonin receptors, is the treatment of choice in this population.

5. Studies Reporting Relationships between Prolactin and Treatment Response

As prolactin elevation is related to D_2 receptor blockade, prolactin may be a useful surrogate marker of the blockade achieved and thereby—in an indirect manner—of the efficacy of antipsychotic medications. Studies that have focused on this association are summarized in Table 4.

The results of the above studies suggest that there is a clear relationship between *changes* in prolactin level and the response to certain antipsychotics, with the best evidence pertaining to risperidone. The equivocal results obtained with other drugs may be related to the observation that prolactin has little predictive value beyond a certain "plateau" level [33] and may also reflect variables such as the effects of gender [34], the use of drugs with low dopamine antagonist activity [35], short treatment durations [36], small sample sizes [36–40], and the use of high doses of depot antipsychotics [38]. The suggestions that challenge tests can be used to assess the serotonergic effects of clozapine [41] and that plasma prolactin can be used to estimate therapeutic doses of dopamine antagonists [33] are both intriguing but require replication. Of note, some of the most relevant positive results have been obtained in male patients [33, 42, 43], suggesting that the utility of prolactin as a biomarker of drug response may be gender-specific.

TABLE 3: Results of studies examining prolactin response to pharmacological challenges in schizophrenia.

Study and authors	Agent used	Patient sample	Results
Spoov et al., 2010 [28]	Thyrotropin-releasing hormone (TRH), 12.5 mcg i.v.	19 drug-naïve patients with schizophrenia	Prolactin response negatively correlated with poverty of speech and inattention
Spoov et al., 1991 [27]	TRH, 12.5 mcg i.v.	20 patients with nonaffective psychosis	Prolactin response to TRH positively correlated with "nonparanoid" symptoms, such as thought disorder
Cabranes et al., 1982 [78]	TRH	Patients with acute and chronic schizophrenia treated with chlorpromazine for 14 days	Increased prolactin response to TRH following chlorpromazine treatment
Brambilla et al., 1976 [79]	TRH, 500 mcg i.v.	20 patients with chronic hebephrenic schizophrenia, off medication for at least 10 days; 8 healthy controls	Enhanced prolactin responses to TRH in patients, despite normal basal prolactin levels
Naber et al., 1980 [80]	TRH, 0.2 mg and luteinizing-hormone releasing hormone (LHRH), 0.025 mg	22 patients with chronic schizophrenia (10 male, 12 female) receiving antipsychotics for 6–21 years	Attenuated prolactin response to TRH with long-term treatment; no relation between TRH response and psychopathology
Mokrani et al., 2000 [13]	Clonidine, 0.35–0.375 mg depending on body weight	134 drug-free in-patients—31 schizophrenia, 16 schizoaffective, 87 major depression—and 22 controls	Blunted prolactin response to clonidine in patients with paranoid schizophrenia, compared to controls and patients with disorganized schizophrenia
Sharma et al., 1999 [25]	Fenfluramine, 60 mg orally	35 drug-free patients—28 schizophrenia, 7 schizoaffective	Significant positive correlation between prolactin response to fenfluramine and negative symptoms, as measured by the BPRS
Monteleone et al., 1999 [30]	Fenfluramine, 30 mg orally	16 drug-free patients with schizophrenia; 16 matched controls	Greater prolactin response to fenfluramine in patients with resistant schizophrenia as per Kane's criteria
Abel et al., 1996 [26]	d-Fenfluramine	13 drug-naïve patients with schizophrenia; 13 matched controls	Greater prolactin response in patients; positive correlation of prolactin response with affective symptoms—anxiety, guilt, and depression—measured on the BPRS
Lerer et al., 1988 [14]	Fenfluramine, 60 mg orally	10 drug-free patients with "chronic schizophrenia"; 10 matched controls	Blunted prolactin response to fenfluramine in patients
Krystal et al., 1993 [81]	m-Chlorophenylpiperazine (m-CPP), 0.1 mg/kg i.v.	12 drug-free patients with schizophrenia; 15 controls	Lower baseline prolactin in patients; no difference in m-CPP response; m-CPP triggered positive symptoms in patients
Iqbal et al., 1991 [15]	m-CPP, 0.25 mg/kg orally	7 male patients with schizophrenia; 8 male controls	Blunted prolactin response to m-CPP in patients; m-CPP worsened positive symptoms in this group
Markianos et al., 2002 [82]	Clomipramine 25 mg i.v.	25 male patients with schizophrenia, pre- and posttreatment with clozapine or olanzapine	Significant increases in prolactin following clomipramine; this response was blocked by both drugs
Cowen et al., 1985 [83]	L-tryptophan, 7.5 g i.v.	18 patients with schizophrenia on treatment and healthy controls	Increased prolactin response to L-tryptophan in patients
Nerozzi et al., 1990 [84]	Growth hormone-releasing hormone (GHRH), 1 mcg/kg	18 drug-free male patients with schizophrenia; 18 matched controls	Transient increase in prolactin following GHRH; no difference between the two groups
Cantalamessa et al., 1985 [85]	Gonadotrophin-releasing hormone (GnRH)	11 male patients with "acute schizophrenia"	Increased prolactin in 2 of 11 patients following GnRH
Keks et al., 1990, 1992 [16, 17]	Haloperidol, 0.5 mg i.v.	44 drug-free male patients with "acute schizophrenia"; 28 healthy controls	Blunted prolactin response to haloperidol in patients; basal prolactin positively correlated with the BPRS depression score. Maximal blunting seen in patients diagnosed with schizophrenia as per Kraepelin's criteria

Table 3: Continued.

Study and authors	Agent used	Patient sample	Results
Copolov et al., 1990 [18]	Low-dose haloperidol, i.v.	46 male in-patients with psychosis (27 schizophrenia, 7 affective, 12 other psychoses); 28 male controls	Lower prolactin response in patients with schizophrenia than in controls, even after correcting for age
Kulkarni et al., 1990 [29]	Haloperidol, 0.5 mg i.v.	24 drug-free male patients with psychosis	Significant inverse correlation between prolactin response and the severity of delusions
Keks et al., 1987 [19]	Haloperidol, 0.5 mg i.v.	14 drug-free male patients with schizophrenia; 14 matched controls	Blunted and slow prolactin response to haloperidol in patients
Nerozzi et al., 1990 [20]	Domperidone, 20 mg	16 drug-free male patients with schizophrenia or schizophreniform disorder; 16 male controls	Blunted prolactin response to domperidone in all patients, more prominently in the schizophreniform group. Basal prolactin was comparable to controls
Nerozzi et al., 1992 [86]	Domperidone, 20 mg	17 elderly, drug-free male patients with schizophrenia; 8 age-matched male controls	Increased prolactin response to domperidone in patients; comparable baseline prolactin
Monteleone et al., 1985 [21][#]	Sodium valproate, 800 mg	18 women with "chronic schizophrenia"; 20 healthy women	Valproate suppressed prolactin in normal women, but failed to do so in those with schizophrenia
Scheinin et al., 1985 [22][#]	Apomorphine, 0.005 mg/kg s.c. and 0.015 mg/kg i.v.	11 patients with schizophrenia on medication; 8 controls	Apomorphine significantly decreased prolactin in controls but not in patients
Whalley et al., 1984 [87][#]	Apomorphine, 0.75 mg	19 drug-free patients with psychosis; 9 healthy controls	Increased suppression of prolactin by apomorphine in patients with schizophrenia compared to controls
Ferrier et al., 1984 [31]	Apomorphine, 0.75 mg s.c.	Unmedicated patients with acute and chronic schizophrenia; healthy controls	No difference in the response to apomorphine across groups; however, basal prolactin was negatively correlated with the severity of positive symptoms
Rotrosen et al., 1978 [23]	Apomorphine and L-dopa	Unmedicated patients with chronic schizophrenia; healthy controls	Slightly blunted suppression of prolactin in patients compared to controls with apomorphine; greater suppression in patients than controls with L-dopa
Kolakowska et al., 1981 [88]	Apomorphine 0.05–0.1 mg/kg	17 patients with schizophrenia on treatment	No relationship between antipsychotic dose and apomorphine-induced prolactin suppression
Tsuchiya 1984 [24]	Experimental stress	Patients with schizophrenia, hypomania, depression, and alcohol dependence; healthy controls	Stress-induced prolactin release significantly greater in patients with schizophrenia than in controls

[#]Study uses an agent that inhibits prolactin release.

6. Studies Reporting Relationships between Prolactin and Tardive Dyskinesia

As tardive dyskinesia (TD) is linked to dopamine receptor supersensitivity [44], alterations in prolactin levels would be expected in these patients. This relationship has been examined by a small number of studies, listed in Table 5.

Because of the small sample sizes involved, the results of these studies must be interpreted with caution. They may indicate dopamine receptor supersensitivity [45] or GABA receptor dysfunction [46], but variables such as gender, duration of illness, the nature of medications used, and the study design (basal prolactin versus challenge tests) must also be taken into account. With the available evidence, the association between prolactin and TD seems slight at best.

7. Studies Linking Prolactin with Circadian Rhythms

Alterations in genes regulating circadian rhythm have been linked to both schizophrenia and the affective disorders [47]. Like other hormones, prolactin shows circadian variations in its rhythm and may be used to track circadian rhythm changes in schizophrenia. These studies are summarized in Table 6.

These studies suggest that there are clear alterations in the circadian rhythm of prolactin in schizophrenia, particularly with regard to sleep [48, 49]. The possibility that schizophrenia has a unique circadian profile of prolactin and sleep changes, distinct from those seen in depression [49], must be seriously considered but requires further replication in larger samples using a consistent study protocol.

TABLE 4: Studies examining the relationship between measures of prolactin and antipsychotic response in schizophrenia.

Study and authors	Patient sample and drug used	Results
Gruen et al., 1978 [89]	15 patients with schizophrenia; high-dose butaperazine or loxapine for 6 weeks	Transient prolactin elevation during the untreated admission period; consistent elevation in all patients following treatment but no relationship between levels and response
Markianos et al., 1991 [90]	12 patients with schizophrenia; haloperidol 30–60 mg for one month	Increases in baseline prolactin were significantly correlated with reduction in the BPRS total score
Zhang et al., 2002 [42]	30 male patients with "chronic schizophrenia"; risperidone 6 mg/day for 12 weeks	A significant association was found between increases in prolactin level and the positive subscore of the Positive and Negative Symptom Scale (PANSS)
Zhang et al., 2005 [91]	78 in-patients with schizophrenia; randomized to risperidone 6 mg/day or haloperidol 20 mg/day for 12 weeks	Change in prolactin levels was significantly related to improvement in the PANSS positive score in patients on risperidone but not haloperidol
Otani et al., 1994 [92]	24 patients with schizophrenia (12 male, 12 female); zotepine 100 mg/day for 1 week, then 200 mg/day for 3 weeks	Significant relationship between increases in prolactin and positive symptom improvement as measured by the BPRS but only in male patients
Kitamura et al., 1988 [93]	100 patients (96 with schizophrenia) receiving fluphenazine decanoate for at least 12 weeks	Higher prolactin to plasma fluphenazine ratio was associated with a better outcome (out-patient versus in-patient status)
Larsson et al., 1984 [94]	4 patients with schizophrenia; thioridazine with or without alpha-methyl tyrosine, 2 g/day	Positive correlation between the antipsychotic response to thioridazine and changes in prolactin
Chou et al., 1998 [95]	23 patients with acute exacerbations of schizophrenia or schizoaffective disorder; haloperidol titrated to achieve "low to moderate" plasma levels for 3 weeks	Increases in prolactin were associated with fewer symptoms at the end of treatment
Van Putten et al., 1991 [33]	73 drug-free male in-patients with schizophrenia; haloperidol 5–20 mg/day for 4 weeks	Posttreatment prolactin levels were significantly related to treatment outcome, but this reached a plateau at levels of 30 ng/mL (achieved with a dose of around 10 mg/day)
Mohr et al., 1998 [96]	23 in-patients (11 male, 12 female) with schizophrenia; haloperidol for 4 weeks	An exaggerated basal prolactin response to TRH predicted a worse response to haloperidol across several domains (positive, negative, anxiety-depression, and total BPRS scores)
Jones et al., 1998 [41]	20 patients with schizophrenia; clozapine	Blunting of the prolactin response to fenfluramine after clozapine treatment was significantly correlated with reductions in total positive symptoms, delusions, and hallucinations as measured by the Scale for the Assessment of Positive Symptoms (SAPS)
Lieberman et al., 1994 [97]	Patients with schizophrenia; clozapine	Blunting of the prolactin response to apomorphine after clozapine treatment was associated with a better response
Meltzer and Busch, 1983 [98]	Drug-free patients with schizophrenia; chlorpromazine 100 mg bid for 1 week and 200 mg bid for 1 week	At doses of 200 mg of chlorpromazine, prolactin elevation was negatively correlated with the severity of hallucinations
Awad et al., 1990 [43]	Patients with schizophrenia; remoxipride (high- and low-dose) and haloperidol	Higher basal prolactin predicted responses to both drugs but only in male patients
Wang et al., 2007 [34]	118 patients with schizophrenia (78 female, 40 male); risperidone 2–8 mg for 8 weeks	No relationship between changes in plasma prolactin and the response to risperidone
Volavka et al., 2004 [35]	157 patients with treatment-resistant schizophrenia (133 male, 24 female); randomized to clozapine, olanzapine, risperidone, or haloperidol for 14 weeks	No relationship between prolactin levels and clinical improvement
Rimon et al., 1985 [37]	28 patients with "acute symptoms" of schizophrenia; fluphenazine for 8 weeks	No correlation between changes in either plasma or CSF prolactin and response to fluphenazine
Smith et al., 1984 [99]	Patients with schizophrenia; haloperidol	No relationship between changes in prolactin level and response to haloperidol
Meltzer et al., 1983 [36]	21 drug-free in-patients with schizophrenia (10 female, 11 male); chlorpromazine 200 mg for 1 week, then 400 mg for 1 week	No relationship between prolactin levels and clinical outcome

TABLE 4: Continued.

Study and authors	Patient sample and drug used	Results
Meco et al., 1983 [38]	23 out-patients (11 male, 12 female) with schizophreniform disorder; haloperidol decanoate 50–250 mg once in 4 weeks for 12 months	No relationship between prolactin levels and clinical improvement
Jørgensen et al., 1982 [39]	9 patients with chronic schizophrenia; flupenthixol decanoate	No correlation between prolactin levels and changes in clinical ratings
Kolakowska et al., 1979 [40]	19 patients with acute psychoses, including schizophrenia; chlorpromazine	Plasma prolactin did not differentiate between patients with a good or poor treatment outcome

TABLE 5: Studies examining the relationship between prolactin and tardive dyskinesia.

Study and authors	Patient sample	Results
Glazer et al., 1981 [100]	19 men with TD; 29 postmenopausal women with TD; 21 men without TD	Prolactin levels were higher in women, but not in men, with severe TD compared to those with mild TD
Csernansky et al., 1986 [75]	33 male patients with schizophrenia on treatment; 8 off treatment; 18 normal male controls	"Prolactin index" (plasma prolactin divided by plasma neuroleptic activity) was negatively correlated with the severity of TD in younger patients
Monteleone et al., 1988 [46]	9 patients with schizophrenia and TD; 7 with schizophrenia alone; 10 healthy controls; challenge with sodium valproate 800 mg	Patients with schizophrenia and TD, but not schizophrenia alone, showed a decrease in prolactin following valproate administration; this decrease was correlated with the severity of TD as measured by the Abnormal Involuntary Movement Scale
Shim et al., 2005 [45]	Patients with schizophrenia with and without TD; challenge with the serotonin agonist and dopamine antagonist buspirone	Prolactin response to buspirone decreased in patients with TD
Asnis et al., 1979 [101]	6 patients with tardive dyskinesia, on and off medication, and following a challenge with haloperidol 0.5 mg i.m.; healthy controls	No difference in prolactin levels between the groups in any of the conditions
Ettigi et al., 1976 [102]	17 patients with "chronic schizophrenia" (4 of whom had oral TD) and 21 normal controls; challenge with apomorphine 0.75 mg s.c.	No difference in prolactin levels between patients and controls, either baseline or after apomorphine challenge

8. Prolactin and Suicide

Suicide attempts and completed suicide are not uncommon in schizophrenia [50]. A link between the prolactin response to a serotonergic challenge and affective symptoms, such as depression and guilt, has been reported in one study [26]; given this, it is logical to examine the association between prolactin levels and suicide. In a study examining 439 patients, 118 of whom were diagnosed as having psychosis, Pompili et al. [51] found slightly reduced prolactin levels in those patients who had attempted suicide.

9. Genetic Studies of Prolactin in Schizophrenia

Two recent studies have examined genetic variants in prolactin in patients with schizophrenia. Rybakowski et al. [52] examined the frequency of the −1149 G/T functional polymorphism of the prolactin gene in 403 patients, compared to 653 healthy controls. They found that the G allele was significantly more common in patients, particularly in males, and pointed out that this variation was similar to that reported in autoimmune diseases. Souza et al. [53] examined the association between the prolactin and prolactin receptor (PRLR) genes and both tardive dyskinesia and treatment response but failed to find a significant association in either case.

10. Summary and Hypothesis

The literature reviewed above, though complex, suggests fruitful lines for further enquiry. First, the association between raised prolactin and acute episodes of schizophrenia needs to be replicated in larger samples. Riecher-Rössler et al. [54] provide an intriguing explanation for this finding. They suggest that stress leads to an increased level of prolactin, which triggers dopamine release by a feedback mechanism; this increase in dopamine transmission may mediate the link between stress and psychosis. There are several lacunae in this hypothesis: (1) neither of the two studies cited above has measured stress or recent life events; (2) while raised prolactin may increase dopamine activity in the tuberoinfundibular

Table 6: Studies of prolactin and circadian rhythm in schizophrenia.

Study and authors	Patient sample	Results
Viganò et al., 2001 [103]	13 patients with schizophrenia (5 drug-free)	Abnormal elevation of diurnal prolactin levels found in 10 of 13 patients
Rao et al., 1994 [104]	115 patients with schizophrenia (90 drug-free, 25 on medication); 34 healthy controls	Significant phase advance in prolactin secretion, similar to that seen in depression
Rao et al., 1993 [105]	Patients with schizophrenia (drug-free and on medication); healthy controls	Lower daily mean and amplitude of prolactin secretion in drug-free female patients with schizophrenia compared to controls
Van Cauter et al., 1991 [48]	9 drug-free male patients with schizophrenia; 9 male controls	Threefold enhancement in the sleep-related increase in prolactin in patients compared to controls
Kemali et al., 1985 [106]	23 in-patients with schizophrenia, off drugs for 2 weeks; control in-patients with "neurotic disorders"	No difference in 24-hour prolactin secretion between the two groups
Appelberg et al., 2002 [49]	17 drug-free patients with nonaffective psychosis	Prolactin strongly correlated with REM latency and negatively correlated with REM sleep in patients

pathway, it is not known if it can produce similar changes in the mesolimbic pathway; (3) this proposal fails to explain why several studies found lower or normal prolactin levels. Despite this, the hypothesis merits further testing, as well as extension to conditions such as acute and transient psychosis, where the role of stress is much clearer. The finding that patients with schizophrenia have an exaggerated prolactin response to stress may be relevant here.

Second, the association of lower prolactin levels with positive symptoms and "paranoid" symptoms in particular are in line with the revised dopamine hypothesis of schizophrenia. This association can certainly be interpreted as suggesting increased dopamine transmission in this subgroup, with the same caveat as above: we do not know how well prolactin correlates with dopamine activity in the mesolimbic pathway. If this finding can be replicated, it provides some support for the notion of subtypes within the broad category of schizophrenia. Given that the most recent edition of the DSM has consciously omitted the traditional subtypes [55], a biomarker for a paranoid subtype could lead to a reversion of this change.

Third, provocation studies provide further support for the idea of blunted or lowered prolactin secretion in patients with "positive" schizophrenia. Whether this relationship holds good for other conditions in which "positive" symptoms are prominent—such as psychotic mood disorders or acute and transient psychosis—needs to be decided by further research. Though alterations in dopamine, serotonin, and GABA activity are all hinted at by individual provocation studies, the true nature of these abnormalities is likely to be slight and subtle, and their significance is unclear. A similar conclusion would apply to the results of studies of circadian rhythm.

Fourth, the association between prolactin and treatment response to antipsychotics, as well as its relationship to tardive dyskinesia, is inconsistent and, in the latter case, unlikely to be of much clinical significance. Given the numerous confounders that can affect prolactin levels, the inconsistency of positive findings and the negative results of recent genetic research, it is unlikely that a consistent association can be made. Changes in prolactin level may be a more sensitive indicator of response in some cases, though these probably reach a plateau at higher doses and may depend crucially on the drug being studied.

Finally, the association of prolactin gene variants with schizophrenia—though preliminary—suggests that there is more to the schizophrenia-prolactin association than simple dopamine-based models. Though Rybakowski et al. [52] invoked the possibility of an autoimmune mechanism, another possibility exists: genetic variations in prolactin are a genuine risk factor for psychosis. As authors writing in other contexts have pointed out, prolactin has a bewildering array of effects on the behaviour of mammals, but its exact behavioural effects in humans are unknown [2]. Given its relationship with parental bonding, an effect of prolactin on social cognition and behavior—both of which are significantly impaired in schizophrenia—is plausible. A tentative model could run as follows. First, genetic variations in prolactin lead to an exaggerated prolactin response to stress, which may further be modulated by childhood adversity or possibly by substance abuse [56, 57]. This is supported by the results of recent research which has found elevated prolactin levels not only in first-episode psychosis, but in over 25% of patients with "at-risk" or prodromal psychosis [58]; the authors of this paper have also suggested, in line with the above model, that this could reflect a stress response. Second, when exposed to further stressors, increases in prolactin levels may indirectly—as in Riecher-Rossler's proposal of a feedback increase in dopamine, which may also be exaggerated—lead to some of the symptoms of psychosis. Third, as a result of subsequent changes, which again may include increased dopamine transmission, prolactin levels decline, and lower prolactin levels may correlate with the development of positive symptoms, such as delusions. This is consistent with both the possibility that prolactin influences social behaviour, and the finding that some forms of stress, such as childhood neglect [59] and social defeat [60], can sensitize the mesolimbic dopamine pathway. Fourth, a moderate increase in prolactin, brought about by antipsychotics, may play a role in alleviating the positive symptoms of schizophrenia. A role for higher cortical centres in modulating prolactin release, which would be consistent with the above, is suggested by the results of studies of lobotomized patients. This hypothesis complements the dopamine model of schizophrenia and is consistent with most of the evidence reviewed above. Further research into the genetic links between prolactin and schizophrenia, the exact relationship between prolactin and central dopamine, the significance of circadian changes in prolactin, and the effects of prolactin on human social behaviour will provide a true test of this proposal.

11. Conclusion

A review of the literature on prolactin and schizophrenia suggests that the relationship between them is complex and not confined to the adverse effects of antipsychotics. Though the above interpretations must be regarded as imperfect and tentative, they do call for a reappraisal of the role of prolactin in the various stages of schizophrenia, particularly with regard to its onset and to the development of positive symptoms. Research in this area may lead to an improved understanding of schizophrenia, as well as a better delineation of the effects of prolactin on social behaviour and cognition in humans.

Conflict of Interests

The author declares that there is no conflict of interests regarding the publication of this paper.

References

[1] I. Gordon, O. Zagoory-Sharon, J. F. Leckman, and R. Feldman, "Prolactin, Oxytocin, and the development of paternal behavior across the first six months of fatherhood," *Hormones and Behavior*, vol. 58, no. 3, pp. 513–518, 2010.

[2] T. H. C. Kruger, B. Leeners, E. Naegeli et al., "Prolactin secretory rhythm in women: immediate and long-term alterations after sexual contact," *Human Reproduction*, vol. 27, no. 4, pp. 1139–1143, 2012.

[3] S. Ranabir and K. Reetu, "Stress and hormones," *Indian Journal of Endocrinology and Metabolism*, vol. 15, pp. 18–22, 2011.

[4] C. Ohta, N. Yasui-Furukori, H. Furukori et al., "The effect of smoking status on the plasma concentration of prolactin already elevated by risperidone treatment in schizophrenia patients," *Progress in Neuro-Psychopharmacology and Biological Psychiatry*, vol. 35, no. 2, pp. 573–576, 2011.

[5] M. Baggaley, "Sexual dysfunction in schizophrenia: focus on recent evidence," *Human Psychopharmacology*, vol. 23, no. 3, pp. 201–209, 2008.

[6] P. M. Haddad and A. Wieck, "Antipsychotic-induced hyperprolactinaemia: mechanisms, clinical features and management," *Drugs*, vol. 64, no. 20, pp. 2291–2314, 2004.

[7] V. O'Keane, "Antipsychotic-induced hyperprolactinaemia, hypogonadism and osteoporosis in the treatment of schizophrenia," *Journal of Psychopharmacology*, vol. 22, no. 2, supplement, pp. 70–75, 2008.

[8] T. Baptista, A. Lacruz, T. Meza et al., "Antipsychotic drugs and obesity: is prolactin involved?" *Canadian Journal of Psychiatry*, vol. 46, no. 9, pp. 829–834, 2001.

[9] J. R. Bostwick, S. K. Guthrie, and V. L. Ellingrod, "Antipsychotic-induced hyperprolactinemia," *Pharmacotherapy*, vol. 29, no. 1, pp. 64–73, 2009.

[10] M. van Bruggen, T. van Amelsvoort, L. Wouters, P. Dingemans, L. de Haan, and D. Linszen, "Sexual dysfunction and hormonal changes in first episode psychosis patients on olanzapine or risperidone," *Psychoneuroendocrinology*, vol. 34, no. 7, pp. 989–995, 2009.

[11] J. Bobes, M. P. García-Portilla, J. Rejas et al., "Frequency of sexual dysfunction and other reproductive side-effects in patients with schizophrenia treated with risperidone, olanzapine, quetiapine, or haloperidol: the results of the EIRE study," *Journal of Sex and Marital Therapy*, vol. 29, no. 2, pp. 125–147, 2003.

[12] M. Segal, A. Avital, S. Berstein, A. Derevenski, S. Sandbank, and A. Weizman, "Prolactin and estradiol serum levels in unmedicated male paranoid schizophrenia patients," *Progress in Neuro-Psychopharmacology and Biological Psychiatry*, vol. 31, no. 2, pp. 378–382, 2007.

[13] M.-C. Mokrani, F. Duval, T. S. Diep, P. E. Bailey, and J. P. MacHer, "Multihormonal responses to clonidine in patients with affective and psychotic symptoms," *Psychoneuroendocrinology*, vol. 25, no. 7, pp. 741–752, 2000.

[14] B. Lerer, A. Ran, M. Blacker et al., "Neuroendocrine responses in chronic schizophrenia. Evidence for serotonergic dysfunction," *Schizophrenia Research*, vol. 1, no. 6, pp. 405–410, 1988.

[15] N. Iqbal, G. M. Asnis, S. Wetzler, R. S. Kahn, S. R. Kay, and H. M. Van Praag, "The MCPP challenge test in schizophrenia: hormonal and behaviral responses," *Biological Psychiatry*, vol. 30, no. 8, pp. 770–778, 1991.

[16] N. A. Keks, D. L. Copolov, J. Kulkarni et al., "Basal and haloperidol-stimulated prolactin in neuroleptic-free men with schizophrenia defined by 11 diagnostic systems," *Biological Psychiatry*, vol. 27, no. 11, pp. 1203–1215, 1990.

[17] N. A. Keks, D. P. McKenzie, L. H. Low et al., "Multidiagnostic evaluation of prolactin response to haloperidol challenge in schizophrenia: maximal blunting in Kraepelinian patients," *Biological Psychiatry*, vol. 32, no. 5, pp. 426–437, 1992.

[18] D. L. Copolov, N. A. Keks, J. Kulkarni et al., "Prolactin response to low-dose haloperidol challenge in schizophrenic, non-schizophrenic psychotic, and control subjects," *Psychoneuroendocrinology*, vol. 15, no. 3, pp. 225–231, 1990.

[19] N. A. Keks, D. L. Copolov, and B. S. Singh, "Abnormal prolactin response to haloperidol challenge in men with schizophrenia," *The American Journal of Psychiatry*, vol. 144, no. 10, pp. 1335–1337, 1987.

[20] D. Nerozzi, A. Magnani, V. Sforza et al., "Plasma prolactin response to domperidone in acute schizophrenia and schizophreniform illness," *Psychiatry Research*, vol. 34, no. 2, pp. 139–147, 1990.

[21] P. Monteleone, G. Zontini, and L. Steardo, "Failure of the gabaergic drug, sodium valproate, to reduce basal plasma prolactin secretion in chronic schizophrenia," *Psychoneuroendocrinology*, vol. 10, no. 4, pp. 475–480, 1985.

[22] M. Scheinin, E. K. Syvälahti, J. Hietala et al., "Effects of apomorphine on blood levels of homovanillic acid, growth hormone and prolactin in medicated schizophrenics and healthy control subjects," *Progress in Neuro-Psychopharmacology and Biological Psychiatry*, vol. 9, no. 4, pp. 441–449, 1985.

[23] J. Rotrosen, B. Angrist, C. Clark, S. Gershon, F. S. Halpers, and E. J. Sachar, "Suppression of prolactin in dopamine agonists in schizophrenics and controls," *The American Journal of Psychiatry*, vol. 135, no. 8, pp. 949–951, 1978.

[24] K. Tsuchiya, "Studies on prolactin in major psychoses—with reference to prolactin response to stress in schizophrenia," *Folia Psychiatrica et Neurologica Japonica*, vol. 38, no. 1, pp. 53–56, 1984.

[25] R. P. Sharma, V. Singh, P. G. Janicak, J. I. Javaid, and G. N. Pandey, "The prolactin response to fenfluramine in schizophrenia is associated with negative symptoms," *Schizophrenia Research*, vol. 39, no. 1, pp. 85–89, 1999.

[26] K. M. Abel, V. O'Keane, and R. M. Murray, "Enhancement of the prolactin response to d-fenfluramine in drug-naive schizophrenic patients," *British Journal of Psychiatry*, vol. 168, pp. 57–60, 1996.

[27] J. Spoov, P.-E. Bredbacka, B. Appelberg et al., "Prolactin response to submaximal stimulation by TRH in nonaffective psychoses," *Biological Psychiatry*, vol. 29, no. 3, pp. 204–210, 1991.

[28] J. Spoov, P.-E. Bredbacka, and U.-H. Stenman, "An abnormal relation between basal prolactin levels and prolactin response to 12.5 microg TRH i.v. in drug-naïve patients with first-episode schizophrenia," *Schizophrenia Research*, vol. 119, no. 1–3, pp. 41–46, 2010.

[29] J. Kulkarni, N. A. Keks, G. Stuart et al., "Relationship of psychotic symptoms to haloperidol-stimulated prolactin release," *Acta Psychiatrica Scandinavica*, vol. 82, no. 4, pp. 271–274, 1990.

[30] P. Monteleone, A. Tortorella, R. Borriello, P. Cassandro, and M. Maj, "Prolactin hyperresponsiveness to D-fenfluramine in drug-free schizophrenic patients: a placebo-controlled study," *Biological Psychiatry*, vol. 45, no. 12, pp. 1606–1611, 1999.

[31] I. N. Ferrier, E. C. Johnstone, and T. J. Crow, "Hormonal effects of apomorphine in schizophrenia," *British Journal of Psychiatry*, vol. 144, no. 4, pp. 349–357, 1984.

[32] M. Segal, A. Avital, M. Rojas et al., "Serum prolactin levels in unmedicated first-episode and recurrent schizophrenia patients: a possible marker for the disease's subtypes," *Psychiatry Research*, vol. 127, no. 3, pp. 227–235, 2004.

[33] T. Van Putten, S. R. Marder, and J. Mintz, "Serum prolactin as a correlate of clinical response to haloperidol," *Journal of Clinical Psychopharmacology*, vol. 11, no. 6, pp. 357–361, 1991.

[34] L. Wang, L. Yu, A.-P. Zhang et al., "Serum prolactin levels, plasma risperidone levels, polymorphism of cytochrome P450 2D6 and clinical response in patients with schizophrenia," *Journal of Psychopharmacology*, vol. 21, no. 8, pp. 837–842, 2007.

[35] J. Volavka, P. Czobor, T. B. Cooper et al., "Prolactin levels in schizophrenia and schizoaffective disorder patients treated with clozapine, olanzapine, risperidone, or haloperidol," *Journal of Clinical Psychiatry*, vol. 65, no. 1, pp. 57–61, 2004.

[36] H. Y. Meltzer, D. A. Busch, and V. S. Fang, "Serum neuroleptic and prolactin levels in schizophrenic patients and clinical response," *Psychiatry Research*, vol. 9, no. 4, pp. 271–283, 1983.

[37] R. Rimon, R. Kampman, R. Laru-Sompa, and L. Heikkila, "Serum and cerebrospinal fluid prolactin patterns during neuroleptic treatment in schizophrenic patients," *Pharmacopsychiatry*, vol. 18, no. 3, pp. 252–254, 1985.

[38] G. Meco, M. Casacchia, M. Attenni, A. Iafrate, F. Castellana, and U. Ecari, "Haloperidol decanoate in schizophreniform disorders. Clinical and neuroendocrine aspects," *Acta Psychiatrica Belgica*, vol. 83, no. 1, pp. 57–68, 1983.

[39] A. Jørgensen, J. Andersen, N. Bjørndal, S. J. Dencker, L. Lundin, and U. Malm, "Serum concentrations of cis(Z)-flupentixol and prolactin in chronic schizophrenic patients treated with flupentixol and cis(Z)-flupentixol decanoate," *Psychopharmacology*, vol. 77, no. 1, pp. 58–65, 1982.

[40] T. Kolakowska, M. Orr, M. Gelder, M. Heggie, D. Wiles, and M. Franklin, "Clinical significance of plasma drug and prolactin levels during acute chlorpromazine treatment: a replication study," *British Journal of Psychiatry*, vol. 135, no. 10, pp. 352–359, 1979.

[41] H. Jones, V. A. Curtis, P. Wright, and J. V. Lucey, "Neuroendocrine evidence that clozapine's serotonergic antagonism is relevant to its efficacy in treating hallucinations and other positive schizophrenic symptoms," *The American Journal of Psychiatry*, vol. 155, no. 6, pp. 838–840, 1998.

[42] X. Y. Zhang, D. F. Zhou, C. L. Yuan, P. Y. Zhang, G. Y. Wu, and Y. C. Shen, "Risperidone-induced increase in serum prolactin is correlated with positive symptom improvement in chronic schizophrenia," *Psychiatry Research*, vol. 109, no. 3, pp. 297–302, 2002.

[43] A. G. Awad, Y. D. Lapierre, K.-G. Jostell et al., "Selective dopamine D2 antagonist and prolactin response in acute schizophrenia—results from remoxipride studies. The Canadian Remoxipride Study Group," *Progress in Neuro-Psychopharmacology and Biological Psychiatry*, vol. 14, no. 5, pp. 769–777, 1990.

[44] H. C. Margolese, G. Chouinard, T. T. Kolivakis, L. Beauclair, and R. Miller, "Tardive dyskinesia in the era of typical and atypical antipsychotics. Part 1: pathophysiology and mechanisms of induction," *Canadian Journal of Psychiatry*, vol. 50, no. 9, pp. 541–547, 2005.

[45] J.-C. Shim, Y.-H. Kim, D. L. Kelly, J.-G. Lee, and R. R. Conley, "Tardive dyskinesia predicts prolactin response to buspirone challenge in people with schizophrenia," *Journal of Neuropsychiatry and Clinical Neurosciences*, vol. 17, no. 2, pp. 221–226, 2005.

[46] P. Monteleone, M. Maj, M. G. Ariano, M. Iovino, L. Fiorenza, and L. Steardo, "Prolactin response to sodium valproate in schizophrenics with and without tardive dyskinesia," *Psychopharmacology*, vol. 96, no. 2, pp. 223–226, 1988.

[47] H. A. Mansour, M. E. Talkowski, J. Wood et al., "Association study of 21 circadian genes with bipolar I disorder, schizoaffective disorder and schizophrenia," *Bipolar Disorders*, vol. 11, pp. 701–710, 2009.

[48] E. Van Cauter, P. Linkowski, M. Kerkhofs et al., "Circadian and sleep-related endocrine rhythms in schizophrenia," *Archives of General Psychiatry*, vol. 48, no. 4, pp. 348–356, 1991.

[49] B. Appelberg, H. Katila, and R. Rimón, "REM sleep and prolactin in patients with non-affective psychoses," *Psychoneuroendocrinology*, vol. 27, no. 6, pp. 661–669, 2002.

[50] B. A. Palmer, V. S. Pankratz, and J. M. Bostwick, "The lifetime risk of suicide in schizophrenia: a reexamination," *Archives of General Psychiatry*, vol. 62, no. 3, pp. 247–253, 2005.

[51] M. Pompili, S. Gibiino, M. Innamorati et al., "Prolactin and thyroid hormone levels are associated with suicide attempts in psychiatric patients," *Psychiatry Research*, vol. 200, pp. 389–394, 2012.

[52] J. K. Rybakowski, M. Dmitrzak-Weglarz, P. Kapelski, and J. Hauser, "Functional -1149 G/T polymorphism of the prolactin gene in schizophrenia," *Neuropsychobiology*, vol. 65, no. 1, pp. 41–44, 2011.

[53] R. P. Souza, H. Y. Meltzer, J. A. Lieberman, A. N. Voineskos, G. Remington, and J. L. Kennedy, "Prolactin as a biomarker

for treatment response and tardive dyskinesia in schizophrenia subjects: old thoughts revisited from a genetic perspective," *Human Psychopharmacology*, vol. 26, no. 1, pp. 21–27, 2011.

[54] A. Riecher-Rössler, J. K. Rybakowski, M. O. Pflueger et al., "Hyperprolactinemia in antipsychotic-naive patients with first-episode psychosis.," *Psychological Medicine*, vol. 43, no. 12, pp. 2571-2582, 2013.

[55] R. Tandon and W. T. Carpenter Jr., "DSM-5 status of psychotic disorders: 1 year prepublication," *Schizophrenia Bulletin*, vol. 38, no. 3, pp. 369–370, 2012.

[56] J. Kaufman, B. Birmaher, J. Perel et al., "Serotonergic functioning in depressed abused children: clinical and familial correlates," *Biological Psychiatry*, vol. 44, no. 10, pp. 973–981, 1998.

[57] G. Gerra, C. Leonardi, E. Cortese et al., "Childhood neglect and parental care perception in cocaine addicts: relation with psychiatric symptoms and biological correlates," *Neuroscience and Biobehavioral Reviews*, vol. 33, no. 4, pp. 601–610, 2009.

[58] J. Aston, E. Rechsteiner, N. Bull, S. Borgwardt, U. Gschwandtner, and A. Riecher-Rössler, "Hyperprolactinaemia in early psychosis-not only due to antipsychotics," *Progress in Neuro-Psychopharmacology and Biological Psychiatry*, vol. 34, no. 7, pp. 1342-1344, 2010.

[59] J. C. Pruessner, F. Champagne, M. J. Meaney, and A. Dagher, "Dopamine release in response to a psychological stress in humans and its relationship to early life maternal care: a positron emission tomography study using [11C] raclopride," *Journal of Neuroscience*, vol. 24, no. 11, pp. 2825–2831, 2004.

[60] J.-P. Selten and E. Cantor-Graae, "Hypothesis: social defeat is a risk factor for schizophrenia?" *British Journal of Psychiatry*, vol. 191, no. 51, pp. s9–s12, 2007.

[61] C. Garcia-Rizo, E. Fernandez-Egea, C. Oliveira et al., "Prolactin concentrations in newly diagnosed, antipsychotic-naïve patients with nonaffective psychosis," *Schizophrenia Research*, vol. 134, no. 1, pp. 16–19, 2012.

[62] M. D. Warner, A. M. Walker, D. C. D'Souza, D. Lee, D. Nasseri, and C. A. Peabody, "Lower prolactin bioactivity in unmedicated schizophrenic patients," *Psychiatry Research*, vol. 102, no. 3, pp. 249–254, 2001.

[63] M. L. Rao, G. Gross, and G. Huber, "Altered interrelationship of dopamine, prolactin, thyrotropin and thyroid hormone in schizophrenic patients," *European Archives of Psychiatry and Neurological Sciences*, vol. 234, no. 1, pp. 8–12, 1984.

[64] A. Kuruvilla, G. Srikrishna, J. Peedicayil, K. Kuruvilla, and A. S. Kanagasabapathy, "A study on serum prolactin levels in schizophrenia: correlation with positive and negative symptoms," *International Clinical Psychopharmacology*, vol. 8, no. 3, pp. 177–179, 1993.

[65] D. Muck-Seler, N. Pivac, M. Mustapic, Z. Crncevic, M. Jakovljevic, and M. Sagud, "Platelet serotonin and plasma prolactin and cortisol in healthy, depressed and schizophrenic women," *Psychiatry Research*, vol. 127, no. 3, pp. 217–226, 2004.

[66] R. Rimon, J. Luera, R. Kampman, and M. Hyyppa, "Prolactin levels in cerebrospinal fluid of patients with chronic schizophrenia," *Neuropsychobiology*, vol. 7, no. 2, pp. 87–93, 1981.

[67] M. T. Hyyppä, J. Liira, R. Kampman, and R. Rimon, "Low prolactin levels in cerebrospinal fluid: an aftereffect of lobotomy in chronic schizophrenia," *Acta Psychiatrica Belgica*, vol. 80, no. 4, pp. 452–457, 1980.

[68] M. Segal, A. Avital, A. Derevenski, S. Berstein, S. Sandbank, and A. Weizman, "Prolactin serum levels in paranoid versus nonparanoid male schizophrenia patients treated with risperidone," *International Clinical Psychopharmacology*, vol. 22, no. 4, pp. 192–196, 2007.

[69] K. Otani, T. Kondo, M. Ishida et al., "Plasma prolactin concentration and psychopathology of schizophrenia," *Progress in Neuro-Psychopharmacology and Biological Psychiatry*, vol. 20, pp. 1369–1374, 1996.

[70] J. W. Newcomer, S. J. Riney, S. Vinogradov, and J. G. Csernansky, "Plasma prolactin and homovanillic acid as markers for psychopathology and abnormal movements during maintenance haloperidol treatment in male patients with schizophrenia," *Psychiatry Research*, vol. 41, no. 3, pp. 191–202, 1992.

[71] S. Akhondzadeh, F. Rezaei, B. Larijani, A.-A. Nejatisafa, L. Kashani, and S. H. Abbasi, "Correlation between testosterone, gonadotropins and prolactin and severity of negative symptoms in male patients with chronic schizophrenia," *Schizophrenia Research*, vol. 84, no. 2-3, pp. 405–410, 2006.

[72] P. Rinieris, M. Markianos, J. Hatzimanolis, and C. Stefanis, "A psychoendocrine study in male paranoid schizophrenics with delusional ideas of homosexual content," *Acta Psychiatrica Scandinavica*, vol. 72, no. 3, pp. 309–314, 1985.

[73] E. C. Johnstone, T. J. Crow, and K. Mashiter, "Anterior pituitary hormone secretion in chronic schizophrenia: an approach to neurohumoral mechanisms," *Psychological Medicine*, vol. 7, no. 2, pp. 223–228, 1977.

[74] J. E. Kleinman, D. R. Weinberger, and A. D. Rogol, "Plasma prolactin concentrations and psychopathology in chronic schizophrenia," *Archives of General Psychiatry*, vol. 39, no. 6, pp. 655–657, 1982.

[75] J. G. Csernansky, E. Prosser, and J. Kaplan, "Possible associations among plasma prolactin levels, tardive dyskinesia, and paranoia in treated male schizophrenics," *Biological Psychiatry*, vol. 21, no. 7, pp. 632–642, 1986.

[76] A. D. Prasad, "Concentration of prolactin in the plasma of schizophrenic patients with positive and negative symptoms," *Zhurnal Nevropatologii i Psikhiatrii Imeni S.S. Korsakova*, vol. 86, no. 9, pp. 1400–1401, 1986 (Russian).

[77] D. J. Luchins, A. G. Robertson, and H. Y. Meltzer, "Serum prolactin, psychopathology, and ventricular size in chronic schizophrenia," *Psychiatry Research*, vol. 12, no. 2, pp. 149–153, 1984.

[78] J. A. Cabranes, F. Fuentenebro, M. N. Recio, M. Borque, and M. I. Almoguera, "Prolactin secretion response to TRH stimulation in acute and chronic schizophrenic patients under neuroleptic treatment," *International Pharmacopsychiatry*, vol. 17, no. 1, pp. 1–7, 1982.

[79] F. Brambilla, A. Guastalla, A. Guerrini et al., "Prolactin secretion in chronic schizophrenia," *Acta Psychiatrica Scandinavica*, vol. 54, no. 4, pp. 275–286, 1976.

[80] D. Naber, M. Ackenheil, and G. Laakmann, "Basal and stimulated levels of prolactin, TSH, and LH in serum of chronic schizophrenic patients long-term treated with neuroleptics: relations to psychopathology," *Advances in Biochemical Psychopharmacology*, vol. 24, pp. 419–423, 1980.

[81] J. H. Krystal, J. P. Seibyl, L. H. Price et al., "m-Chlorophenylpiperazine effects in neuroleptic-free schizophrenic patients: evidence implicating serotonergic systems in the positive symptoms of schizophrenia," *Archives of General Psychiatry*, vol. 50, no. 8, pp. 624–635, 1993.

[82] M. Markianos, J. Hatzimanolis, L. Lykouras, and G. N. Christodoulou, "Prolactin responses to acute clomipramine and

haloperidol of male schizophrenic patients in a drug-free state and after treatment with clozapine or with olanzapine," *Schizophrenia Research*, vol. 56, no. 1-2, pp. 11–17, 2002.

[83] P. J. Cowen, H. Gadhvi, B. Gosden, and T. Kolakowska, "Responses of prolactin and growth hormone to L-tryptophan infusion: effects in normal subjects and schizophrenic patients receiving neuroleptics," *Psychopharmacology*, vol. 86, no. 1-2, pp. 164–169, 1985.

[84] D. Nerozzi, A. Magnani, V. Sforza et al., "Prolactin and growth hormone responses to growth hormone-releasing hormone in acute schizophrenia," *Neuropsychobiology*, vol. 23, no. 1, pp. 15–17, 1990.

[85] L. Cantalamessa, A. Catania, and A. Silva, "Gonadotropin releasing hormone elicits abnormal hormone responses in schizophrenia," *Psychoneuroendocrinology*, vol. 10, no. 4, pp. 481–484, 1985.

[86] D. Nerozzi, A. Magnani, C. Dastoli et al., "Prolactin responses to domperidone in chronic schizophrenia," *Psychiatry Research*, vol. 42, no. 2, pp. 159–169, 1992.

[87] L. J. Whalley, J. E. Christie, S. Brown, and G. W. Arbuthnott, "Schneider's first-rank symptoms of schizophrenia. An association with increased growth hormone response to apomorphine," *Archives of General Psychiatry*, vol. 41, no. 11, pp. 1040–1043, 1984.

[88] T. Kolakowska, M. Gelder, and S. Fraser, "Neuroendocrine tests during treatment with neuroleptic drugs. III. Plasma growth hormone and prolactin responses to apomorphine," *British Journal of Psychiatry*, vol. 139, no. 5, pp. 408–412, 1981.

[89] P. H. Gruen, E. J. Sachar, N. Altman, G. Langer, M. A. Tabrizi, and F. S. Halpern, "Relation of plasma prolactin to clinical response in schizophrenic patients," *Archives of General Psychiatry*, vol. 35, no. 10, pp. 1222–1227, 1978.

[90] M. Markianos, G. Sakellariou, and E. Bistolaki, "Prolactin responses to haloperidol in drug-free and treated schizophrenic patients," *Journal of Neural Transmission—General Section*, vol. 83, no. 1-2, pp. 37–42, 1991.

[91] X. Y. Zhang, D. F. Zhou, L. Y. Cao, P. Y. Zhang, G. Y. Wu, and Y. C. Shen, "Prolactin levels in male schizophrenic patients treated with risperidone and haloperidol: a double-blind and randomized study," *Psychopharmacology*, vol. 178, no. 1, pp. 35–40, 2005.

[92] K. Otani, T. Kondo, S. Kaneko, M. Ishida, and Y. Fukushima, "Correlation between prolactin response and therapeutic effects of zotepine in schizophrenic patients," *International Clinical Psychopharmacology*, vol. 9, no. 4, pp. 287–289, 1994.

[93] T. Kitamura, D. A. McGovern, N. W. Imlah, D. Wiles, and A. A. Schiff, "Plasma levels of fluphenazine and prolactin in psychiatric patients," *European Archives of Psychiatry and Neurological Sciences*, vol. 237, no. 6, pp. 320–326, 1988.

[94] M. Larsson, R. Ohman, L. Wallin, J. Wålinder, and A. Carlsson, "Antipsychotic treatment with α-methyltyrosine in combination with thioridazine: prolactin response and interaction with dopaminergic precursor pools," *Journal of Neural Transmission—General Section*, vol. 60, no. 2, pp. 115–132, 1984.

[95] J. C.-Y. Chou, R. Douyon, P. Czobor, J. Volavka, and T. B. Cooper, "Change in plasma prolactin and clinical response to haloperidol in schizophrenia and schizoaffective disorder," *Psychiatry Research*, vol. 81, no. 1, pp. 51–55, 1998.

[96] P. Mohr, J. Horáček, L. Motlová, J. Libiger, and P. Czobor, "Prolactin response to D-fenfluramine challenge test as a predictor of treatment response to haloperidol in acute schizophrenia," *Schizophrenia Research*, vol. 30, no. 1, pp. 91–99, 1998.

[97] J. A. Lieberman, J. M. Kane, A. Z. Safferman et al., "Predictors of response to clozapine," *Journal of Clinical Psychiatry*, vol. 55, no. 9, pp. 126–128, 1994.

[98] H. Y. Meltzer and D. Busch, "Serum prolactin response to chlorpromazine and psychopathology in schizophrenics: implications for the dopamine hypothesis," *Psychiatry Research*, vol. 9, no. 4, pp. 285–299, 1983.

[99] R. C. Smith, R. Baumgartner, C. H. Misra et al., "Haloperidol. Plasma levels and prolactin response as predictors of clinical improvement in schizophrenia: chemical v radioreceptor plasma level assays," *Archives of General Psychiatry*, vol. 41, no. 11, pp. 1044–1049, 1984.

[100] W. M. Glazer, D. C. Moore, M. B. Bowers Jr., and W. A. Brown, "Serum prolactin and tardive dyskinesia," *The American Journal of Psychiatry*, vol. 138, no. 11, pp. 1493–1496, 1981.

[101] G. M. Asnis, E. J. Sachar, and G. Langer, "Normal prolactin responses in tardive dyskinesia," *Psychopharmacology*, vol. 66, no. 3, pp. 247–250, 1979.

[102] P. Ettigi, N. P. V. Nair, S. Lal, P. Cervantes, and H. Guyda, "Effect of apomorphine on growth hormone and prolactin secretion in schizophrenic patients, with or without oral dyskinesia, withdrawn from chronic neuroleptic therapy," *Journal of Neurology Neurosurgery and Psychiatry*, vol. 39, no. 9, pp. 870–876, 1976.

[103] D. Viganò, P. Lissoni, F. Rovelli et al., "A study of light/dark rhythm of melatonin in relation to cortisol and prolactin secretion in schizophrenia," *Neuroendocrinology Letters*, vol. 22, no. 2, pp. 137–141, 2001.

[104] M. L. Rao, G. Gross, B. Strebel et al., "Circadian rhythm of tryptophan, serotonin, melatonin, and pituitary hormones in schizophrenia," *Biological Psychiatry*, vol. 35, no. 3, pp. 151–163, 1994.

[105] M. L. Rao, G. Gross, A. Halaris et al., "Hyperdopaminergia in schizophreniform psychosis: a chronobiological study," *Psychiatry Research*, vol. 47, no. 2, pp. 187–203, 1993.

[106] D. Kemali, M. Maj, M. G. Ariano, F. Arena, and N. Lovero, "24-hour plasma levels of prolactin, cortisol, growth hormone and catecholamines in schizophrenic patients," *Neuropsychobiology*, vol. 14, no. 3, pp. 109–114, 1985.

2

A Comparative Study between Olanzapine and Risperidone in the Management of Schizophrenia

Saeed Shoja Shafti[1] and Mahsa Gilanipoor[2]

[1] *University of Social Welfare and Rehabilitation Sciences (USWR), Razi Psychiatric Hospital, P.O. Box 18735-569, Tehran, Iran*
[2] *Razi Psychiatric Hospital, P.O. Box 18735-569, Tehran, Iran*

Correspondence should be addressed to Saeed Shoja Shafti; ssshafti@gmail.com

Academic Editor: Robin Emsley

Introduction. Since a variety of comparisons between risperidone and olanzapine have resulted in diverse outcomes, so safety and efficacy of them were compared again in a new trial. *Method.* Sixty female schizophrenic patients entered into one of the assigned groups for random allocation to olanzapine or risperidone ($n = 30$ in each group) in a double-blind, 12-week clinical trial. Scale for Assessment of Positive Symptoms (SAPS) and Scale for Assessment of Negative Symptoms (SANS) were used as the primary outcome measures. Clinical Global Impressions-Severity Scale (CGI-S), Schedule for Assessment of Insight (SAI), and finally Simpson Angus Scale (SAS) as well were employed as secondary scales. *Results.* While both of olanzapine and risperidone were significantly effective for improvement of positive symptoms ($P < 0.0001$), as regards negative symptoms, it was so only by means of olanzapine ($P < 0.0003$). CGI-S and SAI, as well, were significantly improved in both of the groups. SAS increment was significant only in the risperidone group ($P < 0.02$). *Conclusion.* While both of olanzapine and risperidone were equally effective for improvement of positive symptoms and insight, olanzapine showed superior efficacy with respect to negative symptoms, along with lesser extrapyramidal side effects, in comparison with risperidone.

1. Introduction

Schizophrenia is characterized by its chronic recurring course [1]. In addition, as many as 30–40% of such patients may exhibit an insufficient or poor response to conventional antipsychotics [2] and up to 50% of them may experience serious side effects by such treatments [3]. So the focus of new drug development for treatment of schizophrenia has shifted to synthesize compounds capable of alleviating negative symptoms, which are commonly unresponsive to classical antipsychotics, and to synthesize compounds less likely to produce extrapyramidal side effects. At the beginning, atypical antipsychotics seemed to be more efficient than conventional antipsychotics, but in a meta-analysis for comparing the effects of first-generation antipsychotics with second-generation ones, the latter cluster was found to be no more efficacious than the first-generation drugs in schizophrenic patients, even with respect to negative symptoms [4].

Olanzapine is a thienobenzodiazepine with a high affinity for serotonin 5-HT2, histamine H1, α1-adrenergic, D1, and D2 dopamine receptors [5]. Controlled clinical trials have shown that it has better efficacy and healthier side-effect profile than haloperidol and according to some studies seems to be more efficient in the management of negative symptoms [6–8]. Risperidone is a benzisoxazole derivative. Its greatest affinity is for serotonin 5-HT2, histamine H1, α1-adrenergic, and dopamine D2 sites. In some clinical studies, it has been shown to be superior to typical antipsychotics [9]. Both risperidone and olanzapine have been shown to be well tolerated and efficacious in the treatment of psychotic disorders [6, 7, 9, 10]. A variety of assessments for comparing these two atypical antipsychotics have resulted in diverse outcomes. For example, Tran et al. [10] and Gureje et al. [11] had found olanzapine to have a risk-versus-benefit advantage compared to risperidone. In this regard, subjects meeting diagnostic criteria for schizophrenia, schizoaffective or schizophreniform disorder were measured with the Positive and Negative Syndrome

Scale (PANSS). According to Tran, the benefit of olanzapine was due to its greater efficacy, noticeable improvement of negative symptoms, higher response rate, better maintenance of treatment, and finally lower incidence of adverse effects like extrapyramidal side effects, hyperprolactinemia, and sexual dysfunction [10]. Also, Edgell et al. [12] and Rascati et al. [13] found that olanzapine-treated patients were more likely to sustain treatment versus risperidone-treated patients and Feldman et al. [14], as well, had found olanzapine to be more efficacious than risperidone in improvement of negative symptoms in older patients.

But conversely, in parallel comparisons, Taylor et al. [15], Kasper et al. [16], and Conley and Mahmoud [17] generally found equivalent clinical outcome for both of olanzapine- and risperidone-treated patients. So in the present assessment and based on the aforementioned controversies, the safety and efficacy of risperidone and olanzapine were compared once more in a sample of schizophrenic patients, looking for additional convincing proof regarding this important matter.

2. Method

This study was approved by University's Medical Ethics Committee. Sixty female in-patients, as accessible sample in the chronic ward of the hospital, after full explanation of the procedure for them and obtaining signed informed consent, and a minimum of 10–14-day washout period, entered randomly into one of the assigned groups, for random allocation to olanzapine or risperidone ($n = 30$ in each group). Patients were diagnosed as schizophrenic, according to *Diagnostic and Statistical Manual of Mental Disorders*, 4th edition, text revision criteria. Previous drugs of the patients consisted of a series of first-generation antipsychotics, including perphenazine, haloperidol, trifluoperazine, and chlorpromazine. The appraisal had been done through a double-blind, 12-week trial, while the patients, staff, and assessor were unaware of the prescribed drugs that were packed into identical capsules. No other psychotropic drug or psychosocial intervention, during the trial, was administrated for them. Scale for Assessment of Positive Symptoms (SAPS) and Scale for Assessment of Negative Symptoms (SANS) were used as the primary outcome measures [18]. Schedule for Assessment of Insight (SAI) [19], Clinical Global Impressions-Severity Scale (CGI-S) [20], and finally Simpson Angus Scale (SAS) [21] were also employed as secondary scales. The study duration was 12 weeks, and the patients were assessed by means of SAPS and SANS at baseline (week 0) and at weeks 4, 8, and 12. The other scales were scored at baseline and at the end of the assessment. Exclusion criteria included DSM-IV-TR axis I diagnosis other than schizophrenia, documented medical or neurological disease, utilization of atypical neuroleptics or concomitant therapy such as mood stabilizers or antidepressants, and finally any case with depot antipsychotics. Both of these drugs were prescribed according to practice guidelines and standard-titration protocols [22] and in accordance with the following regimen: 1 mg/day of risperidone or 5 mg/day of olanzapine at baseline up to 2 mg/day of risperidone and 10 mg/day olanzapine at the end of the first week. Weekly interval increments of 2 mg for risperidone and 5 mg for olanzapine, individually and according to clinical situation, were up to maximum of 8 mg and 25 mg for risperidone and olanzapine, respectively, at week 5. The 5th week dosage remained constant up to the end of the study.

3. Statistical Analysis

Patients were compared on baseline characteristics by means of t-tests. The primary analysis was carried out according to the mixed-effect model for repeated measure (MMRM), which estimates with comparatively small bias, in comparison with last observation carried forward (LOCF) approach, and controls type I error rates at a nominal level in the presence of missing completely at random (MCAR) or missing at random (MAR) and some possibility of missing not at random (MNAR) data. Treatment efficacy, as well, was analyzed by paired and nonpaired t-tests in intragroup and between-group comparison of means, respectively. Statistical significance was defined as a 2-sided P value < or = to 0.05. Cohen's standard (d) and correlation measures of effect size (r) were used for comparing baseline to end-point changes in primary outcome measures. MedCalc version 9.4.1.0 and OpenStat version 1.0.0.0 were used as statistical software tools for analysis.

4. Results

Analysis for efficacy was based on data from equal number of patients in olanzapine and risperidone groups. Groups were initially comparable and demographic and diagnostic variables were analogous (Table 1). Five patients (16%) in the olanzapine group and 6 patients (20%) in the risperidone group left the experiment in the second half of the trial due to unwillingness or adverse effect of the prescribed drugs.

Clinical improvement, defined as a 20% reduction in total scores of SAPS and SANS, was seen, respectively, in 86.66% and 56.66% of the cases in the olanzapine group and 73.33% and 36.66% of them in the risperidone group at the end of the assessment. Decrement of mean total score of SAPS was around %14.78 and %12.83 for olanzapine and risperidone, respectively. According to the findings, both of olanzapine and risperidone were significantly efficient in the improvement of positive symptoms ($P < 0.0001$). Decrement of mean total score of SANS as well was around %8.62 and %3.91 for olanzapine and risperidone, respectively. Analysis showed that negative symptoms in the present assessment improved significantly by olanzapine ($P < 0.0003$), while it was not so with respect to risperidone ($P < 0.08$) (Table 2).

Between-group analysis as well showed significant benefits of olanzapine versus risperidone at week 12 regarding SANS ($P < 0.0052$), while it was not so with respect to SAPS ($P < 0.11$) (Table 3).

CGI-S, as well, was significantly improved in both of the groups ($P < 0.05$ and $P < 0.03$ for olanzapine and risperidone, resp.) (Table 2). Similarly, SAI showed significant improvement by olanzapine ($P < 0.003$) and risperidone ($P < 0.05$) at week 12. Besides, SAS showed increase

TABLE 1: Demographic characteristics of patients participating in olanzapine and risperidone groups.

Variables	Olanzapine (N = 30)	Risperidone (N = 30)	T	P	95% CI
Age, y	36.89 ± 3.52	38.44 ± 4.91	1.283	0.205	−0.763, 3.481
Age at onset, y	22.48 ± 3.74	23.62 ± 4.91	0.923	0.360	−1.25, 3.17
Duration of illness, y	6.83 ± 1.63	6.39 ± 1.58	0.969	0.337	−2.28, 3.24
Number of prior episodes Mean ± SD	7.18 ± 2.13	6.82 ± 1.51	0.65	0.51	−1.46, 0.74
Baseline SAPS	63.61 ± 3.86	62.19 ± 4.11	1.379	0.1731	−0.64, 3.48
Baseline SANS	46.26 ± 3.37	46.83 ± 3.75	−0.619	0.5382	−2.41, 1.27
Baseline SAI	3.49 ± 0.61	3.51 ± 1.03	−0.092	0.9274	−0.46, 0.42
Baseline SAS	0.35 ± 0.76	0.35 ± 0.76	0.000	1.0000	−0.39, 0.39
Baseline CGI-S	3.65 ± 1.16	3.25 ± 0.12	1.879	0.0653	−0.03, 0.83

SAPS: Scale for Assessment of Positive Symptoms; SANS: Scale for Assessment of Negative Symptoms; CGI-S: Clinical Global Impressions-Severity Scale; SAI: Schedule for Assessment of Insight; and SAS: Simpson Angus Scale.

TABLE 2: Intragroup analysis of different outcome measures between baseline and week 12.

Measure	Olanzapine Baseline	Olanzapine Week 12	T	P	95% CI	Risperidone Baseline	Risperidone Week 12	T	P	95% CI
SAPS	63.61 ± 3.86	54.96 ± 3.42	9.187	0.0001	6.77, 10.53	62.19 ± 4.11	56.31 ± 3.02	6.315	0.0001	4.02, 7.74
SANS	46.26 ± 3.37	42.74 ± 3.69	3.858	0.0003	1.69, 5.35	46.83 ± 3.75	45.28 ± 3.06	1.754	0.08	−0.22, 3.32
CGI-S	3.65 ± 1.16	3.10 ± 1.03	1.942	0.05	−0.02, 1.12	3.25 ± 0.12	3.17 ± 0.16	2.191	0.03	0.01, 0.15
SAI	3.49 ± 0.61	3.83 ± 0.11	−3.004	0.003	−0.57, −0.11	3.51 ± 1.03	3.97 ± 0.74	−1.987	0.05	−0.92, 0.00
SAS	0.35 ± 0.76	0.38 ± 0.02	−0.216	0.82	−0.31, 0.25	0.36 ± 0.11	0.45 ± 0.19	−2.245	0.02	−0.17, −0.01

SAPS: Scale for Assessment of Positive Symptoms; SANS: Scale for Assessment of Negative Symptoms; CGI-S: Clinical Global Impressions-Severity Scale; SAI: Schedule for Assessment of Insight; and SAS: Simpson Angus Scale.

of extrapyramidal symptoms in both of the groups with 13.08% and 32.87% increment by olanzapine and risperidone, respectively, which was only significant in the risperidone group ($P < 0.02$) (Table 2). Between-group analysis, as well, showed significantly poorer state for risperidone vis-à-vis olanzapine ($P < 0.04$) (Table 3).

Since the sample size was small, the effect size (ES) was analyzed for changes on the primary outcome measures at the end of experiment. Results showed a large (d or r = or >0.8 or 0.3, resp.) readily observable improvement of SAPS and SANS by olanzapine and large and small (d or r = or <0.2 or 0.1, resp.) improvement of SAPS and SANS, respectively, by risperidone. The mean modal dose of olanzapine and risperidone during the present assessment was 20.49 ± 4.51 mg/day and 6.32 ± 1.68 mg/day, respectively. Throughout this study, extrapyramidal symptoms, mainly stiffness and tremor, were reported as an adverse event for 48.33% of the cases in the risperidone group and 16.66% of them in the olanzapine group, which was significantly more prevalent in the first group ($P < 0.03$). On the other hand, weight gain was significantly more evident in patients treated with olanzapine (46.66%) in comparison with risperidone (16.66%) ($P < 0.03$). Also, mean weight gain was significantly more in olanzapine group (3.4 +/− 0.8 kg) in comparison with risperidone group (0.7 +/− 0.2 kg) ($P < 0.0001$). Post hoc power analysis showed an intermediary power = 0.60 with respect to this trial.

5. Discussion

The primary objective of this study was to compare once more efficacy and safety of olanzapine and risperidone in schizophrenic patients, since there was no constant deduction so far, based on the results of the previous analogous studies. In essence and according to final outcomes, both of olanzapine and risperidone were significantly effective in reducing the severity of overall psychotic symptoms, while as regards improvement of negative symptoms and extrapyramidal side effects, olanzapine was shown to be more advantageous than risperidone. In this regard, maybe insignificant improvement of negative symptoms by risperidone was a bit due to intensification of secondary negative symptoms, which interfered with or concealed the improvement of primary ones. Anyway, these findings are somewhat comparable to another analogous double-blind, 28-week study on 339 patients who met DSM-IV criteria for schizophrenia, schizophreniform disorder, or schizoaffective disorder [10]. While that study reported a significantly greater proportion of olanzapine-treated patients achieving

Table 3: Between-group analysis of different outcome measures at weeks 4, 8, and 12.

Measures	Olanzapine $N = 30$	Risperidone $N = 30$	T	P	95% CI
SAPS-4th week	61.44 ± 3.92	61.23 ± 3.61	0.216	0.82	−1.74, 2.16
SAPS-8th week	60.27 ± 3.82	60.98 ± 3.58	−0.743	0.46	−2.62, 1.20
SAPS-12th week	54.96 ± 3.42	56.31 ± 3.02	−1.621	0.11	−3.02, 0.32
SANS-4th week	45.19 ± 2.73	45.69 ± 2.29	−0.769	0.44	−1.80, 0.80
SANS-8th week	44.91 ± 3.37	45.76 ± 3.33	−0.983	0.32	−2.58, 0.88
SANS-12th week	42.74 ± 3.69	45.28 ± 3.06	−2.902	0.005	−4.29, −0.79
SAI-12th week	3.83 ± 0.11	3.97 ± 0.74	−1.025	0.30	−0.41, 0.13
SAS-12th week	0.38 ± 0.02	0.45 ± 0.19	−2.007	0.04	−0.14, −0.00
CGI-S-12th week	3.10 ± 1.03	3.17 ± 0.16	−0.368	0.71	−0.45, 0.31

SAPS: Scale for Assessment of Positive Symptoms; SANS: Scale for Assessment of Negative Symptoms; CGI-S: Clinical Global Impressions-Severity Scale; SAI: Schedule for Assessment of Insight; SAS: Simpson Angus Scale.

remarkable improvement in PANSS, better enhancement in SANS, and considerably a lower amount of EPS, in the present assessment there was no significant difference between olanzapine and risperidone with respect to improvement of positive symptoms or insight. There are additional studies as well with varying outcomes. For example, though in an 8-week head-to-head clinical trial comparing olanzapine with risperidone on 377 patients who met DSM-IV criteria for schizophrenia or schizoaffective disorder, there was no significant difference among them with respect to efficacy measures or extrapyramidal side effects [17], in the current appraisal significant worsening of such kind of adverse effects was evident only by risperidone. In the same way, another open-label, head-to-head study of olanzapine versus risperidone concluded that although there was greater improvement in psychotic symptoms in the risperidone group, there was significant increase in akathisia as well in the same group compared to olanzapine-treated cases [23]. Likewise, there are additional studies that have similar assumptions in support of risperidone [14, 15]. Maybe, applying different efficacy measures with various psychometric properties and different samples using unlike diagnostic criteria can explain to some extent these inconsistent results. In addition, since the weight gain was noticeably greater in the olanzapine group and this problem may well be an important trouble, perhaps, especially for women, such an adverse effect and related metabolic side effects, should always be taken into account by clinicians. The same vigilance also could be reasonable regarding extrapyramidal symptoms that were more challenging here with respect to risperidone. Hence, proper prescription of antipsychotics for special target group of patients cannot be independent of their potential side effect. While in comparison with the previous studies, the outcome of the present assessment may not be shown to be more decisive and free from controversy, it may propose the necessity of more parallel trials or meta-analytic studies regarding comparisons between atypical antipsychotics. Also, restriction of diagnosis to only schizophrenia, instead of whole of schizophrenia, schizoaffective and schizophreniform disorders, which was usual in the aforesaid trials, could endorse a more precise tryout in the present assessment. Besides, equal efficacy of these two second-generation antipsychotics regarding improvement of positive symptoms and insight may perhaps weaken any kind of irrational clinical preference regarding picking one of them as first choice, and, then again, significant improvement of negative symptoms by olanzapine may well show a better choice for schizophrenic patients with predominantly negative symptoms in longitudinal course. Also, strengthening of extrapyramidal side effects by risperidone may possibly classify it as antipsychotic that can increase the risk of tardive dyskinesia in susceptible patients. Small sample size, short duration of assessment, gender-based sampling, and lack of placebo arm, which may have significant impact on the assay sensitivity of the study and artificially inflate results in an active comparator trial, were among the weak points of this trial. Further analogous trials in future possibly will improve our knowledge in this regard.

6. Conclusion

While both of olanzapine and risperidone were equally effective for the treatment of patients with schizophrenia, olanzapine showed superior efficacy with respect to negative symptoms, along with lesser extrapyramidal side effects, in comparison with risperidone.

Conflict of Interests

The authors declare that there is no conflict of interests regarding the publication of this paper.

Acknowledgments

The authors gratefully acknowledge their dear colleague S. Akbari (M.D.) and the Department of Research for their practical and financial support of this study.

References

[1] J. M. Kane, "Schizophrenia," *The New England Journal of Medicine*, vol. 334, no. 1, pp. 34–41, 1996.

[2] J. A. Lieberman, "Prediction of outcome in first-episode schizophrenia," *Journal of Clinical Psychiatry*, vol. 54, no. 3, pp. 13–17, 1993.

[3] J. M. Kane and J. A. Lieberman, *Adverse Effects of Psychotropic Drugs*, Guilford Press, New York, NY, USA, 1992.

[4] S. Leucht, C. Corves, D. Arbter, R. R. Engel, C. Li, and J. M. Davis, "Second-generation versus first-generation antipsychotic drugs for schizophrenia: a meta-analysis," *The Lancet*, vol. 373, no. 9657, pp. 31–41, 2009.

[5] N. A. Moore, N. C. Tye, M. S. Axton, and F. C. Risius, "The behavioral pharmacology of olanzapine, a novel "atypical" antipsychotic agent," *Journal of Pharmacology and Experimental Therapeutics*, vol. 262, no. 2, pp. 545–551, 1992.

[6] C. M. Beasley Jr., G. Tollefson, P. Tran, W. Satterlee, T. Sanger, and S. Hamilton, "Olanzapine versus placebo and haloperidol: Acute phase results of the North American Double-Blind Olanzapine Trial," *Neuropsychopharmacology*, vol. 14, no. 2, pp. 111–123, 1996.

[7] G. D. Tollefson, C. M. Beasley Jr., P. V. Tran et al., "Olanzapine versus haloperidol in the treatment of schizophrenia and schizoaffective disorders: results of an international collaborative trial," *The American Journal of Psychiatry*, vol. 154, pp. 457–465, 1997.

[8] M. A. Dellva, P. Tran, G. D. Tollefson, A. L. Wentley, and C. M. Beasley Jr., "Standard olanzapine versus placebo and ineffective-dose olanzapine in the maintenance treatment of schizophrenia," *Psychiatric Services*, vol. 48, no. 12, pp. 1571–1577, 1997.

[9] S. R. Marder and R. C. Meibach, "Risperidone in the treatment of schizophrenia," *American Journal of Psychiatry*, vol. 151, no. 6, pp. 825–835, 1994.

[10] P. V. Tran, S. H. Hamilton, A. J. Kuntz et al., "Double-blind comparison of olanzapine versus risperidone in the treatment of schizophrenia and other psychotic disorders," *Journal of Clinical Psychopharmacology*, vol. 17, no. 5, pp. 407–418, 1997.

[11] O. Gureje, W. Miles, N. Keks et al., "Olanzapine vs risperidone in the management of schizophrenia: a randomized double-blind trial in Australia and New Zealand," *Schizophrenia Research*, vol. 61, no. 2-3, pp. 303–314, 2003.

[12] E. T. Edgell, S. W. Andersen, B. M. Johnstone, B. Dulisse, D. Revicki, and A. Breier, "Olanzapine versus risperidone: a prospective comparison of clinical and economic outcomes in schizophrenia," *PharmacoEconomics*, vol. 18, no. 6, pp. 567–579, 2000.

[13] K. L. Rascati, M. T. Johnsrud, M. L. Crismon, M. J. Lage, and B. L. Barber, "Olanzapine versus risperidone in the treatment of schizophrenia: a comparison of costs among Texas Medicaid recipients," *PharmacoEconomics*, vol. 21, no. 10, pp. 683–697, 2003.

[14] P. D. Feldman, C. J. Kaiser, J. S. Kennedy et al., "Comparison of risperidone and olanzapine in the control of negative symptoms of chronic schizophrenia and related psychotic disorders in patients aged 50 to 65 years," *The Journal of Clinical Psychiatry*, vol. 64, no. 9, pp. 998–1004, 2003.

[15] D. M. Taylor, T. Wright, and S. E. Libretto, "Risperidone compared with olanzapine in a naturalistic clinical study: a cost analysis," *Journal of Clinical Psychiatry*, vol. 64, no. 5, pp. 589–597, 2003.

[16] S. Kasper, M. Jones, and I. Duchesne, "Risperidone olanzapine drug outcomes studies in Schizophrenia (RODOS): health economic results of an international naturalistic study," *International Clinical Psychopharmacology*, vol. 16, no. 4, pp. 189–196, 2001.

[17] R. R. Conley and R. Mahmoud, "A randomized double-blind study of risperidone and olanzapine in the treatment of schizophrenia or schizoaffective disorder," *The American Journal of Psychiatry*, vol. 158, no. 5, pp. 765–774, 2001.

[18] N. Andreasen, *The Scale for the Assessment of Negative Symptoms (SANS)*, University of Iowa, Department of Psychiatry, Iowa City, Iowa, USA, 1981.

[19] A. S. David, "Insight and psychosis," *British Journal of Psychiatry*, vol. 156, pp. 798–808, 1990.

[20] W. Guy, Ed., *Clinical Global Impressions: ECDEU Assessment Manual for Psychopharmacology*, Department of Health, Education, and Welfare, DHEW Publication, Rockville, Md, USA, 1976.

[21] G. M. Simpson and J. W. Angus, "A rating scale for extrapyramidal side effects," *Acta Psychiatrica Scandinavica, Supplement*, vol. 212, supplement 44, pp. 11–19, 1970.

[22] D. P. Van Kammen, S. R. Marder, and V. A. Sadock, "Serotonin-dopamin antagonists," in *Kaplan & Sadock's Comprehensive Textbook of Psychiatry*, B. J. Sadock and V. A. Sadock, Eds., vol. 2, Lippincott Williams & Wilkins, Baltimore, Md, USA, 8th edition, 2005.

[23] B. C. Ho, D. Miller, P. Nopoulos, and N. C. Andreasen, "A comparative effectiveness study of risperidone and olanzapine in the treatment of schizophrenia," *Journal of Clinical Psychiatry*, vol. 60, no. 10, pp. 658–663, 1999.

3

Gender Identity Disorder and Schizophrenia: Neurodevelopmental Disorders with Common Causal Mechanisms?

Ravi Philip Rajkumar

Department of Psychiatry, Jawaharlal Institute of Postgraduate Medical Education and Research (JIPMER), Dhanvantari Nagar, Pondicherry 605 006, India

Correspondence should be addressed to Ravi Philip Rajkumar; ravi.psych@gmail.com

Academic Editor: Luis San

Gender identity disorder (GID), recently renamed gender dysphoria (GD), is a rare condition characterized by an incongruity between gender identity and biological sex. Clinical evidence suggests that schizophrenia occurs in patients with GID at rates higher than in the general population and that patients with GID may have schizophrenia-like personality traits. Conversely, patients with schizophrenia may experience alterations in gender identity and gender role perception. Neurobiological research, including brain imaging and studies of finger length ratio and handedness, suggests that both these disorders are associated with altered cerebral sexual dimorphism and changes in cerebral lateralization. Various mechanisms, such as *Toxoplasma* infection, reduced levels of brain-derived neurotrophic factor (BDNF), early childhood adversity, and links with autism spectrum disorders, may account for some of this overlap. The implications of this association for further research are discussed.

1. Introduction

Gender identity disorder (GID) is a rare condition characterized by an incongruity between gender identity and biological sex. Individuals with this condition experience distress related to their biological sex and frequently express a desire to change it by hormonal or surgical means; in simple terms, they identify themselves as belonging to the opposite gender, and behave accordingly. GID is distinct from disorders of sexual development, such as chromosomal abnormalities or congenital adrenal hyperplasia, in that there is no anatomical or physiological ambiguity regarding the individual's sex; rather, there is a subjective dissatisfaction with it [1, 2]. The central role played by this dissatisfaction and distress has led to the condition being renamed "gender dysphoria" (GD) in the DSM-5, though the term "gender incongruence" (GI) has also been proposed by some authors [1].

Various theories have been proposed to account for GID/GD and related conditions, known as gender identity variants (GIVs) [3]. Abnormalities in genes related to gonadal hormone synthesis and action have been found in these individuals, suggesting that GID/GD is a disorder of sexual brain differentiation caused by exposure to altered hormone levels during a sensitive period [2, 3]; however, evidence for such a viewpoint has not been consistently found, and it fails to account for patients with late-onset GID who have few or no symptoms during childhood [4]. Alternately, GID has been conceptualized as a disorder of cortical representation of sex-specific bodily features, particularly the genitalia [5], but such a proposal does not account for the other behavioural changes seen in this condition. In this paper, I review theoretical and research evidence suggesting that GID is a neurodevelopmental disorder, involving the processes of brain lateralization and sexual differentiation, which is related to schizophrenia. First, the evidence of a symptomatic overlap between the two conditions is reviewed; next, evidence of common causal pathways and mechanisms is outlined and synthesized.

2. Clinical and Phenomenological Overlap between Schizophrenia and GID/GD

2.1. Comorbidity between the Two Disorders. A relationship between two distinct disorders can be inferred if they cooccur at a higher level than would be expected by chance. According to recent estimates, the prevalence of schizophrenia is approximately 1 to 8 per 1,000 population [6], and that of GID is even lower, estimated at around 1 in 10,000 for male-to-female GID and less than 1 in 25,000 for female-to-male GID [7]. Their cooccurrence would therefore be expected to be rare: a crude estimate, obtained by multiplying prevalences, would be less than 1 in 1,000,000 individuals.

Hospital and clinic-based studies of individuals with GID have found rates of schizophrenia far in excess of both this estimate and the general population prevalence; however, comorbid mental illness is likely to have been overrepresented in such samples. A Dutch survey of 186 psychiatrists evaluating patients with GID found that 31 (16.7%) reported seeing patients with comorbid GID and psychotic disorders, including schizophrenia [8]; however, it was not possible to calculate the percentage of patients with schizophrenia from the data provided by the authors, and the study has been criticized on the grounds of response bias, low external validity, and lack of a standardized means of confirming the diagnosis of psychosis [9]. A second Dutch study compared 20 patients who underwent gender-reassignment surgery and 27 in whom this treatment was deferred or delayed; no patient in the former group had schizophrenia, while 2 in the latter (7.4%) received this diagnosis, and a third was reported as having "psychotic episodes" [10]. An earlier clinic-based study obtained similar results; in a sample of 51 individuals with GID referred for psychiatric evaluation, 8% were found to have schizophrenia [11]. An unusual clustering was reported in African-American women with GID at a clinic in the United States; two of these five subjects (40%) were diagnosed with schizophrenia and a third was noted to have a "schizophrenic character" [12].

More modest but still significant results have been obtained in population-based samples. A recent study from Ireland found that 8 of 159 patients with male-to-female gender dysphoria (5%) had comorbid schizophrenia, as opposed to none of 59 patients with female-to-male GD [7]. Psychiatric evaluation of 230 self-referred applicants for gender-reassignment surgery in Spain, after excluding patients with psychosis but no clear diagnosis of GD/GID, identified six cases (2.6%) of psychosis, with equal rates in male and female subjects [13]. Though these figures are lower than those of the referral-based studies, they are likely to be closer to the true prevalence in this population and are still far higher than would be expected by chance alone. A study of Taiwanese students which measured symptoms, rather than diagnoses, found a strong correlation between symptoms of GID and schizophrenia in male students [14], also suggesting an effect of gender on this association.

Taken together, these studies provide indirect evidence for a link between schizophrenia and GID, on the grounds of their greater-than-chance cooccurrence. However, not all studies in adults or adolescents have been positive. A study of 579 subjects with GID from Japan found only one case of schizophrenia (0.17%) in a female-to-male patient, a rate which is comparable to the lower bound of general population values [15]; however, another publication involving the same sample makes it clear that five subjects with schizophrenia were excluded from the first paper, yielding a corrected prevalence of 1.02% [16]. A study of 435 patients attending a gender clinic in Texas found only four (0.92%) cases of schizophrenia [17]. In a sample of 83 Iranian patients with GID, no cases of schizophrenia were reported [18].

2.2. Beliefs Related to Gender Change in Schizophrenia. Beliefs or ideas related to gender change—historically termed *metamorphosis paranoica sexualis* by Richard von Krafft-Ebing—have been documented in schizophrenia for over a century. One of the most influential cases in the early literature on this disorder—Daniel Paul Schreber, whom Freud used as the basis for his psychodynamic formulations of schizophrenia—experienced bizarre delusions in which he believed that he would be transformed into a woman, and that this was part of his mission to redeem the world [19, 20]. Though no study has systematically examined the prevalence of such delusions in schizophrenia, there have been numerous case reports of patients with schizophrenia who had seemingly delusional beliefs related to gender identity [21–27]; in some of these cases, a weakening [21] or resolution [27] of gender dysphoria was reported after antipsychotic treatment, while in others, schizophrenic symptoms resolved and features of GID persisted, suggesting that they were distinct [26]. These reports suggest that there is a grey area between patients with schizophrenia, those with GID/GD, and those whose phenomenology does not clearly fit into either category. This situation is complicated by the fact that many researchers view the two diagnoses as mutually exclusive [15], which may lead to an underestimate of gender-related psychopathology in schizophrenia.

2.3. Gender Identity in Schizophrenia. Leaving aside overt delusions of gender change, are there subtler indications of gender disturbance in schizophrenia? A number of older studies have attempted to address this issue, though they are largely based on projective techniques of psychological assessment [28]. Evidence of disturbed gender role and gender identity in these studies includes distortions or omissions of anatomical features on being asked to draw human figures [29, 30], reduced satisfaction with body parts in male patients with schizophrenia [31], and inappropriate responses on psychological tests of masculinity-femininity [32, 33].

A more recent study of 90 patients with schizophrenia using the Bem Sex Role Inventory found that both men and women had culturally appropriate scores on the feminine role scale and low scores on the masculine role scale [34]. These findings provide evidence for a disturbed or distorted perception of gender identity and role in patients with schizophrenia; however, given the significant impact of culture on gender roles, they need to be replicated in non-Western settings.

2.4. Schizophrenia-Like Traits in Patients with GID/GD. In a similar way, some researchers have assessed schizophrenia-like traits or personality variables in individuals with gender identity disorder. Two studies have used the subscales of the Minnesota Multiphasic Personality Inventory (MMPI) to assess personality dimensions in subjects with GID. In the first, high scores on the femininity subscale were found in men applying for gender-reassignment surgery; however, an elevation in the schizophrenia subscale was found only in those men who were continuing to live as men [35]. In the second, female-to-male transsexuals receiving testosterone therapy as part of the management of GID showed a significant decrease in scores on the paranoia subscale of the MMPI-2 [36]. A study of Taiwanese university students found that gender dysphoria was strongly associated with schizoid personality in both men (OR 4.7; 95% CI 2.2–9.9) and women (OR 3.6; 95% CI 2.1–6.3) [37]. These findings suggest that schizophrenia-linked personality traits may be commoner in persons with GID, though gender and hormonal treatment may moderate this association.

3. Processes and Mechanisms Common to Schizophrenia and GID/GD

3.1. The Role of Prenatal Hormonal Factors in Schizophrenia and GID/GD. An influential model of GID, briefly alluded to above, posits that this condition is due to a disorder of sexual development which specifically involves the brain, but spares the internal and external genitalia [3]. This theory has gained some support from brain imaging studies in which sexually dimorphic brain regions resemble those of the desired rather than the anatomical gender in subjects with GID [38–40]. There is evidence that some brain structures may show a similar variation in schizophrenia, with men showing a "feminized" pattern and women showing a "masculinized" pattern [41, 42], leading to the proposal that schizophrenia itself may be related to gender-atypical brain development, perhaps caused by prenatal hormonal imbalances [43, 44]. However, there are important differences in brain structure across the two disorders: most importantly, the thickness of the cerebral cortex is increased in male-to-female transsexuals [45], while schizophrenia has been consistently associated with decreased cortical thickness, irrespective of gender [46–48]. This suggests that even if both disorders are related to common neurodevelopmental pathways, the changes seen in GID are less severe and more region-specific than those seen in schizophrenia.

Apart from the direct evidence of brain imaging studies, indirect evidence of prenatal hormonal influences can be obtained by studying the ratio of the length of the second and fourth digits (the 2D : 4D ratio) in adults; higher ratios indicate a more "feminized" pattern. In persons with GID, evidence of an altered 2D : 4D ratio has been reported in several studies [49–51], though some researchers have found a specific association only in men [49] or women [50, 51]. These alterations are generally in the direction of individual's self-identified sex, with female-to-male subjects showing a more "masculinized" pattern than control women, and male-to-female subjects showing a more "feminized" ratio. Very similar alterations in the 2D : 4D ratio have been reported in schizophrenia, more specifically in male patients where a reversal of normal sexual dimorphism has been documented [52, 53]. Similar abnormalities are also found in schizotypal disorder, a condition which is genetically and clinically related to schizophrenia [54, 55]. This alteration, especially in male patients with schizophrenia, has also been tentatively linked to abnormalities in prenatal testosterone exposure, a mechanism relevant to GID.

3.2. Cerebral Laterality and Handedness. Besides indicating sexual dimorphism, the finger length ratio is also an indicator of cerebral lateralization [56]. Alterations in cerebral lateralization may result in an excess of atypical hand dominance patterns, such as left-handedness or mixed laterality. A meta-analysis of 40 published studies found that schizophrenia was consistently associated with increased atypical hand dominance, particularly left-handedness [57]. Similarly, both male and female transsexuals have higher rates of non-right-handedness than healthy controls [58], and this has been documented even in young boys with childhood GID [59]. These findings suggest an altered pattern of lateralisation [58], presumably of developmental origin and at least partly linked to genes involved in neurodevelopment [60].

3.3. Toxoplasma Infection, Gender Identity, and Schizophrenia. Prenatal or childhood infection with the parasite *Toxoplasma gondii* has been identified as a risk factor for schizophrenia [61, 62]. Though evidence of this infection is not found in all patients with the disorder, it may be associated with a less favourable outcome [63] and with a higher risk of suicidal behaviour in younger patients with schizophrenia [64]. The exact mechanisms involved in this association are unknown but may include increased dopamine levels [61], alterations in brain development [65], or the activation of endogenous retroviruses [66]. Though there is no direct evidence linking *Toxoplasma* to GID, there is evidence suggesting that prenatal infection can result in "masculinization" of the foetus and even a predominance of male births in infected mothers [67]. In a follow-up study of seven adult patients with congenital toxoplasmosis, one male patient had developed a male-to-female GID and undergone gender-reassignment surgery [68]. It is therefore possible that *Toxoplasma* infection may be a common risk factor for both disorders, though this proposal needs to be tested serologically in individuals with GID. The link between *Toxoplasma* infection and suicidality is also not without relevance, as suicidal and self-injurious behaviour is very common in individuals with GID [15, 17].

3.4. The Role of Brain-Derived Neurotrophic Factor. Brain-derived neurotrophic factor (BDNF) is a nerve growth factor that plays a key role in brain development, as well as in the maintenance of neural plasticity in adult brains. The activity of BDNF can be influenced by several factors, including sex hormones such as oestrogen and testosterone [69]. A meta-analysis of studies conducted in patients with schizophrenia has identified a consistent, moderate decrease in blood BDNF levels compared to healthy controls [70]. A recent study has found evidence of decreased serum BDNF levels in patients with GID [71]. The authors of this paper have suggested that these changes may be due to childhood adversity [71] or stress related to the patients' "minority" status [72]. Yet, it is equally probable that low BDNF levels may signal a defect or deviation in normal brain development in this patient group [73], in the light of what is already known about the role of this molecule in the sexual differentiation of the brain [74]. Moreover, as discussed below, these two explanations are not mutually exclusive.

3.5. The Role of Childhood Attachment and Childhood Adversity. It is now well established that disturbances in parent-child attachment, including severe adverse experiences such as physical and sexual abuse, are associated with an elevated risk of schizophrenia [75]. A variety of biological and psychological mechanisms may underlie this association, including sensitization of dopamine pathways, impaired mentalizing abilities, and distortions of internal representations of the self and others; moreover, childhood adversity can itself alter brain development to some extent [76]. A relationship between disturbed childhood attachment and GID has been recognized for decades [77–81] and has unfortunately led to simplistic, reductionistic approaches to the management of this condition in some cases [82]. Nevertheless, more recent research has also found high rates (25%) of childhood maltreatment in male-to-female transsexuals; patients with a history of maltreatment had greater dissatisfaction with their body and worse mental health [83]. It is possible that, as in the case of schizophrenia, childhood maltreatment interacts with an underlying developmental vulnerability to lead to symptom formation in GID/GD; alternately, trauma-related release of stress hormones may lower BDNF levels [69], affecting childhood brain development.

3.6. Links between Autism, Schizophrenia, and GID/GD. Autism and related conditions, collectively known as autism spectrum disorders (ASD), are neurodevelopmental disorders which are distinct from schizophrenia but also overlap with it substantially on anatomical and neurocognitive grounds [84, 85]. The two conditions are also genetically linked; a family history of schizophrenia is a risk factor for ASD [86], and common genetic vulnerability loci have been identified [87]. Like schizophrenia, autism is linked to abnormalities in prenatal testosterone exposure, which is relevant to the pathogenesis of GID/GD [88, 89]. A study of individuals with ASD identified deviations in gender typicality, particularly lower overall levels of masculinity in both genders and higher levels of "tomboyism" in women with ASD [90]. Individuals of both biological sexes with ASD and comorbid GID/GD have also been reported in the literature [91, 92]. Conversely, studies of individuals with GID have identified high levels of autistic traits [93] and comorbid ASD [94, 95], though some of these results appear to be gender-specific. Deficits in empathising, a feature of ASD, are also associated with GD, especially in female-to-male subjects [96]. Though none of these studies have specifically examined links with schizophrenic symptoms or dimensions, they provide further indirect evidence for an etiological and phenomenological zone of contact between GID/GD and schizophrenia.

4. A Tentative Synthesis

Beginning with the observation that the comorbidity of schizophrenia and GID/GD is greater than would be expected, it is seen that patients with either condition may exhibit symptoms or traits of the other. Several converging lines of evidence, involving cerebral sexual dimorphism, laterality, prenatal infection, and childhood adversity, suggest that both these disorders have their roots in abnormal brain development and that their overlap may be explained by shared risk factors (such as *Toxoplasma* infection) or mechanisms (such as abnormal lateralization and sexual brain differentiation) via common biochemical pathways, such as prenatal hormonal imbalances or reduced BDNF expression and release. Schizophrenia is also associated with disturbances in body image and concept [97–99], which may be mediated through a frontal-limbic-temporal-parietal neural network [100]. Such processes would be relevant to an alternate model of GID, in which disturbances in body image representation, involving suppression or distortion of body maps in the parietal cortex, are considered to be the central feature [5, 101]. In either case, the existence of a link between the two disorders is certainly more than possible. Yet another intriguing possibility is raised by studies showing an association between GID and social cognitive deficits. It has been found by some researchers that individuals with female-to-male GID have deficits in empathising. This leads to difficulties in interacting with people of their own sex, who use empathising as a preferential mode of interaction [93, 96], and may cause them to identify more readily with males, who use "systemizing" more prominently than empathising [96]. Though this possibility was raised in the context of autistic traits, it may also be relevant to the schizoid or schizophrenia-like personality traits seen in individuals with GID/GD [14, 37] and provides a further pathway by which a neurodevelopmental vulnerability can lead to the development of this disorder.

5. Further Directions for Research

The proposal outlined above can be tested in several ways. Structural brain imaging studies can assess similarities and differences in sexually dimorphic structures in both groups and identify areas of overlap. Functional brain imaging and neuropsychological assessment may shed the light on anomalies of cerebral lateralization in these disorders. Clinical studies could focus on identifying body and gender disturbances in patients with schizophrenia and their first-degree relatives and schizotypal-like traits in patients with GID. The contribution of individual risk factors, such as *Toxoplasma* infection, can be assessed serologically. Genetic studies could examine the links between gender dysphoria, schizophrenia spectrum disorders, and related conditions such as autistic spectrum disorders. The consistency of, and correlations between, information obtained through these various methods would either clarify the link between schizophrenia and GID or refute it.

6. Limitations of the above Proposal

The model proposed above is not free of shortcomings. In the first place, it makes the assumption that schizophrenia and GID are both clear-cut syndromes, which is far from the case; schizophrenia is a heterogeneous disorder [102], and some of the clinical and developmental marker studies mentioned above have identified differences between male-to-female and female-to-male GID [7, 49–51]. Second, GID is comorbid with a variety of other psychiatric disorders, particularly mood and anxiety disorders, at rates higher than those reported for comorbid schizophrenia [7, 13, 16, 18]. It is not known if these disorders are the psychological consequence of living with GID, if they reflect shared vulnerabilities that need to be examined in their own right, or if patients with GID are at a nonspecifically elevated risk for a variety of disorders. Third, there are no systematic large-scale studies on gender disturbances in schizophrenia, or schizophrenia-like or schizotypal traits in GID, which would strengthen the case for the association proposed in this paper. Fourth, while the evidence presented earlier points towards a link between these two conditions, it does not explain the large differences between them. Fifth, owing to the relative rarity of comorbid GID and schizophrenia, no study has systematically examined the differences between patients with GID/GD alone, schizophrenia alone, and those with both conditions. Finally, there is evidence that risk factors for schizophrenia and GID/GD, apart from the ones discussed earlier, may be distinct. For example, factors such as migration, urbanicity, obstetric complications, cannabis use, and maternal viral infection are specifically linked to schizophrenia [6], but not to GID. Similarly, developmental antecedents of GID, such as early childhood cross-gender behaviour and same-sex sexual fantasies [103], are not specifically associated within schizophrenia. In the case of birth order, the relationship between GID and schizophrenia seems to be inverse; an earlier birth order is associated with schizophrenia in males [104], while a later birth order is associated with male-to-female GID [105, 106]. These divergences suggest that the two conditions may share certain causal pathways but do not overlap completely.

A further note of caution must be introduced here. The fact that scientific evidence suggests a link between GID and schizophrenia must not be taken to imply that GID is a psychotic disorder, that a wish for gender change is a form of schizophrenic thought disorder [107], or that such individuals must be treated with antipsychotic medication. It is beyond the scope of this paper to address the social and political controversies surrounding the diagnosis of GID [3, 108]. Research in this area should be driven by methodologically sound science rather than personal or political beliefs.

7. Conclusion

The available evidence, though limited, suggests that both gender identity disorder and schizophrenia are neurodevelopmental disorders and that they may share common causal mechanisms and risk factors. Further systematic investigation of these factors may provide a new perspective not only on these quite different conditions but also on the mechanisms and processes involved in normal brain development and sexual differentiation.

Conflict of Interests

The author declares that there is no conflict of interests regarding the publication of this paper.

References

[1] A. A. Lawrence, "Proposed revisions to gender identity disorder diagnoses in the DSM-5," *Archives of Sexual Behavior*, vol. 39, no. 6, pp. 1253–1260, 2010.

[2] A. Michel, C. Mormont, and J. J. Legros, "A psycho-endocrinological overview of transsexualism," *European Journal of Endocrinology*, vol. 145, no. 4, pp. 365–376, 2001.

[3] H. F. L. Meyer-Bahlburg, "From mental disorder to iatrogenic hypogonadism: dilemmas in conceptualizing gender identity variants as psychiatric conditions," *Archives of Sexual Behavior*, vol. 39, no. 2, pp. 461–476, 2010.

[4] T. O. Nieder, M. Herff, S. Cerwenka et al., "Age of onset and sexual orientation in transsexual males and females," *Journal of Sexual Medicine*, vol. 8, no. 3, pp. 783–791, 2011.

[5] V. S. Ramachandran and P. D. McGeoch, "Occurrence of phantom genitalia after gender reassignment surgery," *Medical Hypotheses*, vol. 69, no. 5, pp. 1001–1003, 2007.

[6] R. Tandon, M. S. Keshavan, and H. A. Nasrallah, "Schizophrenia, "just the facts" what we know in 2008. 2. Epidemiology and etiology," *Schizophrenia Research*, vol. 102, no. 1–3, pp. 1–18, 2008.

[7] C. Judge, C. O'Donovan, G. Callaghan, G. Gaoatswe, and D. O'Shea, "Gender dysphoria—prevalence and co-morbidities in an Irish adult population," *Frontiers in Endocrinology*, vol. 5, pp. 1–5, 2014.

[8] J. À Campo, H. Nijman, H. Merckelbach, and C. Evers, "Psychiatric comorbidity of gender identity disorders: a survey among dutch psychiatrists," *The American Journal of Psychiatry*, vol. 160, no. 7, pp. 1332–1336, 2003.

[9] E. J. Giltay, L. J. G. Gooren, P. T. Cohen-Kettenis et al., "Comorbidity of gender identity disorders," *The American Journal of Psychiatry*, vol. 161, no. 5, pp. 934–935, 2004.

[10] Y. L. S. Smith, S. H. M. Van Goozen, and P. T. Cohen-Kettenis, "Adolescents with gender identity disorder who were accepted or rejected for sex reassignment surgery: a prospective follow-up study," *Journal of the American Academy of Child and Adolescent Psychiatry*, vol. 40, no. 4, pp. 472–481, 2001.

[11] S. B. Levine, "Psychiatric diagnosis of patients requesting sex reassignment surgery," *Journal of Sex and Marital Therapy*, vol. 6, no. 3, pp. 164–173, 1980.

[12] L. M. Lothstein and H. Roback, "Black female transsexuals and schizophrenia: a serendipitous finding?" *Archives of Sexual Behavior*, vol. 13, no. 4, pp. 371–386, 1984.

[13] E. Gómez-Gil, A. Trilla, M. Salamero, T. Godás, and M. Valdés, "Sociodemographic, clinical, and psychiatric characteristics of transsexuals from Spain," *Archives of Sexual Behavior*, vol. 38, no. 3, pp. 378–392, 2009.

[14] Y.-L. Chien, S. S.-F. Gau, and K. D. Gadow, "Sex difference in the rates and co-occurring conditions of psychiatric symptoms in incoming college students in Taiwan," *Comprehensive Psychiatry*, vol. 52, no. 2, pp. 195–207, 2011.

[15] M. Hoshiai, Y. Matsumoto, T. Sato et al., "Psychiatric comorbidity among patients with gender identity disorder," *Psychiatry and Clinical Neurosciences*, vol. 64, no. 5, pp. 514–519, 2010.

[16] N. Okabe, T. Sato, Y. Matsumoto, Y. Ido, S. Terada, and S. Kuroda, "Clinical characteristics of patients with gender identity disorder at a Japanese gender identity disorder clinic," *Psychiatry Research*, vol. 157, no. 1-3, pp. 315–318, 2008.

[17] C. M. Cole, M. O'Boyle, L. E. Emory, and W. J. Meyer III, "Comorbidity of gender dysphoria and other major psychiatric diagnoses," *Archives of Sexual Behavior*, vol. 26, no. 1, pp. 13–26, 1997.

[18] A. M. Meybodi, A. Hajebi, and A. G. Jolfaei, "Psychiatric axis I comorbidities among patients with gender dysphoria," *Psychiatry Journal*, vol. 2014, Article ID 971814, 5 pages, 2014.

[19] J. S. Grotstein, "The Schreber case revisited: schizophrenia as a disorder of self-regulation and of interactional regulation," *Yale Journal of Biology and Medicine*, vol. 58, no. 3, pp. 299–314, 1985.

[20] T. H. McGlashan, "Psychosis as a disorder of reduced cathectic capacity: freud's analysis of the schreber case revisited," *Schizophrenia Bulletin*, vol. 35, no. 3, pp. 476–481, 2009.

[21] D. A. Baltieri and A. G. de Andrade, "Schizophrenia modifying the expression of gender identity disorder," *The Journal of Sexual Medicine*, vol. 6, no. 4, pp. 1185–1188, 2009.

[22] M. Urban and J. Rabe-Jabłońska, "Delusion of sex change and body dysmorphic disorder in clinical picture of paranoid schizophrenia—case reports," *Psychiatria Polska*, vol. 44, no. 5, pp. 723–733, 2010.

[23] L. Borras, P. Huguelet, and A. Eytan, "Delusional "pseudotranssexualism" in schizophrenia," *Psychiatry*, vol. 70, no. 2, pp. 175–179, 2007.

[24] C. Caldwell and M. S. Keshavan, "Schizophrenia with secondary transsexualism," *Canadian Journal of Psychiatry*, vol. 36, no. 4, pp. 300–301, 1991.

[25] L. Manderson and S. Kumar, "Gender identity disorder as a rare manifestation of schizophrenia," *Australian and New Zealand Journal of Psychiatry*, vol. 35, no. 4, pp. 546–547, 2001.

[26] S. C. Bhargava and S. Sethi, "Transsexualism and schizophrenia: a case report," *Indian Journal of Psychiatry*, vol. 44, pp. 177–178, 2002.

[27] J. M. Campo, H. Nijman, C. Evers, H. L. Merckelbach, and I. Decker, "Gender identity disorders as a symptom of psychosis, schizophrenia in particular," *Nederlands Tijdschrift voor Geneeskunde*, vol. 145, no. 39, pp. 1876–1880, 2001.

[28] R. A. LaTorre, "The psychological assessment of gender identity and gender role in schizophrenia," *Schizophrenia Bulletin*, vol. 2, no. 2, pp. 266–285, 1976.

[29] A. Burton and B. Sjoberg Jr., "The diagnostic validity of human figure drawings in schizophrenia," *The Journal of Psychology*, vol. 57, pp. 3–18, 1964.

[30] H. A. Ries, M. H. Johnson, H. E. Armstrong Jr., and D. S. Holmes, "The draw-a-person test and process-reactive schizophrenia," *Journal of Projective Techniques & Personality Assessment*, vol. 30, no. 2, pp. 184–186, 1966.

[31] D. C. McClelland and N. F. Watt, "Sex-role alienation in schizophrenia," *Journal of Abnormal Psychology*, vol. 73, no. 3, pp. 226–239, 1968.

[32] H. B. Miller and K. Poey, "An exploratory comparison of sex role-related behaviors in schizophrenics and nonschizophrenics," *Developmental Psychology*, vol. 1, no. 5, p. 629, 1969.

[33] R. Kayton and H. B. Biller, "Sex-role development and psychopathology in adult males," *Journal of Consulting and Clinical Psychology*, vol. 38, no. 2, pp. 208–210, 1972.

[34] M. Sajatovic, J. H. Jenkins, M. E. Strauss, Z. A. Butt, and E. Carpenter, "Gender identity and implications for recovery among men and women with schizophrenia," *Psychiatric Services*, vol. 56, no. 1, pp. 96–98, 2005.

[35] R. P. Greenberg and L. Laurence, "A comparison of the MMPI results for psychiatric patients and male applicants for transsexual surgery," *Journal of Nervous and Mental Disease*, vol. 169, no. 5, pp. 320–323, 1981.

[36] C. L. Keo-Meier, L. I. Herman, S. L. Reisner, S. T. Pardo, C. Sharp, and J. C. Babcock, "Testosterone treatment and MMPI-2 improvement in transgender men: a prospective controlled study," *Journal of Consulting and Clinical Psychology*. In press.

[37] M.-C. Lai, Y.-N. Chiu, K. D. Gadow, S. S.-F. Gau, and H.-G. Hwu, "Correlates of gender dysphoria in Taiwanese university students," *Archives of Sexual Behavior*, vol. 39, no. 6, pp. 1415–1428, 2010.

[38] E. Luders, F. J. Sánchez, C. Gaser et al., "Regional gray matter variation in male-to-female transsexualism," *NeuroImage*, vol. 46, no. 4, pp. 904–907, 2009.

[39] F. P. M. Kruijver, J.-N. Zhou, C. W. Pool, M. A. Hofman, L. J. G. Gooren, and D. F. Swaab, "Male-to-female transsexuals have female neuron numbers in a limbic nucleus," *The Journal of Clinical Endocrinology and Metabolism*, vol. 85, no. 5, pp. 2034–2041, 2000.

[40] G. Rametti, B. Carrillo, E. Gómez-Gil et al., "White matter microstructure in female to male transsexuals before cross-sex hormonal treatment. A diffusion tensor imaging study," *Journal of Psychiatric Research*, vol. 45, no. 2, pp. 199–204, 2011.

[41] R. E. Gur, C. Kohler, B. I. Turetsky et al., "A sexually dimorphic ratio of orbitofrontal to amygdala volume is altered in schizophrenia," *Biological Psychiatry*, vol. 55, no. 5, pp. 512–517, 2004.

[42] P. C. Nopoulos, D. Rideout, B. Crespo-Facorro, and N. C. Andreasen, "Sex differences in the absence of massa intermedia in patients with schizophrenia versus healthy controls," *Schizophrenia Research*, vol. 48, no. 2-3, pp. 177–185, 2001.

[43] A. Mendrek, "Reversal of normal cerebral sexual dimorphism in schizophrenia: evidence and speculations," *Medical Hypotheses*, vol. 69, no. 4, pp. 896–902, 2007.

[44] A. Mendrek and E. Stip, "Sexual dimorphism in schizophrenia: is there a need for gender-based protocols?" *Expert Review of Neurotherapeutics*, vol. 11, no. 7, pp. 951–959, 2011.

[45] E. Luders, F. J. Sanchez, D. Tosun et al., "Increased cortical thickness in male-to-female transsexualism," *Journal of Behavioral and Brain Science*, vol. 2, no. 3, pp. 357–362, 2012.

[46] C. C. Schultz, K. Koch, G. Wagner et al., "Reduced cortical thickness in first episode schizophrenia," *Schizophrenia Research*, vol. 116, no. 2-3, pp. 204–209, 2010.

[47] C. C. Schultz, K. Koch, G. Wagner et al., "Complex pattern of cortical thinning in schizophrenia: results from an automated surface based analysis of cortical thickness," *Psychiatry Research—Neuroimaging*, vol. 182, no. 2, pp. 134–140, 2010.

[48] E. Sprooten, M. Papmeyer, A. M. Smyth et al., "Cortical thickness in first-episode schizophrenia patients and individuals at high familial risk: a cross-sectional comparison," *Schizophrenia Research*, vol. 151, no. 1–3, pp. 259–264, 2013.

[49] B. Kraemer, T. Noll, A. Delsignore, G. Milos, U. Schnyder, and U. Hepp, "Finger length ratio (2D:4D) in adults with gender identity disorder," *Archives of Sexual Behavior*, vol. 38, no. 3, pp. 359–363, 2009.

[50] M. S. Wallien, K. J. Zucker, T. D. Steensma, and P. T. Cohen-Kettenis, "2D:4D finger-length ratios in children and adults with gender identity disorder," *Hormones and Behavior*, vol. 54, no. 3, pp. 450–454, 2008.

[51] S.-I. Hisasue, S. Sasaki, T. Tsukamoto, and S. Horie, "The relationship between second-to-fourth digit ratio and female gender identity," *Journal of Sexual Medicine*, vol. 9, no. 11, pp. 2903–2910, 2012.

[52] A. Divakaran, J. C. Narayanaswamy, S. V. Kalmady, V. Narayan, N. P. Rao, and G. Venkatasubramanian, "Family history correlates of digit ratio abnormalities in schizophrenia," *Indian Journal of Psychological Medicine*, vol. 34, no. 4, pp. 355–359, 2012.

[53] S. L. Collinson, M. Lim, J. H. Chaw et al., "Increased ratio of 2nd to 4th digit (2D:4D) in schizophrenia," *Psychiatry Research*, vol. 176, no. 1, pp. 8–12, 2010.

[54] D. J. Walder, T. L. C. Andersson, A. L. McMillan, S. M. Breedlove, and E. F. Walker, "Sex differences in digit ratio (2D:4D) are disrupted in adolescents with schizotypal personality disorder: altered prenatal gonadal hormone levels as a risk factor," *Schizophrenia Research*, vol. 86, no. 1–3, pp. 118–122, 2006.

[55] Y.-K. Zhu, C.-B. Li, J. Jin et al., "The 2D:4D ratio of the hand and schizotypal personality traits in schizophrenia patients and healthy control persons," *Asian Journal of Psychiatry*, vol. 9, pp. 67–72, 2014.

[56] G. Venkatasubramanian, R. Arasappa, N. P. Rao, and B. N. Gangadhar, "Digit ratio (2D:4D) asymmetry and schneiderian first rank symptoms: implications for cerebral lateralisation theories of schizophrenia," *Laterality*, vol. 16, no. 4, pp. 499–512, 2011.

[57] M. Dragovic and G. Hammond, "Handedness in schizophrenia: a quantitative review of evidence," *Acta Psychiatrica Scandinavica*, vol. 111, no. 6, pp. 410–419, 2005.

[58] R. Green and R. Young, "Hand preference, sexual preference, and transsexualism," *Archives of Sexual Behavior*, vol. 30, no. 6, pp. 565–574, 2001.

[59] K. J. Zucker, N. Beaulieu, S. J. Bradley, G. M. Grimshaw, and A. Wilcox, "Handedness in boys with gender identity disorder," *Journal of Child Psychology and Psychiatry and Allied Disciplines*, vol. 42, no. 6, pp. 767–776, 2001.

[60] W. M. Brandler and S. Paracchini, "The genetic relationship between handedness and neurodevelopmental disorders," *Trends in Molecular Medicine*, vol. 20, no. 2, pp. 83–90, 2014.

[61] R. H. Yolken, F. B. Dickerson, and E. Fuller Torrey, "Toxoplasma and schizophrenia," *Parasite Immunology*, vol. 31, no. 11, pp. 706–715, 2009.

[62] O. Emelia, R. N. Amal, Z. Z. Ruzanna et al., "Seroprevalence of anti-*Toxoplasma gondii* IgG antibody in patients with schizophrenia," *Tropical Biomedicine*, vol. 29, no. 1, pp. 151–159, 2012.

[63] D. Holub, J. Flegr, E. Dragomirecka et al., "Differences in onset of disease and severity of psychopathology between toxoplasmosis-related and toxoplasmosis-unrelated schizophrenia," *Acta psychiatrica Scandinavica*, vol. 127, no. 3, pp. 227–238, 2013.

[64] O. Okusaga, P. Langenberg, A. Sleemi et al., "*Toxoplasma gondii* antibody titers and history of suicide attempts in patients with schizophrenia," *Schizophrenia Research*, vol. 133, no. 1-3, pp. 150–155, 2011.

[65] P. B. Mortensen, B. Nørgaard-Pedersen, B. L. Waltoft, T. L. Sørensen, D. Hougaard, and R. H. Yolken, "Early infections of *Toxoplasma gondii* and the later development of schizophrenia," *Schizophrenia Bulletin*, vol. 33, no. 3, pp. 741–744, 2007.

[66] H. Perron, N. Hamdani, R. Faucard et al., "Molecular characteristics of Human Endogenous Retrovirus type-W in schizophrenia and bipolar disorder," *Translational Psychiatry*, vol. 2, article e201, 2012.

[67] J. Flegr, "Influence of latent *Toxoplasma* infection on human personality, physiology and morphology: pros and cons of the *Toxoplasma*-human model in studying the manipulation hypothesis," *Journal of Experimental Biology*, vol. 216, no. 1, pp. 127–133, 2013.

[68] J.-P. Selten and R. S. Kahn, "Schizophrenia after prenatal exposure to *Toxoplasma gondii*?" *Clinical Infectious Diseases*, vol. 35, no. 5, pp. 633–634, 2002.

[69] D. L. Carbone and R. J. Handa, "Sex and stress hormone influences on the expression and activity of brain-derived neurotrophic factor," *Neuroscience*, vol. 239, pp. 295–303, 2013.

[70] M. J. Green, S. L. Matheson, A. Shepherd, C. S. Weickert, and V. J. Carr, "Brain-derived neurotrophic factor levels in schizophrenia: a systematic review with meta-analysis," *Molecular Psychiatry*, vol. 16, no. 9, pp. 960–972, 2011.

[71] A.-M. V. Fontanari, T. Andreazza, Â. B. Costa et al., "Serum concentrations of brain-derived neurotrophic factor in patients with gender identity disorder," *Journal of Psychiatric Research*, vol. 47, no. 10, pp. 1546–1548, 2013.

[72] A. B. Costa, A.-M. V. Fontanari, T. Andreazza et al., "BDNF: a biomarker for social vulnerability in individuals diagnosed with gender dysphoria," *Journal of Psychiatric Research*, vol. 50, no. 1, pp. 16–17, 2014.

[73] J. Fuss, S. V. Biedermann, G. K. Stalla, and M. K. Auer, "On the quest for a biomechanism of transsexualism: is there a role for BDNF?" *Journal of Psychiatric Research*, vol. 47, no. 12, pp. 2015–2017, 2013.

[74] S. Tobet, J. G. Knoll, C. Hartshorn et al., "Brain sex differences and hormone influences: a moving experience?" *Journal of Neuroendocrinology*, vol. 21, no. 4, pp. 387–392, 2009.

[75] S. Bendall, H. J. Jackson, C. A. Hulbert, and P. D. McGorry, "Childhood trauma and psychotic disorders: a systematic, critical review of the evidence," *Schizophrenia Bulletin*, vol. 34, no. 3, pp. 568–579, 2008.

[76] R. P. Rajkumar, "Childhood attachment and schizophrenia: the "attachment-developmental-cognitive" (ADC) hypothesis," *Medical Hypotheses*, vol. 83, no. 3, pp. 276–281, 2014.

[77] L. M. Lothstein, "Psychodynamics and sociodynamics of gender-dysphoric states," *The American Journal of Psychotherapy*, vol. 33, no. 2, pp. 214–238, 1979.

[78] G. Parker and R. Barr, "Parental representations of transsexuals," *Archives of Sexual Behavior*, vol. 11, no. 3, pp. 221–230, 1982.

[79] P. T. Cohen-Kettenis and W. A. Arrindell, "Perceived parental rearing style, parental divorce and transsexualism: a controlled study," *Psychological Medicine*, vol. 20, no. 3, pp. 613–620, 1990.

[80] K. J. Zucker and S. J. Bradley, "Adoptee overrepresentation among clinic-referred boys with gender identity disorder," *Canadian Journal of Psychiatry*, vol. 43, no. 10, pp. 1040–1043, 1998.

[81] G. A. Rekers and J. J. Swihart, "The association of gender identity disorder with parental separation," *Psychological Reports*, vol. 65, no. 3, pp. 1272–1274, 1989.

[82] G. A. Rekers and O. I. Lovaas, "Behavioral treatment of deviant sex role behaviors in a male child," *Journal of Applied Behavior Analysis*, vol. 7, no. 2, pp. 173–190, 1974.

[83] E. Bandini, A. D. Fisher, V. Ricca et al., "Childhood maltreatment in subjects with male-to-female gender identity disorder," *International Journal of Impotence Research*, vol. 23, no. 6, pp. 276–285, 2011.

[84] C. Cheung, K. Yu, G. Fung et al., "Autistic disorders and schizophrenia: related or remote? An anatomical likelihood estimation," *PLoS ONE*, vol. 5, no. 8, Article ID e12233, 2010.

[85] B. H. King and C. Lord, "Is schizophrenia on the autism spectrum?" *Brain Research*, vol. 1380, pp. 34–41, 2011.

[86] P. F. Sullivan, C. Magnusson, A. Reichenberg et al., "Family history of schizophrenia and bipolar disorder as risk factors for autism," *Archives of General Psychiatry*, vol. 69, no. 11, pp. 1099–1103, 2012.

[87] D. Moreno-De-Luca, S. G. E. N. E. Consortium, J. G. Mulle et al., "Deletion 17q12 is a recurrent copy number variant that confers high risk of autism and schizophrenia," *The American Journal of Human Genetics*, vol. 87, no. 5, pp. 618–630, 2010.

[88] M. Hines, "Sex-related variation in human behavior and the brain," *Trends in Cognitive Sciences*, vol. 14, no. 10, pp. 448–456, 2010.

[89] M. Hines, "Gender development and the human brain," *Annual Review of Neuroscience*, vol. 34, pp. 69–88, 2011.

[90] S. Bejerot and J. M. Eriksson, "Sexuality and gender role in autism spectrum disorder: a case control study," *PLoS ONE*, vol. 9, no. 1, Article ID e87961, 2014.

[91] G. Gallucci, F. Hackerman, and C. W. Schmidt Jr., "Gender identity disorder in an adult male with Asperger's Syndrome," *Sexuality and Disability*, vol. 23, no. 1, pp. 35–40, 2005.

[92] B. Kraemer, A. Delsignore, R. Gundelfinger, U. Schnyder, and U. Hepp, "Comorbidity of Asperger syndrome and gender identity disorder," *European Child and Adolescent Psychiatry*, vol. 14, no. 5, pp. 292–296, 2005.

[93] R. M. Jones, S. Wheelwright, K. Farrell et al., "Brief report: female-to-male transsexual people and autistic traits," *Journal of Autism and Developmental Disorders*, vol. 42, no. 2, pp. 301–306, 2012.

[94] A. L. C. de Vries, I. L. J. Noens, P. T. Cohen-Kettenis, I. A. van Berckelaer-Onnes, and T. A. Doreleijers, "Autism spectrum disorders in gender dysphoric children and adolescents," *Journal of Autism and Developmental Disorders*, vol. 40, no. 8, pp. 930–936, 2010.

[95] V. Pasterski, L. Gilligan, and R. Curtis, "Traits of autism spectrum disorders in adults with gender dysphoria," *Archives of Sexual Behavior*, vol. 43, no. 2, pp. 387–393, 2014.

[96] D. di Ceglie, E. Skagerberg, S. Baron-Cohen, and B. Auyeung, "Empathising and systemising in adolescents with gender dysphoria," *Opticon1826*, vol. 16, no. 6, pp. 1–8, 2014.

[97] S. Priebe and F. Röhricht, "Specific body image pathology in acute schizophrenia," *Psychiatry Research*, vol. 101, no. 3, pp. 289–301, 2001.

[98] R. Koide, S. Iizuka, K. Fujihara, and N. Morita, "Body image, symptoms and insight in chronic schizophrenia," *Psychiatry and Clinical Neurosciences*, vol. 56, no. 1, pp. 9–15, 2002.

[99] J. À Campo, H. Nijman, and H. Merckelbach, "Changes in appearance and schizotypy in normal subjects," *Acta Neuropsychiatrica*, vol. 16, no. 3, pp. 138–141, 2004.

[100] E. F. Torrey, "Schizophrenia and the inferior parietal lobule," *Schizophrenia Research*, vol. 97, no. 1–3, pp. 215–225, 2007.

[101] L. K. Case and V. S. Ramachandran, "Alternating gender incongruity: a new neuropsychiatric syndrome providing insight into the dynamic plasticity of brain-sex," *Medical Hypotheses*, vol. 78, no. 5, pp. 626–631, 2012.

[102] V. Molina and J. A. Blanco, "A Proposal for reframing schizophrenia research," *The Journal of Nervous and Mental Disease*, vol. 201, no. 9, pp. 744–752, 2013.

[103] T. Shechner, "Gender identity disorder: a literature review from a developmental perspective," *The Israel Journal of Psychiatry and Related Sciences*, vol. 47, no. 2, pp. 132–138, 2010.

[104] L. Kemppainen, J. Veijola, J. Jokelainen et al., "Birth order and risk for schizophrenia: a 31-year follow-up of the Northern Finland 1966 Birth Cohort," *Acta Psychiatrica Scandinavica*, vol. 104, no. 2, pp. 148–152, 2001.

[105] R. Green, "Birth order and ratio of brothers to sisters in transsexuals," *Psychological Medicine*, vol. 30, no. 4, pp. 789–795, 2000.

[106] E. Gómez-Gil, I. Esteva, R. Carrasco et al., "Birth order and ratio of brothers to sisters in Spanish transsexuals," *Archives of Sexual Behavior*, vol. 40, no. 3, pp. 505–510, 2011.

[107] V. Siomopoulos, "Transsexualism: disorder of gender identity, thought disorder, or both?" *Journal of the American Academy of Psychoanalysis*, vol. 2, no. 3, pp. 201–213, 1974.

[108] J. Drescher, P. Cohen-Kettenis, and S. Winter, "Minding the body: situating gender identity diagnoses in the ICD-11," *International Review of Psychiatry*, vol. 24, no. 6, pp. 568–577, 2012.

4

Dimensional Information-Theoretic Measurement of Facial Emotion Expressions in Schizophrenia

Jihun Hamm,[1] Amy Pinkham,[2] Ruben C. Gur,[3,4] Ragini Verma,[5] and Christian G. Kohler[3]

[1] *Department of Computer Science and Engineering, The Ohio State University, Columbus, OH 43210, USA*
[2] *Southern Methodist University, Dallas, TX 75205, USA*
[3] *Department of Psychiatry, Neuropsychiatry Section, University of Pennsylvania, Philadelphia, PA 19104, USA*
[4] *Philadelphia Veterans Administration Medical Center, Philadelphia, PA 19104, USA*
[5] *Department of Radiology, Section of Biomedical Image Analysis, University of Pennsylvania, Philadelphia, PA 19104, USA*

Correspondence should be addressed to Christian G. Kohler; kohler@upenn.edu

Academic Editor: Robin Emsley

Altered facial expressions of emotions are characteristic impairments in schizophrenia. Ratings of affect have traditionally been limited to clinical rating scales and facial muscle movement analysis, which require extensive training and have limitations based on methodology and ecological validity. To improve reliable assessment of dynamic facial expression changes, we have developed automated measurements of facial emotion expressions based on information-theoretic measures of expressivity of *ambiguity* and *distinctiveness* of facial expressions. These measures were examined in matched groups of persons with schizophrenia (n = 28) and healthy controls (n = 26) who underwent video acquisition to assess expressivity of basic emotions (happiness, sadness, anger, fear, and disgust) in evoked conditions. Persons with schizophrenia scored higher on *ambiguity*, the measure of conditional entropy within the expression of a single emotion, and they scored lower on *distinctiveness*, the measure of mutual information across expressions of different emotions. The automated measures compared favorably with observer-based ratings. This method can be applied for delineating dynamic emotional expressivity in healthy and clinical populations.

1. Introduction

The ability to communicate emotions through facial expressions is crucial for interpersonal engagement. Altered facial expressions of emotions are viewed as characteristic impairments in schizophrenia [1, 2] that already feature prominently during early illness [3, 4] and may precede the onset of psychosis [5]. Assessment of facial expressions has traditionally relied on observer-based rating scales. The Scale for the Assessment of Negative Symptoms (SANS [2]) and the Positive and Negative Syndrome Scale (PANSS [6]) are commonly used by clinicians to measure facial expressions during interview settings, including the ratings of affective flattening and inappropriate affect. The limited range of quantitative scores obtained during clinical interviews that preferentially focus on positive symptoms without standard prompts to elicit changes in expressivity decrease the ecological validity of facial expression ratings.

An alternative line of investigation of facial expressions of emotions has moved away from clinical assessment of expressions and examined local facial changes based on muscle movements or qualitative assessment of dynamic changes associated with facial expressions. The Facial Action Coding System (FACS [7, 8]) provides detailed descriptions of individual facial muscle movements in multiple facial regions. FACS and some of its adaptations have been applied to schizophrenia [9–13]. However, the FACS procedure requires extensive training and is time-consuming, which makes it difficult to perform in large-scale studies. Due to the prohibitive amount of time to rate videos, the

FACS procedure is usually performed for static emotional displays. The Facial Expression Coding System (FACES [14]) can classify dynamic facial expressions with details such as valence, type, and intensity of emotions as determined by a rater. FACES ratings of videos of evoked emotions in schizophrenia have shown significant flatness and inappropriateness during spontaneous expressions [15, 16], as well as for simulated [17] and evoked expressions [18].

Media for capturing facial expressions have included still photographs [18–20], videotapes [9–13, 15, 17, 21, 22], and electromyographic recordings [23–25]. Videotaped acquisition offers the advantage of capturing duration and frequency of emotion expressions. However, analysis of such lengthy data sets has been limited to more global assessment of positive and negative emotion expressions, rather than changes in specific face regions. Common measurements of emotion expressions have included recognition rates of expressions [19, 21, 26–28] and FACS-derived measures without analysis of specific AUs [9–12, 15, 17]. Other methods have included computerized face morphometry [25, 27] and electromyographic measurements [23–25, 29, 30] that can measure minute muscle activations, albeit limited to select face regions, for example, zygomatic and corrugator muscles that are typically utilized in frowning and smiling expressions. An interesting and frequent finding arising from these investigations has been the possible disconnectedness between emotion expressions and subjective emotion experience [18, 30, 31], which in turn may affect social interactions in schizophrenia.

In an effort to derive more objective and scalable measurement of facial expressivity, we have pursued computerized measurement of facial expressions that were obtained during standardized procedures to elicit emotion expressions. Initial efforts based on manually defined face regions from still images in healthy actors [32] and persons with schizophrenia [33] showed significant group differences in expressions of happiness, sadness, anger, and fear. Wang et al. [34] refined the method to allow automated analysis of videos and demonstrated different frequencies of four emotions in three exemplar participants. To account for low intensity and ambiguous expressions of emotions, Hamm et al. [35] proposed automated measurement of individual facial muscles using FACS parameters and demonstrated the differences of facial muscle activities in four patients and controls. However, the implications of altered individual facial muscle movements on global expressivity and respective differences in schizophrenia, where facial expressions are commonly impaired, remain to be better elucidated. In this paper, we present novel measures of facial expressivity, based on individual muscle movements that are derived from information theory [36] and applied these measures to matched groups of schizophrenia and control subjects. Information theory originated in the 1950s from the field of applied mathematics to analyze the capacity of communication channels. The method has provided powerful tools to analyze human performance measures in psychological experiments [37] and a framework for understanding emotional communications [38]. Information theory has also been successfully used in biomedical investigations, such as processing capacity of neural coding [39], complexity in electrocardiogram sequences [40], and electroencephalography in Alzheimer's disease [41] and schizophrenia [42].

As an extension of our previous work that examined both observer-based and computerized measurements of facial expressivity of emotions, we tested sensitivity of the information-theoretic measures in characterizing and quantifying affective expression deficits in schizophrenia, and we examined their relationship with observer-based ratings of inappropriate and flattened emotion expressions. We applied two-dimensional measures of facial expressivity that can be computed objectively from videos of facial expressions without requiring observer-based ratings: (1) *ambiguity* of facial expressions within a single emotion and (2) *distinctiveness* of facial expressions across separate emotions. These measures correspond to the two most important information-theoretic quantities of (1) *conditional entropy* and (2) *mutual information*. Briefly, *ambiguity* is the amount of uncertainty in a person's facial muscle patterns during expression of a single emotion as contrasted with consistency of the pattern. A person whose facial muscle pattern is only brief or is variable during emotion expression will be less effective in communicating his or her intended emotion to another person. *Distinctiveness* is the capacity of a person to express different emotions succinctly through facial muscles. A person who is unable to produce distinct facial patterns for different emotions will also be less effective in communicating a specific emotion. We anticipated that *ambiguity* and *distinctiveness* measures can be applied to large data sets of dynamic expressions and they can capture aspects of expressivity deficits that would improve our understanding of emotion expression abilities in persons with schizophrenia. In addition, although representing different theoretical constructs, we examined whether information-theoretic measures correlate with observer-based ratings such as inappropriate and flattened affect.

2. Methods

2.1. Subjects. We collected videos of healthy controls and persons with schizophrenia for a neuropsychiatric study of emotions under an approved IRB protocol at the University of Pennsylvania. After describing the study to the subjects, we obtained written informed consents, including consent to publish pictures. There were 28 outpatients with a DSM-IV diagnosis of schizophrenia and 26 healthy controls balanced in gender, race, age, and parental education. All patients were clinically stable without hospitalization for at least 3 months prior to research assessment and had been maintained on their present medication for the past month. Presence of significant acute extrapyramidal symptoms as evidenced by a score of 1 or higher on at least 2 of the rigidity or tremor items (items 2, 3, 4, 5, and 9) was exclusionary. Likewise presence of significant tardive extrapyramidal symptoms as evidenced by a score of 2 or higher on items 1–4 (facial and oral movements) was exclusionary. All patients were treated

Table 1: Demographic and clinical characteristics.

	Patient group	Control group
Gender (M : F)	14 : 14	16 : 10
Ethnicity		
(Caucasian : African-American : other)	9 : 16 : 3	8 : 15 : 3
Age		
Mean	32.3 ± 9.0	33.0 ± 8.6
Range	20–47 yrs	20–48 yrs
Duration of illness	13.00 ± 8.3	N/A
Range	2–33	N/A
Symptoms		
Positive (SAPS-total)	6.00 ± 8.5	N/A
Negative (SANS-total)	13.00 ± 8.3	N/A
Antipsychotics		
Chlorpromazine-equivalents (n = 28)	225 mg ± 247	N/A
Olanzapine-equivalents (n = 2)	13.6 mg ± 7.6	N/A

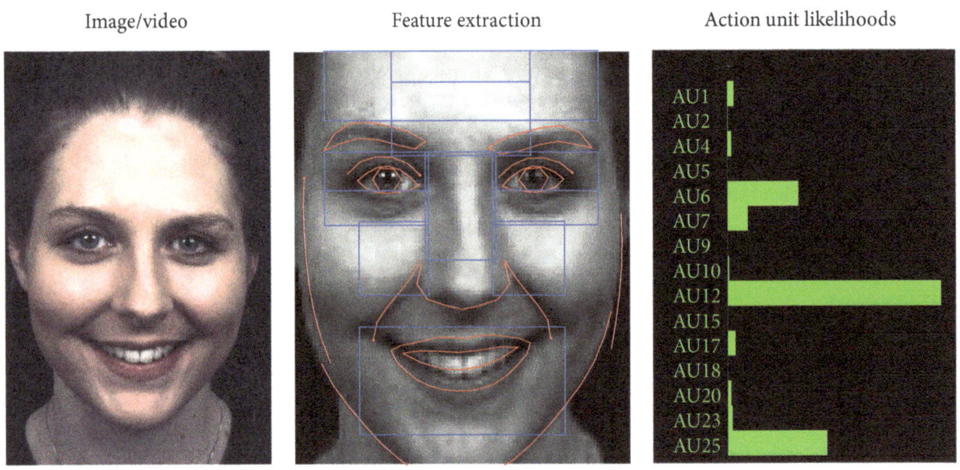

Figure 1: Automated Action Unit recognition system. For each frame of a video, geometric changes in facial components (red curves) are automatically tracked, and textural changes due to temporary wrinkles are detected in multiple regions of interest (blue boxes). These extracted features are fed through pattern classifiers to yield activity of each Action Unit (green bars: longer bar means higher activity).

with second-generation antipsychotics that were converted to dosages equivalent to olanzapine (OLZ); two patients were also treated with first-generation antipsychotics that were converted to dosages equivalent to chlorpromazine (CPZ). All medication dosages were stable for the past month prior to testing and no patient was treated with anticholinergic medications. Pertinent demographic and clinical information is summarized in Table 1.

2.2. Emotion Elicitation Procedure and Video Acquisition. To test emotion expression ability, we followed the emotion elicitation procedure previously described [43] and adapted it for use in schizophrenia [13]. Videos were obtained for neutral expressions and for five universal emotions (happiness, sadness, anger, fear, and disgust). Before recording, participants were asked to describe biographical emotional situations, when each emotion was experienced in mild, moderate, and high intensities, and these situations were summarized as vignettes. Subsequently, subjects were seated in a brightly lit room where recordings took place, and emotional vignettes were recounted to participants in a narrative manner using exact wording derived from the vignettes. The spontaneous facial expressions of the subjects were recorded as videos. Before and between the five emotion sessions, the subjects were asked to relax and return to a neutral state. The duration of each session was about two minutes (110 ± 54 sec).

2.3. Video Processing and Automated FACS. Our group has developed an automated facial coding procedure that can score intensity of facial muscle activity known as Action Units (AUs [7, 8]) by computerized analysis of videos. The details of the system and the validation of accuracy appeared in Hamm et al. [35], and here we describe key components of the system and how we used it to measure information (see Figure 1). Videos acquired in evoked emotions were analyzed frame by frame. For each frame, geometric changes in facial components such as eyes, eyebrows, nasolabial line, and lips were automatically tracked, and textural changes due to temporary wrinkles were detected in multiple regions of the face. To increase the reliability of the tracking, a small fraction (~3%) of frames from videos in which the face leaves the screen (i.e., nonfrontal) were automatically discarded from analysis. Extracted geometric and texture features were then passed through pattern classifiers to yield intensity of the following 15 AUs: AU1 (Inner Brow Raiser), AU2 (Outer Brow Raiser), AU4 (Brow Lowerer), AU5 (Upper Lid Raiser), AU6 (Cheek Raise), AU7 (Lid Tightener), AU9 (Nose Wrinkler), AU10 (Upper Lip Raiser), AU12 (Lip Corner Puller), AU15 (Lip Corner Depressor), AU17 (Chin Raiser), AU18 (Lip Puckerer), AU20 (Lip Stretcher), AU23 (Lip Tightener) and AU25-27 (Lips Part and Mouth Open). The other AUs than these 15 AUs were not used since they were too infrequently in the recorded videos.

2.4. Computation of Ambiguity and Distinctiveness of Facial Expressions. From the distribution of 15-dimensional continuous variables collected from videos, we computed information-theoretic measures of expressivity for each subject. Specifically, we measure *ambiguity* of facial expression patterns within each emotion and *distinctiveness* of facial expression patterns across emotions. These two measures correspond to conditional entropy and mutual information, which are the fundamental variables of information theory [36]. Interpretations of the two information-theoretic measures depend on the experiments being conducted, and *ambiguity* and *distinctiveness* are specific interpretations of our experimental results with the spontaneous expression of emotions. In psychology, the two measures have been called equivocation and information transmission, respectively, in the context of absolute judgment tasks [44].

Computation of *ambiguity* and *distinctiveness* requires estimation of differential entropy from facial muscles. Differential entropy is the amount of uncertainty in continuous probabilistic distributions from which we derive mutual information and conditional entropy. Let x denote the (discrete) emotional state of an individual and y denote the (continuous and multivariate) facial muscle activity. Differential entropy is then defined by $H(p(y)) = E[-\log p(y)] = -\int_{\mathbb{R}^d} p(y)\log p(y)dy$. Unlike discrete entropy, differential entropy is a relative measure and can have negative values; a univariate Gaussian distribution with $\sigma = (2\pi e)^{-1/2}$ has zero differential entropy, and Gaussians with narrower or wider peaks have negative or positive entropy, respectively. Since we do not know $p(y)$ *a priori*, the differential entropy has to be estimated from samples, much like estimation of mean and variance. Several estimation methods have been proposed, including adaptive partitioning, kernel density estimation, and nearest neighbor estimation (see Beirlant et al. [45] for a review). We used a k-nearest neighbor estimator of entropy [46–48].

$H(p(y)) \approx (d/n)\sum_i^n \log\rho + v_d - \psi(k) + \log n$. The $v_d = \pi^{d/2}/\Gamma(d/2+1)$ is the volume of a d-dimensional unit sphere, where Γ is the gamma function $\Gamma(z) = \int_0^\infty t^{z-1}e^{-t}dt$ and $\psi(z)$ is the digamma function $\psi(z) = \Gamma(z)'/\Gamma(z)$. The only free parameter of nearest-neighbor estimate is the size of the neighbors k for which we used the heuristic rule [47].

$k = round\ (n^{1/2} + 0.5)$, where n is the number of samples. For numerical stability, we also added negligible amount (= 10^{-8}) of random noise to the data while computing entropy.

In our experiments, the conditional entropy is defined as $H(y \mid x) = \sum_{x=x_i} p(x_i)H(y \mid x_i) = \sum_{x=x_i} p(x_i)\int -p(y \mid x_i)\log(p(y \mid x_i))dy$, which is the average entropy of facial expression per emotion computed from facial muscle activity y in the video of each emotion x with equal priors for each emotion ($p(x) = 1/5$). We refer to this conditional entropy as *ambiguity* in the following context: when an individual's facial expression is consistent within each emotion, the conditional entropy is low, and when the expression is varying and ambiguous within each emotion, the conditional entropy is high.

The mutual information $I(x, y)$ can be computed from $I(x; y) = H(y) - H(y \mid x)$. Mutual information between discrete and continuous variables, as in our case, is also known as Jensen-Shannon divergence [49, 50] and is nonnegative and bounded. By reformulating $I(x; y)$ as the average KL-divergence [51] between conditional $p(y \mid x)$ and marginal $p(y)$ distributions $I(x; y) = KL(p(x, y)\|p(x)p(y)) = \sum_x p(x)\int p(y \mid x)\log(p(yx)/p(y))dy = \sum_x p(x)KL(p(y \mid x)\|p(y))$, we notice that mutual information measures the average distance of emotion-specific facial expression pattern ($p(x \mid y)$) from the patterns of all emotions combined ($p(x)$). Hence our choice of the term *distinctiveness* is for mutual information.

2.5. Interpretation of Ambiguity and Distinctiveness Measures. In this paper, we report the *ambiguity* and the *distinctiveness* as z-scores ($= (x - m)/s$) instead of their raw values for an easier interpretation, where the mean and the standard deviation are computed using all subjects and conditions. We do this because these values are unitless and dependent on the experimental setting and therefore meaningful only in a relative sense. For example, if we use six basic emotions including "surprise" instead of five, the absolute values of *ambiguity* and *distinctiveness* will change. However, the difference of values in diagnostic groups or conditions still measures the relative amount of the *ambiguity* and *distinctiveness* of facial expressions and provides meaningful information. Note that the standardization of raw values using z-scores does not affect the subsequent statistical analysis.

Lastly, the *ambiguity* and the distinctiveness are computed across all emotions and not for individual emotions. While it is possible to analyze *ambiguity* for each emotion, pooling the values across emotions results in more reliable measures.

2.6. Observer-Based Measures

Validation of Ambiguity and Distinctiveness. To verify that the information-theoretic measures agree with an observer's interpretation of *ambiguity* and *distinctiveness* from videos, the following criteria for manual scores from 0 to 4 were defined, and each video was rated by an observer blind to the diagnosis of subjects. For *ambiguity*, which was rated for videos of each emotion, 0 meant very consistent (with only single facial expression pattern in the single video of an emotion) and 4 meant very ambiguous (with more than four different facial expression patterns in the video of an emotion). Scores 1 to 3 corresponded to intermediate levels of *ambiguity* (with 1, 2, and 3 major facial expression patterns in a video, resp.). For *distinctiveness*, which was rated across videos of five emotions of a single subject, 0 meant the five emotional videos were totally indistinguishable in representing the target emotions, and 4 meant all five videos were distinctive and representative of the target emotions. Scores 1 to 3 corresponded to intermediate levels of *distinctiveness* (with 1, 2, and 3 videos of distinctive emotions, resp.).

Observer-Based Ratings of Facial Expressions. To compare information measures with previous observer-based ratings, flatness and inappropriateness of facial expression from the Scale for the Assessment of Negative Symptoms (SANS) were adapted to video-based ratings [33]. Two raters scored each video with separate scores for flat and inappropriate affect, ranging from 0 (none) to 4 (extremely flat or inappropriate). SANS raters knew the intended emotion of the video but not the diagnosis of subjects. Video-based SANS was based on a 5-point rating, similar to observer-based SANS. Ratings that differed by 2 or more points were reviewed for consensus and final ratings were averaged.

2.7. Statistical Analysis. The following data analysis was performed to demonstrate applicability and validity of the measures of *ambiguity* and *distinctiveness*. Group-based comparisons for *ambiguity* and *distinctiveness* of expressions involved were carried out via two-way ANOVA of *ambiguity* and *distinctiveness* separately, using sex and diagnosis as grouping factors. We also measured the effect size of diagnosis by Cohen's d $(= (m_1 - m_2)/(0.5(s_1^2 + s_2^2))^{1/2})$. Validation of computerized measures of *ambiguity* and *distinctiveness* against observer-based measures was performed by Pearson correlations, where higher values meant better agreement between the computerized and observer-based measures. For observer-based ratings of inappropriateness and flatness of expressions we performed separate two-way ANOVA using sex and diagnosis as grouping factors. We also measured the effect size of diagnosis by Cohen's d. For the purposes of interpretability and comparison with alternative measures of symptom severity, we performed multiple regression analysis to study the explanatory power of the computerized measures of *ambiguity* and *distinctiveness* for observer-based ratings of inappropriate and flat affects, in which computerized measures were used as independent variables and each of the observer-based ratings was used as a dependent variable. We performed multiple regression also in the other direction, in which observer-based ratings were used as independent variables and each of the computerized measures was used as a dependent variable.

3. Results

3.1. Ambiguity and Distinctiveness of Emotion Expressions. *Ambiguity* of expression, averaged across emotions, showed a strong effect of diagnosis ($F = 12$, $df = 1, 53$, $P = 0.0012$), but no effect of sex ($F < 0.001$, $df = 1, 53$, $P = 0.99$) nor interaction ($F = 0.78$, $df = 1, 53$, $P = 0.38$) by two-way ANOVA. Patients showed higher *ambiguity* (0.41 ± 1.0) than controls (-0.44 ± 0.79), with a large effect size of 0.93 (Cohen's d). Likewise, *distinctiveness* of expression showed a strong effect of diagnosis ($F = 8.3$, $df = 1, 53$, $P = 0.0057$), but no effect of sex ($F = 0.056$, $df = 1, 53$, $P = 0.81$) nor interaction ($F = 0.26$, $df = 1, 53$, $P = 0.61$) by two-way ANOVA. Patients showed lower *distinctiveness* (-0.37 ± 0.88) than controls (0.40 ± 0.98) with a large effect size of Cohen's $d = 0.83$.

The characteristics of *ambiguity* and *distinctiveness* measures are demonstrated with sample videos of subjects in Figures 2–5 that illustrate the expressions of subjects with ratings for low *ambiguity*/high *distinctiveness*, in contrast to subjects with ratings for low *ambiguity*/low *distinctiveness*, high *ambiguity*/low *distinctiveness*, and high *ambiguity*/high *distinctiveness*.

3.2. Observer-Basted Measures

Validation of Ambiguity and Distinctiveness. The computerized measures of *ambiguity* and *distinctiveness* were well correlated with the observer's scores of *ambiguity* ($r = 0.71$, $P < 0.01$) and *distinctiveness* ($r = 0.60$, $P < 0.01$). These correlations supported the notion of agreement between the computerized measures from information theory and the observer-rated measures from visual examination of the videos.

Observer-Based Ratings of Facial Expressions. For video-based expert SANS ratings, flatness of expression showed a moderate effect of diagnosis ($F = 4.6$, $df = 1, 53$, $P = 0.038$), but no effect of sex ($F = 3.9$, $df = 1, 53$, $P = 0.055$) nor interaction ($F = 0.19$, $df = 1, 53$, $P = 0.66$) by two-way ANOVA. Patients were more flat (2.0 ± 0.93) than controls (1.5 ± 0.91), with a medium effect size of 0.57. The inappropriateness of expression showed a strong effect of diagnosis ($F = 9.6$, $df = 1, 53$, $P = 0.0033$), but no effect of sex ($F = 0.99$, $df = 1, 53$, $P = 0.33$) nor interaction ($F = 0.0047$, $df = 1, 53$, $P = 0.95$) by two-way ANOVA. Patients were rated higher on inappropriate affect (1.1 ± 0.65) than controls (0.63 ± 0.37)with a large effect size of 0.92.

3.3. Relationship between Computerized and Observer-Based Measures. We examined the relationships between information-theoretic measures of *ambiguity* and *distinctiveness* and observer-based measures of inappropriate and flattened facial expressions of emotions. Regression of *ambiguity* on observer-based measures was moderately predictive ($R^2 = 0.13$, $F = 3.4$, $P = 0.040$), and the coefficients from flatness and inappropriateness were −0.14 ($P = 0.30$) and 0.50 ($P = 0.032$), respectively. Regression of *distinctiveness* on observer-based measures was highly predictive ($R^2 = 0.19$, $F = 5.8$, $P = 0.0056$), and the coefficients from flatness and inappropriateness were −0.32 ($P = 0.027$) and −0.65 ($P = 0.0063$), respectively. Regression of flatness on computerized measures was moderately predictive ($R^2 = 0.15$, $F = 4.3$, $P = 0.019$), and the coefficients from *ambiguity* and *distinctiveness* were −0.33 ($P = 0.025$) and −0.34 ($P = 0.013$) respectively. Lastly, regression of inappropriateness on computerized measures was moderately predictive ($R^2 = 0.15$, $F = 4.3$, $P = 0.018$), and the coefficients from *ambiguity* and *distinctiveness* were 0.14 ($P = 0.11$) and −0.14 ($P = 0.11$), respectively.

4. Discussion and Conclusions

Impaired abilities of facial expression of emotions are common dysfunctions in schizophrenia that are associated with worse quality of life and poorer outcome [52, 53]. Clinical assessment of emotion expression abilities is typically obtained using observer-based rating scales administered during interviews that are not standardized to elicit emotion expressions and with limited potential to compare data across different studies and populations. More advanced observer-based measurements of facial expressions have been challenged by the complexity inherent in rating regional and global changes in dynamic facial expressions and their applications have been mainly limited to research. Nevertheless these investigations using standardized observer based ratings and electromyography have underscored that persons with schizophrenia exhibit altered expressions of volitional and of more fleeting spontaneous facial emotions that do not necessarily reflect their internal emotional state. Another challenge of measuring emotion expressions has been the importance to obtain emotion expressions that are genuine and naturalistic and not obscured by the artifice of the testing setting and methodology or influenced by rater fatigue. This is where automated computerized measurement offers an advantage over other methods to investigate dynamic expressions.

Our group has developed computerized assessment of emotion expression abilities that allows for objective measurement of facial expressions that are obtained in a standardized setting [32–35]. As an extension to these efforts, we have applied computerized assessments of facial expressivity to patients with schizophrenia and healthy controls to examine whether the novel methodology can elucidate differences in facial expression of emotions. Computerized information-theoretic measures focus on differences in *ambiguity*, which represents the measure of variability within the expression of a single emotion, and *distinctiveness*, which represents the measure of how distinctive facial expressions are for a particular emotion in comparison to other emotions. The computerized approach was validated by observer-based ratings of *ambiguity* and *distinctiveness*. In addition when computerized measures were predicted by observer-based ratings, *ambiguity* was positively related to inappropriateness, and *distinctiveness* was negatively related to both flatness and inappropriateness. Conversely, when observer-based ratings were predicted by computerized measures, flatness was negatively related to both *ambiguity* and *distinctiveness*, while inappropriateness was not significantly related with either measure alone, although it was significantly predicted by overall *ambiguity* and *distinctiveness*. As illustrated in Figures 2–5, computerized measures of *ambiguity* and *distinctiveness* were associated with facial expressions that, in the combination of low *ambiguity*/high *distinctiveness* (Figure 2), were well recognizable within each emotion and also different across emotions. High *ambiguity* with either low (Figure 3) or high (Figure 4) *distinctiveness* values appeared as inappropriate expressions that were either similar or different across emotions. The computerized measures also indicate flatness, as when facial expressions are not variable within an emotion (low *ambiguity*) and also indistinguishable across emotions (low *distinctiveness*) (Figure 5). These results suggest that the information-theoretic measures of emotion expressions are related to the observer-based ratings and computerized measures may provide quantifiable information on different causes of observed inappropriate affect. Specifically, inappropriateness of expression may result either from ambiguous and inconsistent facial expressions in each emotion regardless of distinctiveness across emotions. Flat affect, on the other hand, was mainly related to emotion expressions being indistinct across emotions.

Our computerized method employing information-theoretic measures offers several methodological advantages over currently available observer-based rating scales and FACS-based rating instruments, for example, our method being more objective and repeatable for any number of subjects, at the same time being less labor intensive and time-consuming. It is more objective than FACES since the method does not involve observer-judgment of emotions expressed and is less labor/time intensive than FACS and FACES since it is fully automated similar to EMG, without the inconvenience of physically placing electrodes on the participants' faces.

While we demonstrated the feasibility and applicability of these measures with schizophrenia patients and healthy controls, we are applying the analysis to a larger sample that can better reflect the range of individual differences in the respective populations. A major limitation of our approach is based on the fact that no computerized determination was made regarding emotional valence and such qualitative information could have enhanced the results based on information-theoretic measures of expressivity. Another limitation of the current study is that the induction procedure within the laboratory, while standardized, may lack ecological

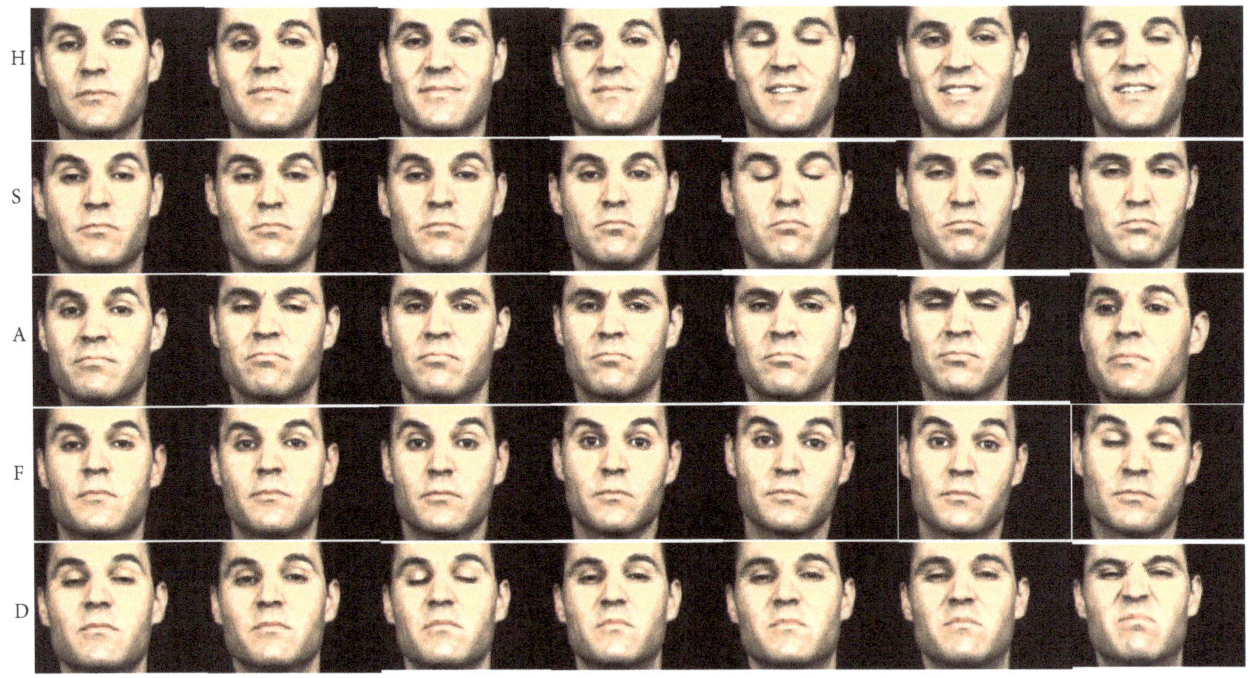

FIGURE 2: Sample videos of a subject with low *ambiguity* and high *distinctiveness*. H, S, A, F, and D stand for happiness, sadness, anger, fear, and disgust. Each row shows sample images evenly chosen from a video of the emotion. Facial expressions of low *ambiguity* and high *distinctiveness* are consistent within each emotion and also different across emotions, which makes each emotion well recognizable.

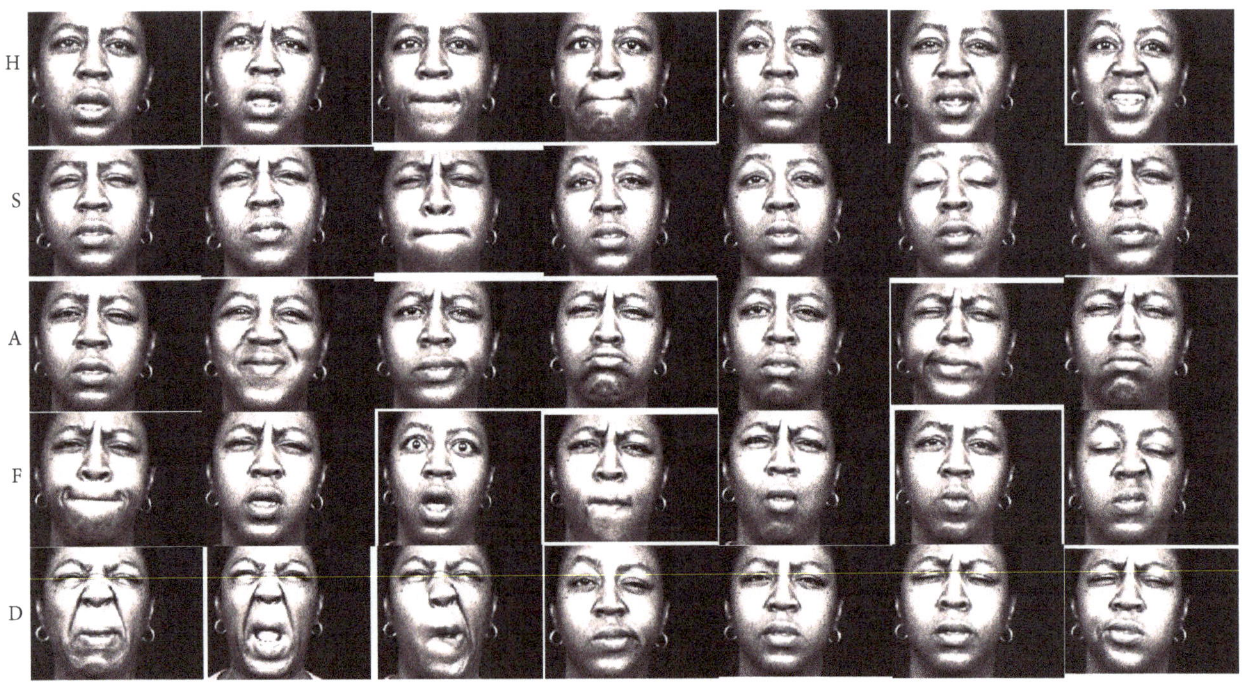

FIGURE 3: Sample videos of a subject with high *ambiguity* and low *distinctiveness*. High *ambiguity* and low *distinctiveness* appear as inappropriate facial expressions, due to the lack of consistent patterns within each emotion and the overlap of patterns across emotions.

validity. A more naturalistic setting would include filming participants while they recount their own experiences. Unfortunately at the present state of this methodology, facial movements on account of speech would generate too much noise for our algorithms to overcome.

In conclusion, our method offers an automated means for quantifying individual differences in emotional expressivity, similar to what has been accomplished in the area of emotion recognition. This capability opens new venues for delineating emotional expressivity in healthy people and across clinical

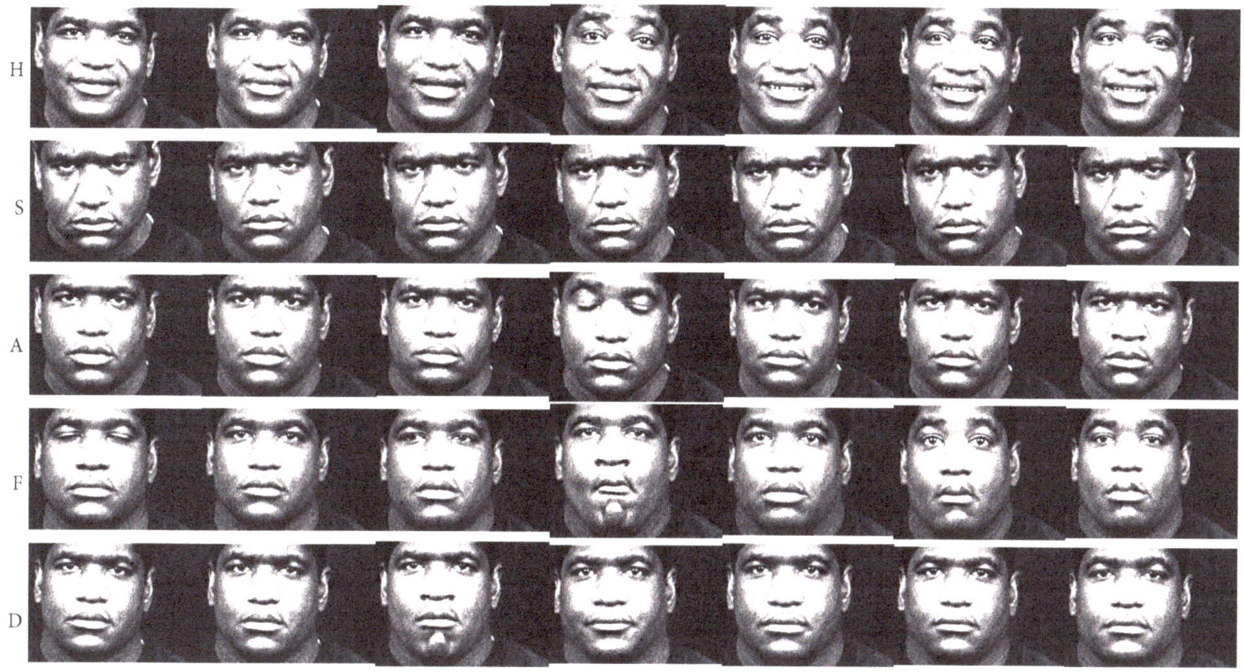

Figure 4: Sample videos of a subject with high *ambiguity* and high *distinctiveness*. High *ambiguity* and high *distinctiveness* also appear as inappropriate facial expressions due to the lack of consistent patterns within each emotion.

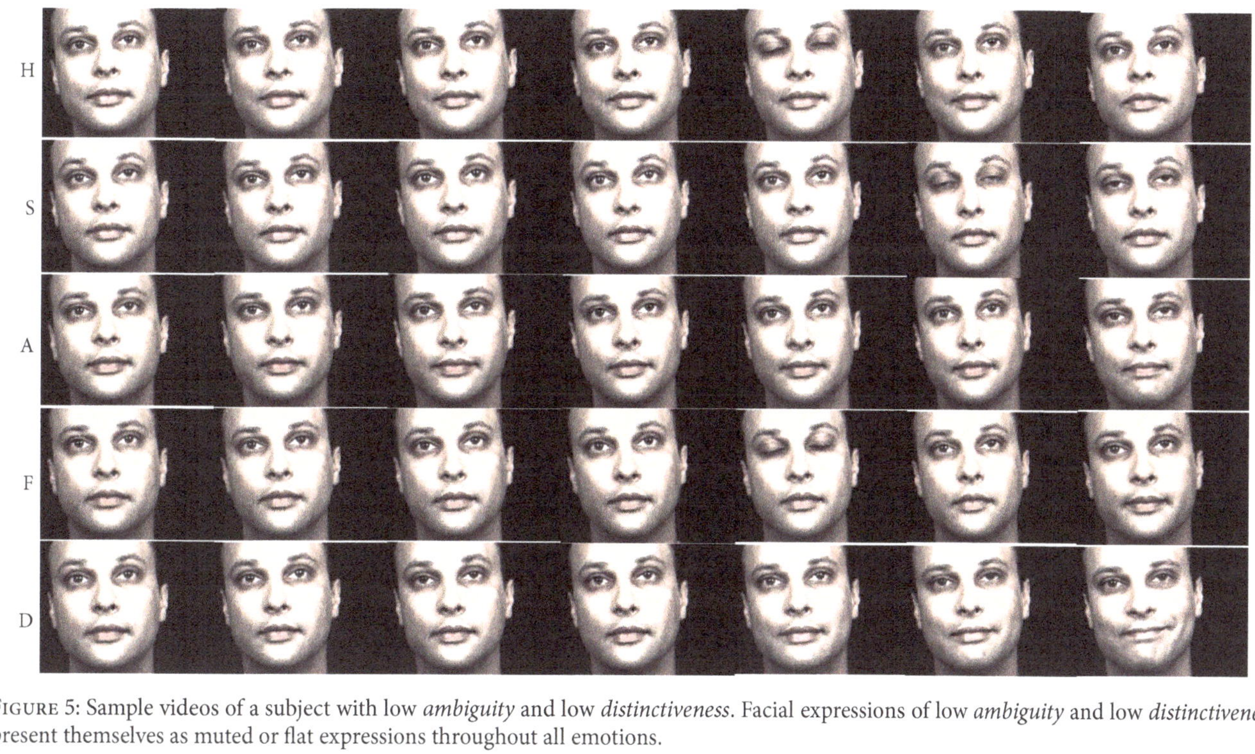

Figure 5: Sample videos of a subject with low *ambiguity* and low *distinctiveness*. Facial expressions of low *ambiguity* and low *distinctiveness* present themselves as muted or flat expressions throughout all emotions.

populations. As for investigations in healthy population, the automated procedure is well suited to examine both age and gender related changes in emotion expression abilities. Potential clinical applications may include repeated monitoring of facial expressions to investigate effects of disease progression and more general treatment effects or to measure targeted efforts to remediate emotion expression abilities. Automated comparisons need not be limited to select clinical populations and may allow for effective comparisons of emotion expressivity across different psychiatric disorders.

Conflict of Interests

The authors declare that there is no conflict of interests regarding the publication of this paper.

Acknowledgments

This work was supported by the National Institutes of Health (R01-MH073174 and R01-MH060722) and by Stanley Foundation Grant. The authors thank Elizabeth Martin and Kristin Healey for their assistance in data acquisition.

References

[1] E. Bleuler, "Dementia praecox oder die gruppe der schizophrenien," 1911.

[2] N. C. Andreasen, *The Scale for the Assessment of Negative Symptoms (SANS). The Scale for the Assessment of Positive Symptoms (SAPS)*, The University of Iowa, Iowa City, Iowa, USA, 1984.

[3] A. K. Malla, J. J. Takhar, R. M. G. Norman et al., "Negative symptoms in first episode non-affective psychosis," *Acta Psychiatrica Scandinavica*, vol. 105, no. 6, pp. 431–439, 2002.

[4] J. Mäkinen, J. Miettunen, M. Isohanni, and H. Koponen, "Negative symptoms in schizophrenia—a review," *Nordic Journal of Psychiatry*, vol. 62, no. 5, pp. 334–341, 2008.

[5] E. F. Walker, K. E. Grimes, D. M. Davis, and A. J. Smith, "Childhood precursors of schizophrenia: facial expressions of emotion," *American Journal of Psychiatry*, vol. 150, no. 11, pp. 1654–1660, 1993.

[6] S. R. Kay, A. Fiszbein, and L. A. Opler, "The positive and negative syndrome scale (PANSS) for schizophrenia," *Schizophrenia Bulletin*, vol. 13, no. 2, pp. 261–276, 1987.

[7] P. Ekman and W. Friesen, *Facial Action Coding System: Investigators Guide*, Consulting Psychologists Press, Palo Alto, Calif, USA, 1978.

[8] P. Ekman and W. Friesen, *Manual of the Facial Action Coding System (FACS)*, Consulting Psychologists Press, Palo Alto, Calif, USA, 1978.

[9] H. Berenbaum, "Posed facial expressions of emotion in schizophrenia and depression," *Psychological Medicine*, vol. 22, no. 4, pp. 929–937, 1992.

[10] H. Berenbaum and T. F. Oltmanns, "Emotional experience and expression in schizophrenia and depression," *Journal of Abnormal Psychology*, vol. 101, no. 1, pp. 37–44, 1992.

[11] W. Gaebel and W. Wölwer, "Facial expressivity in the course of schizophrenia and depression," *European Archives of Psychiatry and Clinical Neuroscience*, vol. 254, no. 5, pp. 335–342, 2004.

[12] F. Trémeau, D. Malaspina, F. Duval et al., "Facial expressiveness in patients with schizophrenia compared to depressed patients and nonpatient comparison subjects," *American Journal of Psychiatry*, vol. 162, no. 1, pp. 92–101, 2005.

[13] C. G. Kohler, E. A. Martin, N. Stolar et al., "Static posed and evoked facial expressions of emotions in schizophrenia," *Schizophrenia Research*, vol. 105, no. 1–3, pp. 49–60, 2008.

[14] A. M. Kring and D. M. Sloan, "The facial expression coding system (FACES): development, validation, and utility," *Psychological Assessment*, vol. 19, no. 2, pp. 210–224, 2007.

[15] A. M. Kring, S. L. Kerr, D. A. Smith, and J. M. Neale, "Flat affect in schizophrenia does not reflect diminished subjective experience of emotion," *Journal of Abnormal Psychology*, vol. 102, no. 4, pp. 507–517, 1993.

[16] A. M. Kring and J. M. Neale, "Do schizophrenic patients show a disjunctive relationship among expressive, experiential, and psychophysiological components of emotion?" *Journal of Abnormal Psychology*, vol. 105, no. 2, pp. 249–257, 1996.

[17] M. A. Aghevli, J. J. Blanchard, and W. P. Horan, "The expression and experience of emotion in schizophrenia: a study of social interactions," *Psychiatry Research*, vol. 119, no. 3, pp. 261–270, 2003.

[18] C. G. Kohler, E. A. Martin, M. Milonova et al., "Dynamic evoked facial expressions of emotions in schizophrenia," *Schizophrenia Research*, vol. 105, no. 1–3, pp. 30–39, 2008.

[19] E. Gottheil, C. C. Thornton, and R. V. Exline, "Appropriate and background affect in facial displays of emotion. Comparison of normal and schizophrenic males," *Archives of General Psychiatry*, vol. 33, no. 5, pp. 565–568, 1976.

[20] B. L. Schwartz, J. Mastropaolo, R. B. Rosse, G. Mathis, and S. I. Deutsch, "Imitation of facial expressions in schizophrenia," *Psychiatry Research*, vol. 145, no. 2-3, pp. 87–94, 2006.

[21] K. M. Putnam and A. M. Kring, "Accuracy and intensity of posed emotional expressions in unmedicated schizophrenia patients: vocal and facial channels," *Psychiatry Research*, vol. 151, no. 1-2, pp. 67–76, 2007.

[22] E. Steimer-Krause, R. Krause, and G. Wagner, "Interaction regulations used by schizophrenic and psychosomatic patients: studies on facial behavior in dyadic interactions," *Psychiatry*, vol. 53, no. 3, pp. 209–228, 1990.

[23] K. S. Earnst, A. M. Kring, M. A. Kadar, J. E. Salem, D. A. Shepard, and P. T. Loosen, "Facial expression in schizophrenia," *Biological Psychiatry*, vol. 40, no. 6, pp. 556–558, 1996.

[24] A. M. Kring, S. L. Kerr, and K. S. Earnst, "Schizophrenic patients show facial reactions to emotional facial expressions," *Psychophysiology*, vol. 36, no. 2, pp. 186–192, 1999.

[25] R. M. Mattes, F. Schneider, H. Heimann, and N. Birbaumer, "Reduced emotional response of schizophrenic patients in remission during social interaction," *Schizophrenia Research*, vol. 17, no. 3, pp. 249–255, 1995.

[26] E. Gottheil, A. Paredes, R. V. Exline, and R. Winkelmayer, "Communication of affect in schizophrenia," *Archives of General Psychiatry*, vol. 22, no. 5, pp. 439–444, 1970.

[27] F. Schneider, H. Heimann, W. Himer, D. Huss, R. Mattes, and B. Adam, "Computer-based analysis of facial action in schizophrenic and depressed patients," *European Archives of Psychiatry and Clinical Neuroscience*, vol. 240, no. 2, pp. 67–76, 1990.

[28] B. L. Schwartz, J. Mastropaolo, R. B. Rosse, G. Mathis, and S. I. Deutsch, "Imitation of facial expressions in schizophrenia," *Psychiatry Research*, vol. 145, no. 2-3, pp. 87–94, 2006.

[29] K. Wolf, R. Mass, F. Kiefer, K. Wiedemann, and D. Naber, "Characterization of the facial expression of emotions in schizophrenia patients: preliminary findings with a new electromyography method," *Canadian Journal of Psychiatry*, vol. 51, no. 6, pp. 335–341, 2006.

[30] M. Iwase, K. Yamashita, K. Takahashi et al., "Diminished facial expression despite the existence of pleasant emotional experience in schizophrenia," *Methods and Findings in Experimental and Clinical Pharmacology*, vol. 21, no. 3, pp. 189–194, 1999.

[31] C. E. Sison, M. Alpert, R. Fudge, and R. M. Stern, "Constricted expressiveness and psychophysiological reactivity in schizophrenia," *Journal of Nervous & Mental Disease*, vol. 184, no. 10, pp. 589–597, 1996.

[32] R. Verma, C. Davatzikos, J. Loughead et al., "Quantification of facial expressions using high-dimensional shape transformations," *Journal of Neuroscience Methods*, vol. 141, no. 1, pp. 61–73, 2005.

[33] C. Alvino, C. Kohler, F. Barrett, R. E. Gur, R. C. Gur, and R. Verma, "Computerized measurement of facial expression of emotions in schizophrenia," *Journal of Neuroscience Methods*, vol. 163, no. 2, pp. 350–361, 2007.

[34] P. Wang, F. Barrett, E. Martin et al., "Automated video-based facial expression analysis of neuropsychiatric disorders," *Journal of Neuroscience Methods*, vol. 168, no. 1, pp. 224–238, 2008.

[35] J. Hamm, C. G. Kohler, R. C. Gur, and R. Verma, "Automated facial action coding system for dynamic analysis of facial expressions in neuropsychiatric disorders," *Journal of Neuroscience Methods*, vol. 200, no. 2, pp. 237–256, 2011.

[36] C. E. Shannon, "A mathematical theory of communication," *Bell System Technical Journal*, vol. 27, no. 4, Article ID 379423, pp. 623–656, 1948.

[37] W. R. Garner, *Uncertainty and Structure as Psychological Concepts*, John Wiley & Sons, New York, NY, USA, 1962.

[38] A. T. Dittman, *Interpersonal Messages of Emotion*, Springer, New York, NY, USA, 1972.

[39] A. Borst and F. E. Theunissen, "Information theory and neural coding," *Nature Neuroscience*, vol. 2, no. 11, pp. 947–957, 1999.

[40] M. Costa, A. L. Goldberger, and C. K. Peng, "Multiscale entropy analysis of biological signals," *Physical Review E*, vol. 71, no. 2, part 1, Article ID 021906, 2005.

[41] J. Jeong, J. C. Gore, and B. S. Peterson, "Mutual information analysis of the EEG in patients with Alzheimer's disease," *Clinical Neurophysiology*, vol. 112, no. 5, pp. 827–835, 2001.

[42] S. H. Na, S. H. Jin, S. Y. Kim, and B. J. Ham, "EEG in schizophrenic patients: mutual information analysis," *Clinical Neurophysiology*, vol. 113, no. 12, pp. 1954–1960, 2002.

[43] R. C. Gur, R. Sara, M. Hagendoorn et al., "A method for obtaining 3-dimensional facial expressions and its standardization for use in neurocognitive studies," *Journal of Neuroscience Methods*, vol. 115, no. 2, pp. 137–143, 2002.

[44] W. R. Garner and H. W. Hake, "The amount of information in absolute judgments," *Psychological Review*, vol. 58, no. 6, pp. 446–459, 1951.

[45] J. Beirlant, E. J. Dudewicz, L. Gyoerfi, and E. C. Meulen, "Nonparametric entropy estimation: an overview," *International Journal of Mathematical and Statistical Sciences*, vol. 6, pp. 17–39, 1997.

[46] L. F. Kozachenko and N. N. Leonenko, "Sample estimate of the entropy of a random vector," *Problemy Peredachi Informatsii*, vol. 23, no. 2, pp. 9–16, 1987.

[47] M. N. Goria, N. N. Leonenko, V. V. Mergel, and P. L. N. Inverardi, "A new class of random vector entropy estimators and its applications in testing statistical hypotheses," *Journal of Nonparametric Statistics*, vol. 17, no. 3, pp. 277–297, 2005.

[48] R. M. Mnatsakanov, N. Misra, S. Li, and E. J. Harner, "Kn-nearest neighbor estimators of entropy," *Mathematical Methods of Statistics*, vol. 17, no. 3, pp. 261–277, 2008.

[49] J. Lin, "Divergence measures based on the Shannon entropy," *IEEE Transactions on Information Theory*, vol. 37, no. 1, pp. 145–151, 1991.

[50] D. M. Endres and J. E. Schindelin, "A new metric for probability distributions," *IEEE Transactions on Information Theory*, vol. 49, no. 7, pp. 1858–1860, 2003.

[51] S. Kullback and R. A. Leibler, "On Information and Sufficiency," *Annals of Mathematical Statistics*, vol. 22, no. 1, pp. 79–86, 1951.

[52] B. C. Ho, P. Nopoulos, M. Flaum, S. Arndt, and N. C. Andreasen, "Two-year outcome in first-episode schizophrenia: predictive value of symptoms for quality of life," *American Journal of Psychiatry*, vol. 155, no. 9, pp. 1196–1201, 1998.

[53] R. E. Gur, C. G. Kohler, J. D. Ragland et al., "Flat affect in schizophrenia: relation to emotion processing and neurocognitive measures," *Schizophrenia Bulletin*, vol. 32, no. 2, pp. 279–287, 2006.

5

Pomaglumetad Methionil (LY2140023 Monohydrate) and Aripiprazole in Patients with Schizophrenia: A Phase 3, Multicenter, Double-Blind Comparison

David H. Adams, Lu Zhang, Brian A. Millen, Bruce J. Kinon, and Juan-Carlos Gomez

Lilly Research Laboratories, Eli Lilly and Company, Lilly Corporate Center, Indianapolis, IN 46285, USA

Correspondence should be addressed to David H. Adams; adams_david_henry@lilly.com

Academic Editor: Robin Emsley

We tested the hypothesis that long-term treatment with pomaglumetad methionil would demonstrate significantly less weight gain than aripiprazole in patients with schizophrenia. In this 24-week, multicenter, randomized, double-blind, Phase 3 study, 678 schizophrenia patients were randomized to either pomaglumetad methionil ($n = 516$) or aripiprazole ($n = 162$). Treatment groups were also compared on efficacy and various safety measures, including serious adverse events (SAEs), discontinuation due to adverse events (AEs), treatment-emergent adverse events (TEAEs), extrapyramidal symptoms (EPS), and suicide-related thoughts and behaviors. The pomaglumetad methionil group showed significantly greater weight loss at Week 24 (Visit 12) compared with the aripiprazole group (-2.8 ± 0.4 versus 0.4 ± 0.6; $P < 0.001$). However, change in Positive and Negative Syndrome Scale (PANSS) total scores for aripiprazole was significantly greater than for pomaglumetad methionil (-15.58 ± 1.58 versus -12.03 ± 0.99; $P = 0.045$). The incidences of SAEs (8.2% versus 3.1%; $P = 0.032$) and discontinuation due to AEs (16.2% versus 8.7%; $P = 0.020$) were significantly higher for pomaglumetad methionil compared with aripiprazole. No statistically significant differences in the incidence of TEAEs, EPS, or suicidal ideation or behavior were noted between treatment groups. In conclusion, long-term treatment with pomaglumetad methionil resulted in significantly less weight gain than aripiprazole. This trial is registered with ClinicalTrials.gov NCT01328093.

1. Introduction

All of the current antipsychotics target dopamine receptors as their common mechanism of action [1, 2]. Due to differences in the affinities to the dopamine receptors and interactions with other biogenic monoamine receptors, therapeutic profiles and limitations of individual drugs vary [1]. The conventional/typical antipsychotic drugs are effective in treating positive symptoms of schizophrenia [3, 4]. However, they are associated with extrapyramidal symptoms (EPS) and hyperprolactinemia [3, 4]. The newer generation atypical antipsychotics not only improve positive and, to some extent, negative symptoms of schizophrenia [5, 6] but also have a lower propensity to cause EPS [3, 4, 7, 8] and hyperprolactinemia [3, 4]. However, these agents may still be associated with other adverse events (AEs), such as body weight gain, lipid abnormalities [9, 10], and glucose dysregulation [3, 4] in some patients. Furthermore, drug-induced weight gain may affect long-term compliance, which directly influences the likelihood of successfully managing the course of disease [11, 12]. Hence, a significant need exists to develop treatments for schizophrenia that are not associated with these and other AEs.

Pomaglumetad methionil (LY2140023 monohydrate), a methionine prodrug of the active compound LY404039, is a specific and potent metabotropic glutamate 2/3 (mGlu2/3) receptor agonist. It is devoid of affinity to all biogenic amine receptors, including dopamine receptors [1], but demonstrates a preclinical pharmacological profile similar to that of clinically effective atypical antipsychotic drugs [13, 14]. Unlike currently approved antipsychotic medications, pomaglumetad methionil was not expected to be associated with weight gain, EPS, or metabolic side effects because of its selective receptor binding profile [14] and hence has been suggested as an alternative treatment for schizophrenia [15]. Previous studies—a proof-of-concept study [15], a Phase 2, inpatient, dose-ranging study [13], a Phase 2 long-term safety study [16], and an acute, fixed-dose, Phase 2 study [17]—showed that treatment with pomaglumetad methionil was well-tolerated and demonstrated a low incidence of AEs, such as weight gain, EPS, and hyperprolactinemia, that are typically observed with currently available dopaminergic antipsychotic treatments. Efficacy results were as follows: positive in the proof-of-concept study [15], inconclusive in the Phase 2, inpatient, dose-ranging study, [13] and negative in the acute, fixed-dose, Phase 2 registration study [17].

Aripiprazole, a quinolinone derivative, is a novel atypical antipsychotic drug which has a mechanism of action distinct from other atypical antipsychotic drugs as it is a partial dopamine D_2 receptor agonist with a lower association with weight gain [3]. Because pomaglumetad methionil also has a low likelihood of inducing weight gain and may even be associated with weight loss in patients previously treated with antipsychotics [16], aripiprazole was selected as an appropriate comparator in this weight gain study to demonstrate a potentially unique weight profile for pomaglumetad methionil.

The present study was part of a Phase 3 clinical development program for pomaglumetad methionil in the treatment of schizophrenia. The purpose of the present study was to compare the mean weight gain in flexibly dosed pomaglumetad methionil (20, 40, or 80 mg, twice daily [BID]) with flexibly dosed aripiprazole (10, 15, or 30 mg/day) in patients with schizophrenia after 24 weeks of double-blind treatment. The study was intended to help characterize the benefits and risks of pomaglumetad methionil for a broad population of patients with schizophrenia but was stopped early when the pomaglumetad methionil schizophrenia monotherapy development program was stopped, based on lack of efficacy in an acute placebo-controlled efficacy study [17] as well as early stopping of a second acute trial due to futility [18]. This early stopping had minimal impact on the double-blind active treatment phase results of the present study, however, since enrollment was complete and 97% of patients had already completed or discontinued the double-blind active treatment phase of the study at the time of the termination.

2. Materials and Methods

2.1. Participants. This study was conducted at 57 centers in 10 countries. Male and female outpatients, aged 18 to 65 years (inclusive) with a diagnosis of schizophrenia, as defined by the *Diagnostic and Statistical Manual of Mental Disorders, Fourth Edition, Text Revision* (DSM-IV-TR) [19] and confirmed by Structural Clinical Interview for DSM-IV-TR (SCID), were enrolled into the study. Patients were excluded for the following reasons: (1) if they had other current Axis I psychiatric diagnoses (as defined in DSM-IV-TR) in addition to schizophrenia, (2) if they had a history of inadequate clinical response, in the opinion of the investigator, to antipsychotic treatment for schizophrenia (inadequate clinical response for this study was defined as persistent and moderately severe hallucinations, delusions, or thought disorder after completion of 2 or more antipsychotic medication trials of at least 8 weeks duration in the past 12 months prior to Visit 1), (3) if they had aripiprazole treatment within the past 2 months, (4) if they had a DSM-IV-TR diagnosis of substance abuse or dependence, (5) if they had a substance-induced psychosis by DSM-IV-TR criteria, or (6) if they were pregnant or breast-feeding. Written informed consent was obtained from the participants at the screening visit.

2.2. Study Design. This was a multicenter, randomized, double-blind, Phase 3 study to assess the safety and efficacy of pomaglumetad methionil (flexibly dosed between 20 and 80 mg BID) in patients with schizophrenia. An active control, aripiprazole (flexibly dosed between 10 and 30 mg/day), was included for comparison.

This study was divided into 3 study periods. Study Period I was a screening and antipsychotic drug taper/discontinuation phase (3–10 days). During this period, all screening procedures were completed and previous antipsychotic medications were stopped. Study Period II was the double-blind active treatment phase. Patients who met enrollment criteria during Study Period I continued into Study Period II and were randomized in 3 : 1 ratio to either pomaglumetad methionil or aripiprazole. The duration of the double-blind active treatment phase (24 weeks) enabled assessment of the safety of pomaglumetad methionil over a longer period of time than acute efficacy studies. Patients who completed Study Period II continued into Study Period III, which was an open-label active treatment phase. The duration of the open-label active treatment phase (28 weeks) enabled collection of additional safety data.

2.3. Ethical Considerations. The study was conducted in accordance with consensus ethics principles derived from international ethics guidelines, including the Declaration of Helsinki and Council for International Organizations of Medical Sciences International Ethical Guidelines, International Conference on Harmonization Guideline for Good Clinical Practice E6, and applicable laws and regulations.

2.4. Safety Measures. Safety measures that were monitored at every visit included weight, AEs, vital signs, suicidality as measured by the Columbia Suicide Severity Rating Scale (C-SSRS) [20], results of a neurological examination, and waist circumference (except at screening). Weight was assessed using a calibrated digital scale and investigator sites were instructed to assess patient's weight at a consistent time of day in light consistent clothing and by the same person at each visit. All serious adverse events (SAEs) and treatment-emergent adverse events (TEAEs) were reported according to terminology in the Medical Dictionary for Regulatory Activities (MedDRA), version 15.1. Other safety parameters that were monitored throughout the study were electrocardiogram (ECG) intervals and laboratory analytes, as well as EPS and abnormal movements, which were evaluated using the Barnes Akathisia Scale (BAS) [21], the Simpson-Angus Scale (SAS) [22], and the Abnormal Involuntary Movement Scale (AIMS) [23].

2.5. Efficacy Measures. Efficacy scales which were assessed/collected throughout the study were the Positive and Negative Syndrome Scale (PANSS) [24], Clinical Global Impression-Severity (CGI-S) [25], and the 16-Item Negative Symptom Assessment (NSA-16) [26].

2.6. Statistical Analysis. An expected sample size of at least 450 patients in the pomaglumetad methionil group and 150 patients in the aripiprazole group provided at least an 88% chance to demonstrate that the pomaglumetad methionil group had about 1.8 kilograms (kg) less mean body weight increase from baseline compared with the aripiprazole group at a 1-sided 0.025 alpha level. Sample size was based on a 2-sample t-test, assuming that the standard deviation of body weight change from baseline would be approximately 6 kg. The sample ratio of 3 : 1 was chosen to maximize exposure to pomaglumetad methionil.

The analyses were conducted on the intent-to-treat (ITT) population that included all patients according to the treatment group to which they were assigned and received at least 1 dose. The ITT set was modified prior to data lock, excluding patients ($n = 3$) from a site with an International Conference on Harmonisation Good Clinical Practices noncompliance issue. Analyses of the double-blind active treatment phase included comparisons between treatment groups with 2-sided tests conducted at the 0.05 alpha level. Data collected during the open-label active treatment phase were summarized.

The primary objective was evaluated with a mixed-model repeated measures (MMRM) analysis. The model included the fixed categorical effects of treatment, gender, pooled site, visit, treatment-by-visit interaction, and prior olanzapine use (yes or no, where "yes" was defined as usage of olanzapine for >7 cumulative days during the 6 weeks prior to screen), as well as the continuous, fixed covariates of baseline and baseline-by-visit interaction. The within-patient errors were modeled according to an unstructured covariance matrix. The Kenward-Roger approximation was used to estimate denominator degrees of freedom. The primary contrast was the pomaglumetad methionil versus aripiprazole comparison at Week 24 (Visit 12). Based on the visitwise treatment contrasts from the primary analysis, a sequential testing procedure was used to determine (with appropriate type I error control) the earliest time point at which the treatments differed statistically in mean weight change. The incidence of patients meeting criteria for potentially clinically significant weight gain (i.e., ≥7% increase from baseline) or weight loss (i.e., ≥7% decrease from baseline) at endpoint or any time during the double-blind active treatment phase was compared between treatment groups using the Cochran-Mantel-Haenszel test [27], controlling for baseline body mass index (BMI) and prior olanzapine use.

Incidence rates of safety categorical variables were summarized and compared between treatment groups using Fisher's exact test. The change from baseline in vital signs, ECG, SAS total score, AIMS total score (items 1–7), and BAS global score was assessed using an MMRM analysis with a model similar to that used for the efficacy analysis. The change from baseline to the last observed measure in the laboratory analytes was ranktransformed prior to analysis and was assessed using an analysis of variance (ANOVA) model with treatment as a fixed effect.

All the efficacy variables were evaluated with MMRM analysis. The model included the fixed, categorical effects of treatment, gender, pooled site, visit, treatment-by-visit interaction, and predefined subpopulation (yes/no), as well as the continuous, fixed covariates of baseline and baseline-by-visit interaction.

Reason for discontinuation, baseline characteristics, baseline efficacy, and baseline EPS measures along with illness characteristics were summarized by treatment group. Continuous measures were analyzed with a single factor ANOVA model with fixed effect of treatment and Fisher's exact test was used to compare categorical data between treatment groups. Time-to-discontinuation (due to AEs, lack of efficacy, and for any reason) was analyzed separately with Kaplan-Meier estimated survival curves [28], and the log-rank test was used for comparisons. All statistical analyses were performed using SAS, version 9.2 (SAS Institute, Inc., Cary, NC, USA).

3. Results

3.1. Patient Characteristics and Disposition. Of the 962 patients screened, 678 were randomized in an approximately 3 : 1 ratio (516 in the pomaglumetad methionil group and 162 in the aripiprazole group) during the double-blind active treatment phase, with 672 patients (511 in the pomaglumetad methionil group and 161 in the aripiprazole group) making up the ITT population (Figure 1). Baseline patient characteristics were comparable between the treatment groups (Table 1). Most of the patients were male (64.3%), white (52.4%), and from the United States (67.4%). The mean (standard deviation [SD]) for age was 42.45 (10.88) years, for baseline weight 89.90 (22.21) kg, for BMI 30.44 (7.39) kg/m^2, and for waist circumference −101.11 (17.10) cm. The major reasons for discontinuation across treatment arms during the double-blind active treatment phase were as follows: AE-subject decision (8.3%), subject decision-consent withdrawn (8.2%), lost to follow-up (7.7%), protocol violation (6.0%), AE-physician decision (5.4%), perceived lack of efficacy-physician decision (5.4%), and perceived lack of efficacy-subject decision (4.6%). Reasons for discontinuation were comparable between pomaglumetad methionil and aripiprazole groups except for AE-physician decision (6.7% versus 1.2%, resp.; $P = 0.005$).

A total of 313 patients completed the double-blind active treatment phase (229 in pomaglumetad methionil arm and 84 in aripiprazole arm) from which 272 patients enrolled into the open-label active treatment phase. Of 83 patients who completed the open-label active treatment phase, 60

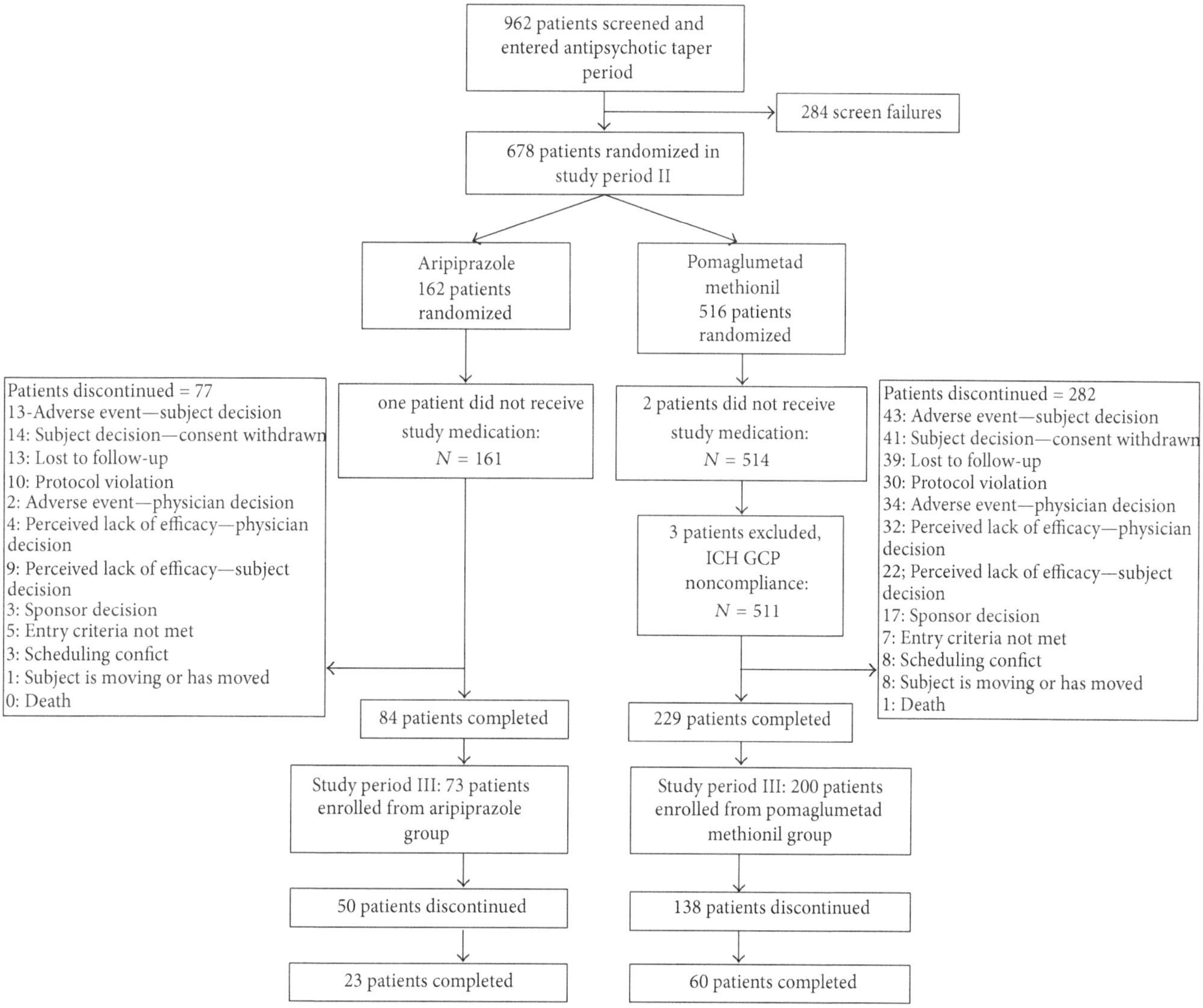

FIGURE 1: Patient disposition.

had taken pomaglumetad methionil during the double-blind active treatment phase. The most common reason for discontinuation during the open-label active treatment phase was sponsor decision (48.9%), reflecting early termination of the study following negative efficacy of an acute (Phase 2) registration trial [17], as well as early stopping of a second (Phase 3) registration trial due to futility [18].

There were no statistically significant differences between the pomaglumetad methionil and aripiprazole treatment groups in time-to-discontinuation (all causality) and time-to-discontinuation due to lack of efficacy. However, time-to-discontinuation due to AEs through the double-blind active treatment phase was significantly shorter for patients in the pomaglumetad methionil group than for those in the aripiprazole group ($P = 0.043$; Figure 2).

3.2. Safety Measures

3.2.1. Body Weight. A statistically significant difference was observed between pomaglumetad methionil and aripiprazole groups in least-squares (LS) mean change for weight at Week 24 (Visit 12 LS mean change [SE]: −2.8 [0.4] kg versus 0.4 [0.6] kg, resp.; $P < 0.001$). The onset of statistically different mean weight changes between pomaglumetad methionil and aripiprazole treatment group was at Week 2 (Visit 4 LS mean change [SE]: −0.5 [0.1] kg versus −0.1 [0.2] kg; $P = 0.016$; Figure 3). A significantly larger percentage of pomaglumetad methionil-treated than aripiprazole-treated patients reported ≥7% loss of baseline body weight at endpoint (13.1% versus 3.2%; $P < 0.001$) and at any time (15.6% versus 4.5%; $P < 0.001$) during the double-blind active treatment phase, while no significant findings were reported between pomaglumetad methionil-treated and aripiprazole-treated patients for ≥7% weight gain at endpoint (4.1% versus 7.1%, resp.) and at any time (5.1% versus 8.4%, resp.).

3.2.2. Serious Adverse Events (SAEs). In total, 47 of 672 (7.0%) patients experienced at least 1 SAE during the double-blind active treatment phase. There was a significant difference in

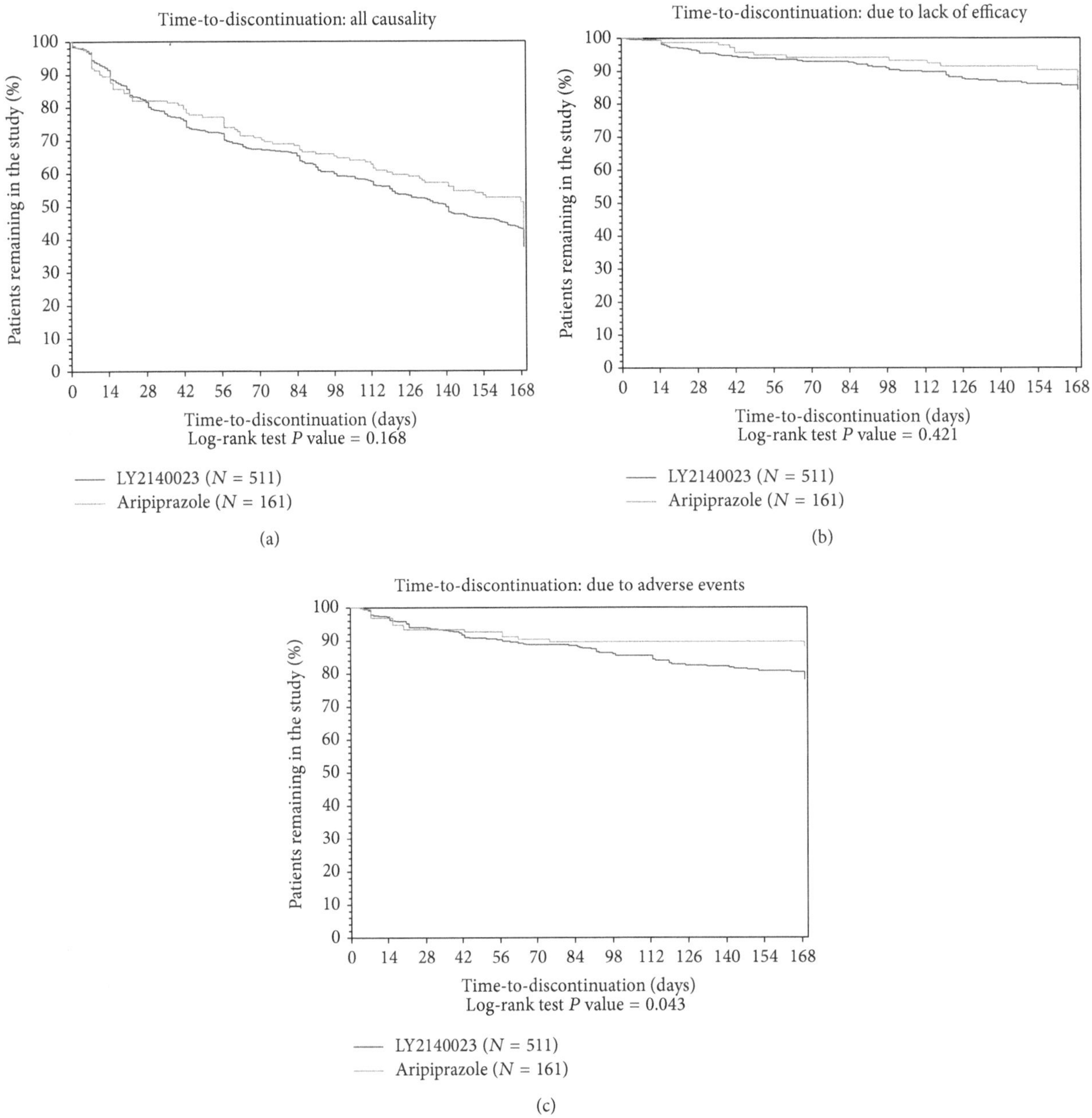

FIGURE 2: Kaplan-Meier plots showing time-to-discontinuation (all causality, due to lack of efficacy, and due to adverse events) for intent-to-treat (ITT) patients with schizophrenia in pomaglumetad methionil ($N = 511$) and aripiprazole ($N = 161$) treatment groups for 24 weeks of double-blind treatment.

the incidence of SAEs between pomaglumetad methionil-treated and aripiprazole-treated patients (8.2% versus 3.1%, resp.; $P = 0.032$; Table 2); however, no significant differences were reported between the treatment groups in the incidence of individual SAEs. The most common SAE among pomaglumetad methionil-treated and aripiprazole-treated patients was schizophrenia (2.9% versus 1.2%, resp.). One death (completed suicide) was reported in the pomaglumetad methionil treatment group but was judged by the investigator not to be treatment-related. During the open-label active treatment phase, 12 (4.4%) patients experienced at least 1 SAE.

3.2.3. Discontinuations due to Adverse Events (AEs). A total of 97 patients (14.4%) discontinued due to AEs, with significantly more patients discontinuing in the pomaglumetad methionil treatment group than in the aripiprazole treatment group due to AEs (16.2% versus 8.7%; $P = 0.020$; Table 2). The most common AE that resulted in discontinuation among both pomaglumetad methionil-treated and aripiprazole-treated patients was schizophrenia (2.9% and 1.2%, resp.). No significant difference was reported between the treatment groups in the incidence of any individual AEs that resulted in discontinuation. A total of 14 (5.2%) patients

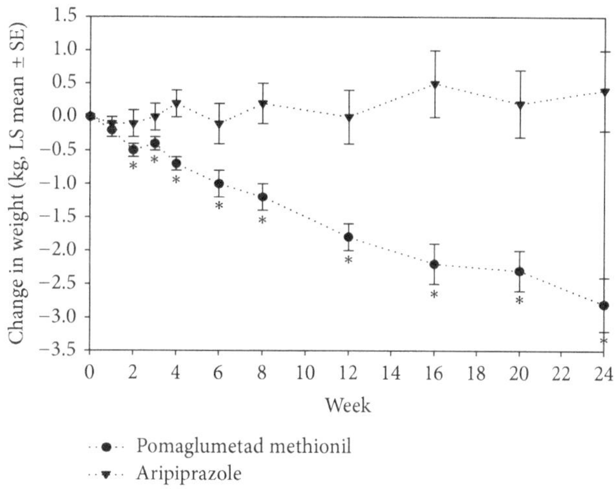

FIGURE 3: Least-squares mean change of the weight from mixed-effects model repeated measures among intent-to-treat (ITT) patients with schizophrenia in pomaglumetad methionil ($N = 511$) and aripiprazole ($N = 161$) treatment groups for 24 weeks of double-blind treatment. $^{*}P \leq 0.05$. P values are from type III tests of LS mean differences between treatments at each visit from MMRM. LS mean: least-squares means, MMRM: mixed-effects model with repeated measures, and SE: standard error.

TABLE 1: Patient demographics and baseline characteristics.

Variable	Double-blind treatment phase Pomaglumetad methionil $N = 511$	Aripiprazole $N = 161$	Total $N = 672$	P value[a]
Sex				
Female, n (%)	185 (36.2)	55 (34.2)	240 (35.7)	0.706
Male, n (%)	326 (63.8)	106 (65.8)	432 (64.3)	
Age				
Mean, year (SD)	42.29 (10.86)	42.95 (10.95)	42.45 (10.88)	0.500
Range, year	18.4–64.4	21.3–65.0	18.4–65.0	
Ethnicity, n (%)				
Hispanic or Latino	73 (14.3)	23 (14.3)	96 (14.3)	>0.999
Not Hispanic or Latino	438 (85.7)	138 (85.7)	576 (85.7)	
Race, n (%)				
American Indian or Alaskan Native	6 (1.2)	0 (0.0)	6 (0.9)	0.130
Asian	3 (0.6)	0 (0.0)	3 (0.4)	
Black or African American	238 (46.6)	64 (39.8)	302 (44.9)	
Multiple	5 (1.0)	4 (2.5)	9 (1.3)	
White	259 (50.7)	93 (57.8)	352 (52.4)	
Weight				
Mean, kg (SD)	89.8 (22.04)	90.18 (22.80)	89.90 (22.21)	0.851
BMI				
Mean, kg/m^2 (SD)	30.35 (7.32)	30.72 (7.63)	30.44 (7.39)	0.575
Waist circumference				
Mean, cm (SD)	100.90 (16.82)	101.80 (18.01)	101.11 (17.10)	0.559

[a]P value is from Fisher's exact test for categorical data and is from a single-factor analysis of variance model (ANOVA) with fixed effect of treatment for continuous variable.
BMI: body mass index; cm: centimeter; N: total number of patients in each treatment group; n: number of patients in each category; kg: kilogram; kg/m^2: kilogram per square meter; SD: standard deviation.

discontinued the open-label active treatment phase due to AEs.

3.2.4. Treatment-Emergent Adverse Events (TEAEs). A total of 479 (71.3%) patients experienced ≥1 TEAE during the double-blind active treatment phase. AEs reported with ≥3% incidence are shown in Table 3. Nausea, reported by 17.3% of patients, was the most frequent TEAE; however, only 1.3% of all patients discontinued the study because of nausea. Significantly more pomaglumetad methionil-treated patients reported nausea compared with aripiprazole-treated patients (19.2% versus 11.2%; $P = 0.023$). Significantly more aripiprazole-treated patients compared with pomaglumetad methionil-treated patients reported akathisia (7.5% versus 2.5%; $P = 0.007$), dyspepsia (3.7% versus 1.0%; $P = 0.027$), pyrexia (2.5% versus 0.4%; $P = 0.032$), and nasal congestion (1.9% versus 0.2%; $P = 0.045$). During the open-label active treatment phase, 114 (42.2%) patients experienced ≥1 TEAE (compared to the maximum severity observed during the double-blind phase). Headache (5.9%), nausea (5.6%), and insomnia (3.0%) were the most frequent TEAEs (≥3%) during the open-label phase.

3.2.5. Extrapyramidal Symptoms (EPS). Baseline EPS were comparable between the treatment groups (Table 4). No significant differences were found between treatment groups at the end of the double-blind active treatment phase. There were also no statistically significant differences based on categorical analysis of EPS scales (data not shown).

3.2.6. Suicidality. There were no statistically significant differences between treatment groups in measures of suicidal ideation and suicidal behavior, as assessed with the CSSRS during the double-blind active treatment phase. Forty-six (9.4%) patients in the pomaglumetad methionil group and 7 (4.5%) patients in the aripiprazole group had treatment-emergent suicidal ideation ($P = 0.064$), and 7 (1.4%) patients in the pomaglumetad methionil group and no patients in the aripiprazole group had suicidal behavior ($P = 0.205$) compared to baseline.

3.2.7. Additional Safety Measures. There were no significant differences between treatment groups in the incidence of treatment-emergent neurological exam findings, except abnormal gait, which was significantly higher in the aripiprazole treatment group than the pomaglumetad methionil group (2.5% versus 0.4%; $P = 0.032$) during the double-blind active treatment phase.

There were no clinically relevant laboratory findings for the pomaglumetad methionil group, and there were no clinically significant findings on vital signs or ECGs for the pomaglumetad methionil group compared with the aripiprazole group during the double-blind active treatment phase. Both treatment groups had significant within-group decreases in cholesterol and small but significant within-group increases in fasting glucose, but there were no significant differences between treatment groups. There was no significant change from baseline in triglycerides for either of the treatment groups. Based on the National Cholesterol Education Program (NCEP) [29] criteria, the percentage of patients exhibiting a shift from normal/borderline to high triglycerides was statistically significantly lower for the pomaglumetad methionil group than for the aripiprazole group at any time (11.6% versus 21.3%; $P = 0.010$) and at endpoint (4.5% versus 10.7%; $P = 0.026$). There were no other significant treatment differences in shifts in the NCEP criteria. There was a significantly greater mean decrease from baseline in prolactin for the pomaglumetad methionil group compared with the aripiprazole group (−2.25 versus −1.82, resp.; $P = 0.047$). The percentage of patients with treatment-emergent high prolactin at any time (10.7% versus 4.5%, resp.) or endpoint (4.9% versus 3.6%, resp.) was not significantly different between treatment groups.

Significant decreases in the pomaglumetad methionil treatment group compared with the aripiprazole treatment group were reported for BMI [standard error: SE] (−1.0 [0.1] versus 0.2 [0.2] kg/m^2; $P < 0.001$) and waist circumference (SE) (−2.3 [0.3] versus 0.4 [0.6] cm; $P < 0.001$) (Table 4).

3.3. Efficacy Measures. There was a significant improvement within the pomaglumetad methionil and aripiprazole treatment groups in all the efficacy scores at Week 24 (Visit 12) when compared with baseline scores. However, the change in PANSS total scores for the aripiprazole treatment group was statistically significantly greater than the change for the pomaglumetad treatment group during the double-blind active treatment phase, as measured by the LS mean (SE) change from baseline (−15.58 [1.58] versus −12.03 [0.99]; $P = 0.045$) at Week 24 (Visit 12). Similarly, the change in positive symptoms (−4.62 [0.50] versus −3.40 [0.32]; $P = 0.032$) and general psychopathology symptoms (−7.85 [0.89] versus −5.80 [0.56]; $P = 0.040$) for the aripiprazole treatment group was statistically significantly greater than the change for the pomaglumetad treatment group. There were no significant differences reported between treatment groups in the improvement of negative symptoms as measured by the PANSS negative scale and the NSA-16 scale at Week 24 (Visit 12). No significant differences were reported between treatment groups at Week 24 (Visit 12) on the CGI-S scale (Table 5).

At the end of the double-blind active treatment phase, significantly more responders (defined as those having ≥30% decrease in PANSS total scores from baseline) were noted in the aripiprazole treatment group compared with the pomaglumetad methionil group (16.1% versus 9.1%; $P = 0.017$).

4. Discussion

Weight gain prevention has become a major research interest since drug-induced weight gain is a risk factor for diabetes and cardiovascular problems and is a significant cause of antipsychotic treatment noncompliance [30]. Aripiprazole has generally been considered to have a lower propensity for weight gain than some other antipsychotics [3] but may still be associated with weight increase in some populations,

TABLE 2: Incidence of serious adverse events, discontinuations due to adverse events, and treatment-emergent adverse events during the double-blind treatment phase.

Safety measure	Double-blind treatment phase			
	Pomaglumetad methionil $N = 511$	Aripiprazole $N = 161$	Total $N = 672$	P value[a]
SAEs	42 (8.2)	5 (3.1)	47 (7.0)	0.032*
Discontinuations due to AEs	83 (16.2)	14 (8.7)	97 (14.4)	0.020*
TEAEs	370 (72.4)	109 (67.7)	479 (71.3)	0.272

* $P < 0.05$.
[a] P values are from Fisher's exact test.
AE: adverse event; N: total number of patients in each treatment group; SAE: serious adverse event; TEAE: treatment-emergent adverse event.

TABLE 3: Incidence of most common treatment-emergent adverse events ≥3% in any treatment group and/or with statistically significant treatment difference, by preferred term.

MedDRA preferred term	Double-blind treatment phase			
	Pomaglumetad methionil $N = 511$ n (%)	Aripiprazole $N = 161$ n (%)	Total $N = 672$ n (%)	P value[a]
Nausea	98 (19.2)	18 (11.2)	116 (17.3)	0.023*
Insomnia	50 (9.8)	19 (11.8)	69 (10.3)	0.459
Headache	57 (11.2)	10 (6.2)	67 (10.0)	0.071
Vomiting	41 (8.0)	12 (7.5)	53 (7.9)	>0.999
Nasopharyngitis	38 (7.4)	8 (5.0)	46 (6.8)	0.371
Blood creatine phosphokinase increased	29 (5.7)	4 (2.5)	33 (4.9)	0.141
Anxiety	22 (4.3)	9 (5.6)	31 (4.6)	0.519
Decreased appetite	22 (4.3)	6 (3.7)	28 (4.2)	>0.999
Diarrhea	20 (3.9)	8 (5.0)	28 (4.2)	0.651
Schizophrenia	24 (4.7)	2 (1.2)	26 (3.9)	0.058
Dizziness	17 (3.3)	8 (5.0)	25 (3.7)	0.343
Akathisia	13 (2.5)	12 (7.5)	25 (3.7)	0.007*
Dry mouth	15 (2.9)	5 (3.1)	20 (3.0)	>0.999
Fatigue	14 (2.7)	6 (3.7)	20 (3.0)	0.594
Back pain	9 (1.8)	5 (3.1)	14 (2.1)	0.341
Dyspepsia	5 (1.0)	6 (3.7)	11 (1.6)	0.027*
Pyrexia	2 (0.4)	4 (2.5)	6 (0.9)	0.032*
Nasal congestion	1 (0.2)	3 (1.9)	4 (0.6)	0.045*

* $P < 0.05$.
[a] P values are from Fisher's exact test.
N: total number of patients in each treatment group; MedDRA: Medical Dictionary for Regulatory Activities; TEAE: treatment-emergent adverse event.

depending upon previous antipsychotic exposure [31, 32]. The significant separation of pomaglumetad methionil and aripiprazole on weight outcome offers the opportunity to demonstrate a unique weight attribute of pomaglumetad methionil. In the current study, the aripiprazole group showed a very small increase in weight from baseline (0.4 kg), consistent with previous reports. In contrast, the pomaglumetad methionil group showed significant weight loss from baseline (−2.8 kg), and significantly more pomaglumetad methionil-treated patients reported a ≥7% decrease in weight from baseline compared with aripiprazole-treated patients at endpoint and at any time during the double-blind study. It is not clear from the present results whether any of the reported weight loss was a consequence of the discontinuation of previous antipsychotic treatment, resulting in shedding of excess weight gained during that treatment, was due to anticraving effects of pomaglumetad methionil treatment, or both [33]. Regardless, the results suggest that the weight profile for pomaglumetad is unique compared with current antipsychotics.

Most AEs were reported at similar incidence rates in both treatment groups. However, nausea occurred more often in the pomaglumetad methionil group, and there was a significantly higher incidence of akathisia, dyspepsia, pyrexia, and nasal congestion in the aripiprazole treatment group. The higher incidence of akathisia in the aripiprazole group

Table 4: Least-squares mean change from baseline to Week 24 (Visit 12) in the safety measures.

Measure total score	Double-blind Treatment Phase: Pomaglumetad methionil (N = 511)		Aripiprazole (N = 161)		LS mean difference between pomaglumetad methionil and aripiprazole (SE)	P value[a]
	Baseline mean (SD)	Δ to Week 24 (Visit 12) LS mean (SE)	Baseline mean (SD)	Δ to Week 24 (Visit 12) LS mean (SE)		
Weight (kg)	89.80 (22.04)	−2.8 (0.4)	90.18 (22.80)	0.4 (0.6)	−3.2 (0.7)	<0.001*
BMI (kg/m^2)	30.35 (7.32)	−1.0 (0.1)	30.72 (7.63)	0.2 (0.2)	−1.1 (0.2)	<0.001*
Waist circumference (cm)	100.9 (16.8)	−2.3 (0.3)	101.8 (18.0)	0.4 (0.6)	−2.7 (0.6)	<0.001*
EPS						
BAS	0.1 (0.5)	0.00 (0.03)	0.1 (0.4)	−0.04 (0.04)	0.04 (0.04)	0.353
SAS	0.5 (1.7)	−0.17 (0.06)	0.4 (1.2)	−0.20 (0.08)	0.03 (0.09)	0.698
AIMS	0.3 (1.2)	−0.11 (0.05)	0.3 (1.1)	−0.10 (0.07)	−0.01 (0.07)	0.924

*$P < 0.001$.
[a] P values are from type III tests of LS mean differences between treatments at each visit from MMRM.
Δ: change from baseline; LS mean: least-squares means; AIMS: Abnormal Involuntary Movement Scale; BAS: Barnes Akathisia Scale; cm: centimeter; EPS: extrapyramidal symptoms; kg: kilogram; kg/m^2: kilogram per square meter; MMRM: mixed-effects model with repeated measures; N: number of patients; SAS: Simpson-Angus Scale; SD: standard deviations; SE: standard error.

Table 5: Least-squares mean change from baseline to Week 24 (Visit 12) in the efficacy measures.

Measure	Double-blind treatment phase: Pomaglumetad methionil (N = 511)		Aripiprazole (N = 161)		LS mean difference between pomaglumetad methionil and aripiprazole (SE)	P value[a]
	Baseline mean (SD)	Δ to Week 24 (Visit 12) LS mean (SE)	Baseline mean (SD)	Δ to Week 24 (Visit 12) LS mean (SE)		
PANSS						
Total score	77.9 (24.15)	−12.03 (0.99)	79.5 (22.19)	−15.58 (1.58)	3.55 (1.77)	0.045*
Positive	19.1 (6.75)	−3.40 (0.32)	19.5 (6.31)	−4.62 (0.50)	1.21 (0.56)	0.032*
Negative	20.4 (7.13)	−2.98 (0.31)	21.2 (7.10)	−3.34 (0.48)	0.36 (0.54)	0.509
General psychopathology	38.4 (13.08)	−5.80 (0.56)	38.7 (12.10)	−7.85 (0.89)	2.05 (1.00)	0.040*
CGI-S score	4.1 (0.79)	−0.51 (0.05)	4.1 (0.74)	−0.69 (0.08)	0.17 (0.09)	0.055
NSA-16 total score	46.3 (13.34)	−6.22 (0.68)	47.5 (13.48)	−6.37 (1.03)	0.15 (1.11)	0.891

*$P < 0.05$.
[a] P values are from type III tests of LS mean differences between treatments at each visit from MMRM.
Δ: change from baseline; LS mean: least-squares mean; N: number of patients; CGI-S: Clinical Global Impression-Severity; MMRM: mixed-effects model with repeated measures; NSA-16: 16-Item Negative Symptom Assessment; PANSS: Positive and Negative Syndrome Scale; SD: standard deviations; SE: standard error.

is consistent with previously reported outcomes for this compound [34, 35]. Nausea and vomiting have been observed in other pomaglumetad methionil trials, and aripiprazole has also been previously associated with gastrointestinal-related AEs. The observed decrease in weight for the pomaglumetad methionil group does not appear to be a consequence of nausea and vomiting because for most patients the gastrointestinal events occurred only during the first weeks of treatment, whereas the time course of weight changes was gradual and persistent across the 24 weeks. Suicidal ideation (40% to 50%) and behavior (20% to 50%) are frequent in patients with schizophrenia [36]. In the present study, rates of suicidal ideation and behavior were not significantly different between the treatment groups during the double-blind active treatment phase, with 1.4% of patients in the pomaglumetad methionil group exhibiting suicidal behavior.

There were no clinically relevant laboratory findings, and there were no clinically significant findings on vital signs or ECGs for the pomaglumetad methionil group compared with the aripiprazole group. Analysis of fasting lipids and glucose generally did not show significant treatment differences, although there were significantly fewer patients with a shift from normal/borderline triglycerides to high triglycerides at any time in the pomaglumetad methionil group. It is possible that a longer duration of observation may be needed to observe further differences in metabolic parameters as a result of the decreases in weight.

The overall greater number of SAEs and discontinuations due to AEs in the pomaglumetad methionil group appeared to be primarily driven by disease state-related AEs (psychosis and schizophrenia) and may be related to inferior efficacy compared with aripiprazole as well as manifestations of the underlying disease state.

The lack of placebo in the current study limits our interpretation of efficacy, so efficacy outcomes were secondary. However, the efficacy of pomaglumetad methionil was inferior compared with aripiprazole in this trial. Definitive placebo-controlled efficacy studies were being conducted in parallel to this study. The present study was stopped early when the pomaglumetad methionil schizophrenia monotherapy development program was stopped, based on lack of efficacy in an acute placebo-controlled efficacy study [17] as well as early stopping of a second acute trial due to futility [18]. This early stopping had minimal impact on the double-blind active treatment phase results of the present study, however, since enrollment was complete and 97% of patients had already completed or discontinued the double-blind active treatment phase of the study at the time of termination. (As noted in the Results Section, the most common reason for discontinuation during the open-label active treatment phase was sponsor decision (48.9%), reflecting early termination of the study.) Subgroups defined by clinical parameters, markers that may reflect an underlying hyperglutamatergic tone, or genotype are currently being explored across the completed pomaglumetad methionil studies to understand if there may be a more responsive subgroup of patients.

5. Conclusions

Treatment for 24 weeks with pomaglumetad methionil resulted in significantly less weight gain compared with aripiprazole. However, inferior efficacy in this longer term study along with the recent results of acute placebo-controlled pivotal efficacy studies suggests that pomaglumetad methionil is not effective in a broad schizophrenia patient population. More research is needed to determine whether a targeted patient population may be responsive to a glutamatergic treatment for the treatment of schizophrenia.

Disclosure

All authors are employees and minor stockholders of Eli Lilly and Company.

Conflict of Interests

The authors declare that there is no conflict of interest regarding the publication of this paper.

Acknowledgments

This research was supported by Eli Lilly and Company, Indianapolis, IN, USA. The authors would like to thank Pavan K. Yenduri (inVentiv Health Clinical, funded by Eli Lilly and Company) for his assistance in drafting the paper.

References

[1] P. J. Harrison, "Metabotropic glutamate receptor agonists for schizophrenia," *The British Journal of Psychiatry*, vol. 192, no. 2, pp. 86–87, 2008.

[2] P. Seeman, "Atypical antipsychotics: mechanism of action," *Canadian Journal of Psychiatry*, vol. 47, no. 1, pp. 27–38, 2002.

[3] T. S. Harrison and C. M. Perry, "Aripiprazole: a review of its use in schizophrenia and schizoaffective disorder," *Drugs*, vol. 64, no. 15, pp. 1715–1736, 2004.

[4] R. Bridler and D. Umbricht, "Atypical antipsychotics in the treatment of schizophrenia," *Swiss Medical Weekly*, vol. 133, no. 5-6, pp. 63–76, 2003.

[5] S. W. Lewis, L. Davies, P. B. Jones et al., "Randomised controlledtrials of conventional antipsychotic versus new atypicaldrugs, and new atypical drugs versus clozapine, in people withschizophrenia responding poorly to, or intolerant of, currentdrug treatment," *Health Technology Assessment*, vol. 10, no. 17, pp. 1–165, 2006.

[6] J. M. Kane, "Utilization of long-acting antipsychotic medication in patient care," *CNS Spectrums*, vol. 11, supplement 14, no. 12, pp. 1–8, 2006.

[7] J. Geddes, N. Freemantle, P. Harrison, and P. Bebbington, "Atypical antipsychotics in the treatment of schizophrenia: systematic overview and meta-regression analysis," *British Medical Journal*, vol. 321, no. 7273, pp. 1371–1376, 2000.

[8] S. Leucht, G. Pitschel-Walz, D. Abraham, and W. Kissling, "Efficacy and extrapyramidal side-effects of the new antipsychotics olanzapine, quetiapine, risperidone, and sertindole compared to conventional antipsychotics and placebo. A meta-analysis of randomized controlled trials," *Schizophrenia Research*, vol. 35, no. 1, pp. 51–68, 1999.

[9] K. A. Stigler, M. N. Potenza, D. J. Posey, and C. J. McDougle, "Weight gain associated with atypical antipsychotic use in children and adolescents: prevalence, clinical relevance, and management," *Pediatric Drugs*, vol. 6, no. 1, pp. 33–44, 2004.

[10] D. J. Müller and J. L. Kennedy, "Genetics of antipsychotic treatment emergent weight gain in schizophrenia," *Pharmacogenomics*, vol. 7, no. 6, pp. 863–887, 2006.

[11] I. Kurzthaler and W. W. Fleischhacker, "The clinical implications of weight gain in schizophrenia," *Journal of Clinical Psychiatry*, vol. 62, supplement 7, pp. 32–37, 2001.

[12] D. O. Perkins, "Predictors of noncompliance in patients with schizophrenia," *Journal of Clinical Psychiatry*, vol. 63, no. 12, pp. 1121–1128, 2002.

[13] B. J. Kinon, L. Zhang, B. A. Millen et al., "A multicenter, inpatient, phase 2, double-blind, placebo-controlled dose-ranging study of LY2140023 monohydrate in patients with DSM-IV schizophrenia," *Journal of Clinical Psychopharmacology*, vol. 31, no. 3, pp. 349–355, 2011.

[14] M. Mezler, H. Geneste, L. Gault, and G. J. Marek, "LY-2140023, a prodrug of the group II metabotropic glutamate receptor agonist LY-404039 for the potential treatment of schizophrenia," *Current Opinion in Investigational Drugs*, vol. 11, no. 7, pp. 833–845, 2010.

[15] S. T. Patil, L. Zhang, F. Martenyi et al., "Activation of mGlu2/3 receptors as a new approach to treat schizophrenia: a randomized Phase 2 clinical trial," *Nature Medicine*, vol. 13, no. 9, pp. 1102–1107, 2007.

[16] D. H. Adams, B. J. Kinon, S. Baygani et al., "A long-term, phase 2, multicenter, randomized, open-label, comparative safety study of pomaglumetad methionil (LY2140023 monohydrate) versus atypical antipsychotic standard of care in patients with schizophrenia," *BMC Psychiatry*, vol. 13, no. 1, article 143, 2013.

[17] B. Kinon, B. A. Millen, A. C. Downing et al., "LY, 2140023 monohydrate in the treatment of patients with schizophrenia: results of 2 clinical trials assessing efficacy in treating acutely ill patients and those with prominent negative symptoms," *Schizophrenia Bulletin*, vol. 39, supplement 1, p. S338, 2013.

[18] Eli Lilly, "A Study of LY2140023 in Patients with Schizophrenia," NLM identifier: NCT01307800, ClinicalTrials.gov, 2013, http://clinicaltrials.gov/show/NCT01307800.

[19] [APA] American Psychiatric Association, *Diagnostic and Statistical Manual of Mental Disorders*, American Psychiatric Association, Washington, DC, USA, 4th edition, 2000.

[20] K. Posner, G. A. Melvin, B. Stanley, M. A. Oquendo, and M. Gould, "Factors in the assessment of suicidality in youth," *CNS Spectrums*, vol. 12, no. 2, pp. 156–162, 2007.

[21] T. R. E. Barnes, "A rating scale for drug-induced akathisia," *British Journal of Psychiatry*, vol. 154, pp. 672–676, 1989.

[22] G. M. Simpson and J. W. Angus, "A rating scale for extrapyramidal side effects," *Acta Psychiatrica Scandinavica*, vol. 45, supplement 212, pp. 11–19, 1970.

[23] W. Guy, *ECDEU Assessment Manual for Psychopharmacology, Revised 1976*, pp. 534–537, National Institute of Mental Health, Early Clinical Drug Evaluation, Psychopharmacology Research Branch, Rockville, Md, USA, 1976.

[24] S. R. Kay, A. Fiszbein, and L. A. Opler, "The positive and negative syndrome scale (PANSS) for schizophrenia," *Schizophrenia Bulletin*, vol. 13, no. 2, pp. 261–276, 1987.

[25] W. Guy, *ECDEU Assessment Manual for Psychopharmacology, Revised 1976*, pp. 217–222, National Institute of Mental Health, Early Clinical Drug Evaluation, Psychopharmacology Research Branch, Rockville, Md, USA, 1976.

[26] L. D. Alphs, A. Summerfelt, H. Lann, and R. J. Muller, "The negative symptom assessment: a new instrument to assess negative symptoms of schizophrenia," *Psychopharmacology Bulletin*, vol. 25, no. 2, pp. 159–163, 1989.

[27] R. J. Landis, E. R. Heyman, and G. G. Koch, "Average partial association in three-way contingency tables: a review and discussion of alternative tests," *International Statistical Review*, vol. 46, no. 3, pp. 237–254, 1978.

[28] E. L. Kaplan and P. Meier, "Nonparametric estimation from incomplete observations," *Journal of American Statistical Association*, vol. 53, no. 282, pp. 457–481, 1958.

[29] National Cholesterol Education Program, "Third Report of the National Cholesterol Education Program (NCEP) Expert Panel on Detection, Evaluation, and Treatment of High Blood Cholesterol in Adults (Adult Treatment Panel III) Final Report," *Circulation*, vol. 106, no. 25, pp. 3143–3421, 2002.

[30] P. K. Narula, H. S. Rehan, K. E. S. Unni, and N. Gupta, "Topiramate for prevention of olanzapine associated weight gain and metabolic dysfunction in schizophrenia: a double-blind, placebo-controlled trial," *Schizophrenia Research*, vol. 118, no. 1–3, pp. 218–223, 2010.

[31] R. L. Findling, A. Robb, M. Nyilas et al., "A multiple-center, randomized, double-blind, placebo-controlled study of oral aripiprazole for treatment of adolescents with schizophrenia," *American Journal of Psychiatry*, vol. 165, no. 11, pp. 1432–1441, 2008.

[32] S. G. Potkin, A. R. Saha, M. J. Kujawa et al., "Aripiprazole, an antipsychotic with a novel mechanism of action, and risperidone vs placebo in patients with schizophrenia and schizoaffective disorder," *Archives of General Psychiatry*, vol. 60, no. 7, pp. 681–690, 2003.

[33] Z. A. Rodd, D. L. McKinzie, R. L. Bell et al., "The metabotropic glutamate 2/3 receptor agonist LY404039 reduces alcohol-seeking but not alcohol self-administration in alcohol-preferring (P) rats," *Behavioural Brain Research*, vol. 171, no. 2, pp. 207–215, 2006.

[34] R. Kerwin, B. Millet, E. Herman et al., "A multicentre, randomized, naturalistic, open-label study between aripiprazole and standard of care in the management of community-treated schizophrenic patients Schizophrenia Trial of Aripiprazole: (STAR) study," *European Psychiatry*, vol. 22, no. 7, pp. 433–443, 2007.

[35] R. Tandon, R. N. Marcus, E. G. Stock et al., "A prospective, multicenter, randomized, parallel-group, open-label study of aripiprazole in the management of patients with schizophrenia or schizoaffective disorder in general psychiatric practice: Broad Effectiveness Trial with Aripiprazole (BETA)," *Schizophrenia Research*, vol. 84, no. 1, pp. 77–89, 2006.

[36] J. Kasckow, K. Felmet, and S. Zisook, "Managing suicide risk in patients with schizophrenia," *CNS Drugs*, vol. 25, no. 2, pp. 129–143, 2011.

6

Vascular Endothelial Growth Factor and Brain-Derived Neurotrophic Factor in Quetiapine Treated First-Episode Psychosis

Brendan P. Murphy,[1,2] Terence Y. Pang,[3] Anthony J. Hannan,[3] Tina-Marie Proffitt,[4] Mirabel McConchie,[4] Melissa Kerr,[4] Connie Markulev,[4] Colin O'Donnell,[5] Patrick D. McGorry,[4] and Gregor E. Berger[6]

[1] *Early in Life Mental Health Service, Southern Health, Melbourne, VIC 3175, Australia*
[2] *School of Psychology and Psychiatry, Monash University, Melbourne, VIC 3800, Australia*
[3] *Howard Florey Institute, Florey Neuroscience Institutes, University of Melbourne, Melbourne, VIC 3052, Australia*
[4] *Orygen Youth Health Research Centre, University of Melbourne, Melbourne, VIC 3052, Australia*
[5] *St. Davnet's Hospital, Monaghan, County Monaghan, Ireland*
[6] *Department of Child and Adolescent Psychiatry, University of Zurich, 8032 Zurich, Switzerland*

Correspondence should be addressed to Brendan P. Murphy; brendan.murphy@monash.edu

Academic Editor: Robin Emsley

Objective. It has been suggested that atypical antipsychotics confer their effects via brain-derived neurotrophic factor (BDNF). We investigated the effect of quetiapine on serum levels of BDNF and vascular endothelial growth factor (VEGF) in drug-naive first-episode psychosis subjects. *Methods.* Fifteen patients drawn from a larger study received quetiapine treatment for twelve weeks. Baseline levels of serum BDNF and VEGF were compared to age- and sex-matched healthy controls and to levels following treatment. Linear regression analyses were performed to determine the relationship of BDNF and VEGF levels with outcome measures at baseline and week 12. *Results.* The mean serum BDNF level was significantly higher at week 12 compared to baseline and correlated with reductions in Brief Psychiatric Rating Scale (BPRS) and general psychopathology scores. Changes in serum VEGF levels also correlated significantly with a reduction in BPRS scores, a significant improvement in PANNS positive symptoms scores, and displayed a positive relationship with changes in BDNF levels. *Conclusions.* Our findings suggest that BDNF and VEGF are potential biomarkers for gauging improvement of psychotic symptoms. This suggests a novel neurotrophic-based mechanism of the drug effects of quetiapine on psychosis. This is the first report of VEGF perturbation in psychosis.

1. Introduction

The precise molecular mechanisms mediating the actions of antipsychotic drugs remain poorly understood [1]. It has been proposed that atypical antipsychotics confer some of their benefits through neuroprotective effects [2]. Evidence from rodent studies suggests that this protective effect is mediated by an upregulation of brain-derived neurotrophic factor (BDNF) in the brain [3–5]. A review of animal studies concluded that, with the exception of risperidone, atypical antipsychotics might increase BDNF expression while conventional antipsychotics might decrease expression [6]. Risperidone's inability to alter expression of BDNF or to even increase it at higher doses (Favelli) suggests differential effects of atypical antipsychotics on BDNF expression. Olanzapine and risperidone significantly increase D2 binding in the medial prefrontal cortex and hippocampus, whilst quetiapine does not. Similarly, olanzapine and risperidone produce significant up-regulation of D4 receptors in the hippocampus, caudate-putamen, and nucleus accumbens, whilst quetiapine does not [7]. Quetiapine's inability to adjust dopamine receptors suggests that nondopaminergic mechanisms may contribute more to its efficacy than with other atypical antipsychotics. Quetiapine has been shown to attenuate stress-induced reductions in BDNF expression in rats [5].

A previous study of drug-naive first-episode psychosis patients reported that serum BDNF levels are lower in this patient group and were increased toward healthy control levels following olanzapine treatment, in association with a reduction of positive symptoms [8].

Brain-Derived Neurotrophic Factor. BDNF is the most widely distributed neurotrophin in the central nervous system (CNS) [9] and is highly expressed in the prefrontal cortex and hippocampus [10]. It serves a variety of essential functions during development including neurogenesis, neuronal differentiation and survival, and normal maturation of neurodevelopmental pathways [11, 12]. In the adult, it continues to play a crucial role in neuronal integrity, promoting synaptic plasticity [13] as well as modulating synthesis, metabolism, and release of dopamine, GABA, serotonin and glutamate [14] and moderating use-dependent plasticity processes including long-term potentiation, learning, and memory [15, 16]. Perturbations in BDNF are likely to have widespread psychopathological consequences leading to altered brain development and functioning [17], and there is accumulating evidence that abnormal BDNF signalling may be involved in the pathophysiology of a range of psychiatric disorders including depression [18], bipolar affective disorder [19], and schizophrenia [20].

There are several lines of evidence pointing to a possible role in schizophrenia. Firstly, BDNF is known to be important both in the neurodevelopment of dopaminergic-related systems and in ongoing dopaminergic function [21], particularly exerting its effects through the mesolimbic pathway [22]. Secondly, as mentioned, BDNF regulates other neurotransmitters putatively involved in the aetiology of schizophrenia, including glutamate, GABA, and serotonin [14]. Thirdly, BDNF principally exercises its influence through neuroanatomical areas known to be associated with symptom domains in schizophrenia, including the prefrontal cortex and hippocampus [10].

Evidence for disturbed BDNF functioning in schizophrenia comes from several different sources. Several studies have found alterations in postmortem levels of BDNF in the brains of schizophrenic subjects: decreased levels in the prefrontal cortex [23–25] and hippocampus [26] and increased levels in the hippocampus [27, 28], anterior cingulate cortex [28], and cerebral cortex [26]. Another study reported deceased gene expression of BDNF and TrkB receptors in postmortem schizophrenic brains [29]. BDNF is known to mediate its effects through binding to TrkB receptors, which in turn activate intracellular survival pathways [17].

BDNF crosses the blood-brain barrier [30] and serum concentrations strongly correlate with brain levels [31]. Reports of BDNF levels in the serum of schizophrenic patients have proven inconsistent. The majority demonstrate a significant reduction in serum BDNF in chronic and medicated schizophrenics compared to healthy controls [32–38], though there have been reverse findings [39–41]. Similarly, amongst first-episode and drug-naive cohorts, significant reductions relative to healthy subjects have been reported more often [42–49] than not [50–53]. Unlike postmortem samples or chronic cohorts, FEP populations—especially drug-naïve ones—are beneficial to study as the effects of chronicity, medication, and medical comorbidities are attenuated. A recent systematic review and meta-analysis concluded that there was moderate evidence for reduced serum BDNF levels in medicated and drug-naive schizophrenia, with an association between reduced levels and increasing age, but no effects of medication dosage [54]. However, the reviewers were unable to account for the heterogeneity across studies, though gender and body mass are known to affect BDNF levels, as are stage of illness, subtype of schizophrenia and medication [52], substance misuse [53] and diet [54].

Vascular Endothelial Growth Factor. The cytokine vascular endothelial growth factor (VEGF) is critical for blood vessel growth during embryonic development and in adults, promoting vasculogenesis and playing a central role in wound healing [55]. As well as indirectly promoting neurogenesis by regulating brain angiogenesis, VEGF is also believed to have direct trophic effects on neurons and glia in the CNS, supporting neuronal migration in the developing CNS and displaying essential neuroprotective properties in the adult. While VEGF is believed to have significant effects on hippocampal morphology [56] and its role in treating depression has been explored [57], there has been little research with respect to schizophrenia. There has been one study that reported decreased VEGF mRNA levels in the dorsolateral prefrontal cortex of schizophrenic subjects [58]. In rats, VEGF levels are increased in the hippocampus after 14 days of treatment with haloperidol and olanzapine. Upon continuing with daily drug administration, it was found that the effect of haloperidol was lost after 45 days of treatment while VEGF levels continued to rise in the olanzapine-treated rats. That difference was suggested to reflect the increased efficacy in treating cognitive and negative symptoms that second generation antipsychotics demonstrate [59]. In support of this, chlorpromazine has been shown to reduce VEGF secretion *in vitro* [60].

VEGF levels have not been measured in schizophrenic subjects though there have been several studies in depression. One study found raised plasma VEGF levels in 16 depressed subjects [61] while another found raised levels in 35 depressed subjects and 35 manic subjects compared to healthy controls. The latter study also reported that there was no correlation of VEGF levels to symptoms and the authors suggested that the raised levels may be serving a neuroprotective function [62]. VEGF levels were not significantly altered by antidepressant therapy in 25 depressed subjects [63], though one study demonstrated significant increases in 19 depressed subjects one month after ECT treatment that correlated with an improvement in depression scores [64].

Aims. There have been no previous studies investigating the effects of quetiapine on serum BDNF levels in FEP. We therefore sought to compare baseline BDNF levels in drug-naive FEP subjects with age- and sex-matched healthy controls and then to determine whether there was a change in levels in FEP subjects following 12 weeks of treatment with quetiapine. We hypothesised that baseline subjects would have lower BDNF levels than healthy controls but that levels would improve with treatment. We also hypothesised that there would be a negative correlation between BDNF levels and a number of outcome measures, including positive and negative symptoms.

There has been no exploration of VEGF in schizophrenia or other psychoses. We therefore sought to measure VEGF levels in our sample. We hypothesised that baseline subjects would have lower VEGF levels than healthy controls, which would increase following quetiapine treatment. We also hypothesized that changes to VEGF levels would be negatively correlated to a number of outcome measures. Finally, we proposed that there would be a positive correlation between BDNF and VEGF levels.

2. Materials and Methods

2.1. Subjects. 15 subjects (10 males/5 females; mean age = 18.6 ± 3.3 years) were drawn from a prospective, randomized, double-blind cohort study (Trial Registration: clinicaltrials.gov Identifier: NCT00449397) that compared 4-weeks of 200 mg/day versus 400 mg/day of quetiapine for efficacy, tolerability, and safety in 141 drug-naive first-episode psychosis patients aged 15–25 [65]. All subjects who had provided sufficient samples at baseline and week 12 had their serum assayed. Eight subjects were completely drug-naive, two subjects had received 3 days of quetiapine, four had received 4 days of quetiapine, and one had received 7 days of quetiapine prior to serum collection. Five subjects were randomized to 200 mg, ten to 400 mg. The control group consisted of a group of fifteen healthy volunteers with no history of psychiatric disorder (18.5 ± 3.1 years). Subjects were age- and sex-matched to controls because of the known effects of age and gender [66]. The serum for all subjects was separated in a centrifuge and stored at −80°C until assayed. A first episode of psychosis was defined as daily psychotic symptoms for longer than a week that could not be explained by other factors (e.g., organic in the context of temporal lobe epilepsy or drug-induced psychotic episodes that remitted within 7 days without antipsychotic medication. Subjects were recruited from the Early Psychosis Prevention and Intervention Centre (EPPIC), a subprogram of Orygen Youth Health [67]. Exclusion criteria included having received more than one week of previous treatment with an antipsychotic, a concurrent manic episode, and a history of neurological disease. Subjects were randomly allocated to either 200 mg or 400 mg of quetiapine and treated for four weeks. Following this, subjects remained on quetiapine for a further eight weeks and had their doses adjusted according to clinical need. No other antipsychotic was permitted during the twelve week study. Subjects were assessed using SCID-IV, Research Version, Patient Edition (2002), and symptomatology ratings included the BPRS extended version 4, the Scale for the Assessment of Negative Symptoms (SANS) and the Positive and Negative Syndrome Scale (PANSS). Adverse events were assessed using the Udvalg for Kliniske Undersogelser (UKU). All raters undertook systematic psychopathology training in the context of annual rater workshops at the Orygen Research Centre; the ratings demonstrated good reliability, with intraclass coefficients of agreement ≥0.8, and all were within 20% of the standard scores. All raters were blind to BDNF levels. The research was approved by the relevant Research and Ethics Committees and both subjects and controls provided written informed consent.

2.2. BDNF Measurement. BDNF concentrations of serum samples were quantified using the BDNF Emax Immunoassay system (Promega, Madison, WI, USA) according to manufacturer's instructions. Briefly, each sample was diluted with sample buffer to obtain two dilutions (1/10 and 1/50) and each was assayed in triplicate. Technical replicates with greater than 10% variance were repeated. After adjusting for dilution factors, samples with greater than 25% variance were repeated. The average serum concentration of BDNF of both dilutions was determined and used for subsequent data analysis.

2.3. VEGF Measurement. VEGF concentrations of serum samples were quantified using MILLIPLEX MAP human cytokine/chemokine panel (Cat. number MPXHCYTO-60 K, Millipore, Billerica, MA, USA) in conjunction with a Luminex 100 system (Austin, TX, USA). Undiluted samples were assayed in duplicate and technical replicates with greater than 10% variance were repeated. The serum concentration of VEGF from both readouts was averaged and used for subsequent data analysis.

2.4. Statistical Analyses. Data was analysed using GraphPad Prism Version 6.1 (GraphPad Software, La Jolla, California, USA). Data sets were separated according to sex and drug dosage for analysis by one-way ANOVA using Bonferroni adjusted α-values of 0.0167. 95% confidence intervals were calculated and r^2 values determined.

3. Results

3.1. BDNF. Serum BDNF levels of males and females in the control group were similar, and this was also observed in patient groups at week 0 and week 12 (data not shown). Therefore, sexes were pooled for subsequent analyses. There was no other significant effect of quetiapine dose on BDNF levels in the patient group (data not shown) so both dosages were pooled for subsequent analyses.

One-way ANOVA found a significant difference in the mean serum BDNF levels between the groups ($F_{(2,51)} = 7.797$; $P = 0.0011$; Figure 1(a)), and post hoc testing revealed that this was significantly higher in the Week 12 patient group compared to baseline (Wk12 versus Wk0: $P = 0.012$) but not compared to the control group ($P = 0.0256$).

Linear regression analysis found no significant relationship between Week 0 serum BDNF levels and BPRS, UKU, or SANS scores (see *Supplementary Figures 1(a)–1(c)* available online at http://dx.doi.org/10.1155/2014/719395). There was

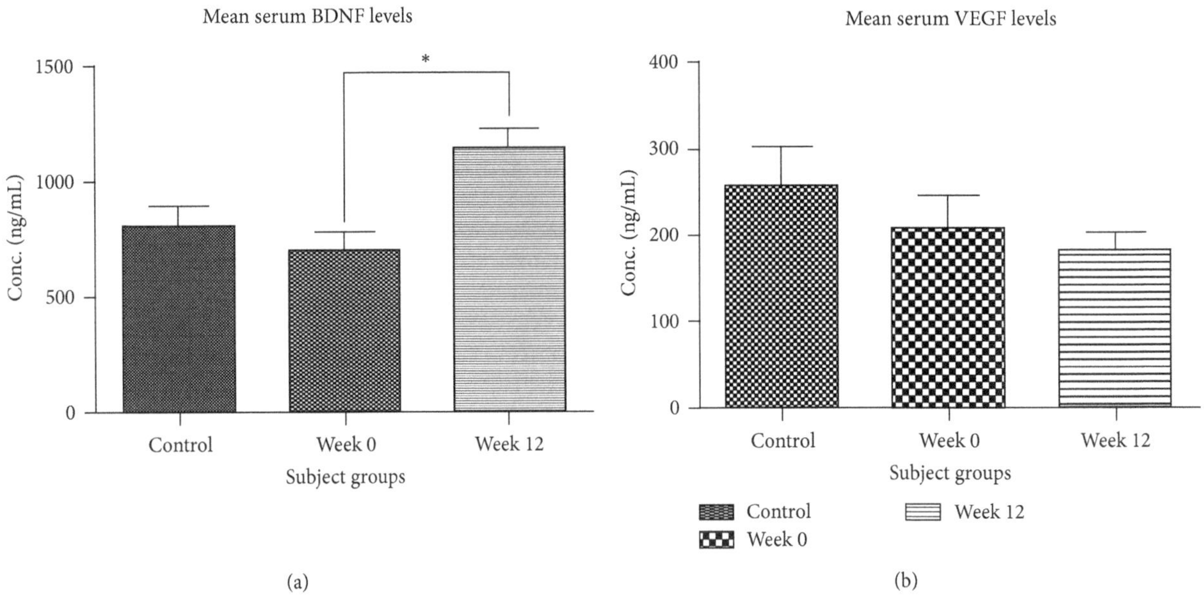

Figure 1: Serum neurotrophin levels. Grouped analysis of serum BDNF levels (a) revealed a greater mean BDNF level of the FEP patient group at week 12 compared to week 0. There was no overall difference in VEGF levels between the three subject groups (b). *One-way ANOVA followed by post hoc t-test $P < 0.05$.

also no relationship between serum BDNF levels and PANSS negative, positive, or general psychopathology scores at Week 0 (see *Supplementary Figures 1(d)-1(e)*). At Week 12, there was no significant relationship between serum BDNF levels and outcome scores (see *Supplementary Figure 2*).

The difference in serum BDNF levels at weeks 0 and 12 was determined and analysed against the change in evaluative test scores. There was a significant positive relationship with reduction in BPRS scores and change in BDNF levels ($r^2 = 0.3656$, $P = 0.0131$) (Figure 2(a)), though there was no significant relationship between the change in serum BDNF levels and changes in UKU ($r^2 = 0.08078$, $P = 0.2861$; Figure 2(b)) or SANS scores ($r^2 = 0.0569$, $P = 0.3637$; Figure 2(c)).

The extent of the reduction in PANSS general psychopathology scores displayed a positive relationship with the change in BDNF levels ($r^2 = 0.4176$, $P = 0.0068$; Figure 2(d)) but there was no significant relationship between the change in BDNF levels and change in PANSS positive ($r^2 = 0.1867$, $P = 0.0946$; Figure 2(e)) or negative scores ($r^2 = 0.1037$, $P = 0.2239$; Figure 2(f)).

3.2. VEGF. Mean serum VEGF levels of males and females in all three groups (control group, T0, and T12) did not differ significantly (data not shown); therefore sexes were pooled for subsequent analyses. There was no significant difference in VEGF levels between patients allocated to dosage 1 and dosage 2 at both week 0 and week 12 timepoints and patient data for both dosages were pooled for subsequent analyses. One-way ANOVA analysis of the pooled data revealed no significant difference in the mean serum VEGF levels ($F_{(2,45)} = 1.095$, $P = 0.3437$; Figure 1(b)).

Linear regression analysis found no significant relationship between Week 0 serum VEGF levels and BPRS, UKU, or SANS scores (*Supplementry Figures 3(a)–3(c)*). There was also no relationship between serum BDNF levels and PANSS negative, positive, or general psychopathology scores at Week 0 (*Supplementry Figures 3(d)–3(f)*). Similarly, at Week 12, there was no significant relationship between serum VEGF levels and outcome scores (*Supplementry Figure 4*).

The difference in serum VEGF levels at weeks 0 and 12 was determined and analysed against the change in evaluative test scores. There was a significant positive relationship with reduction in BPRS scores and change in VEGF levels ($r^2 = 0.3820$, $P = 0.0244$; Figure 3(a)), though there was no significant relationship between change in UKU ($r^2 = 0.03133$, $P = 0.5629$; Figure 3(b)) or SANS scores ($r^2 = 0.0035$, $P = 0.8473$; Figure 3(c)) and the change in serum VEGF levels. The change in VEGF levels displayed a significant positive relationship with the reduction in PANSS positive symptom scores ($r^2 = 0.4847$, $P = 0.0082$; Figure 3(d)). However there was no significant relationship between the change in VEGF levels and change in PANSS negative ($r^2 = 0.01708$, $P = 0.6704$; Figure 3(e)) or general scores ($r^2 = 0.2457$, $P = 0.0849$; Figure 3(f)).

3.3. Relationship between BDNF and VEGF. We examined the data set for a possible association between BDNF and VEGF levels. Linear regression revealed that at Week 0, VEGF levels were significantly associated with BDNF levels ($r^2 = 0.2833$, $P = 0.0338$; Figure 4(a)) but this relationship was lost at the Week 12 timepoint ($r^2 = 0.04886$, $P = 0.4285$; Figure 4(b)). Furthermore, the change in BDNF levels from Week 0 to Week 12 was significantly associated with changes in VEGF levels ($r^2 = 0.2758$, $P = 0.0444$; Figure 4(c)).

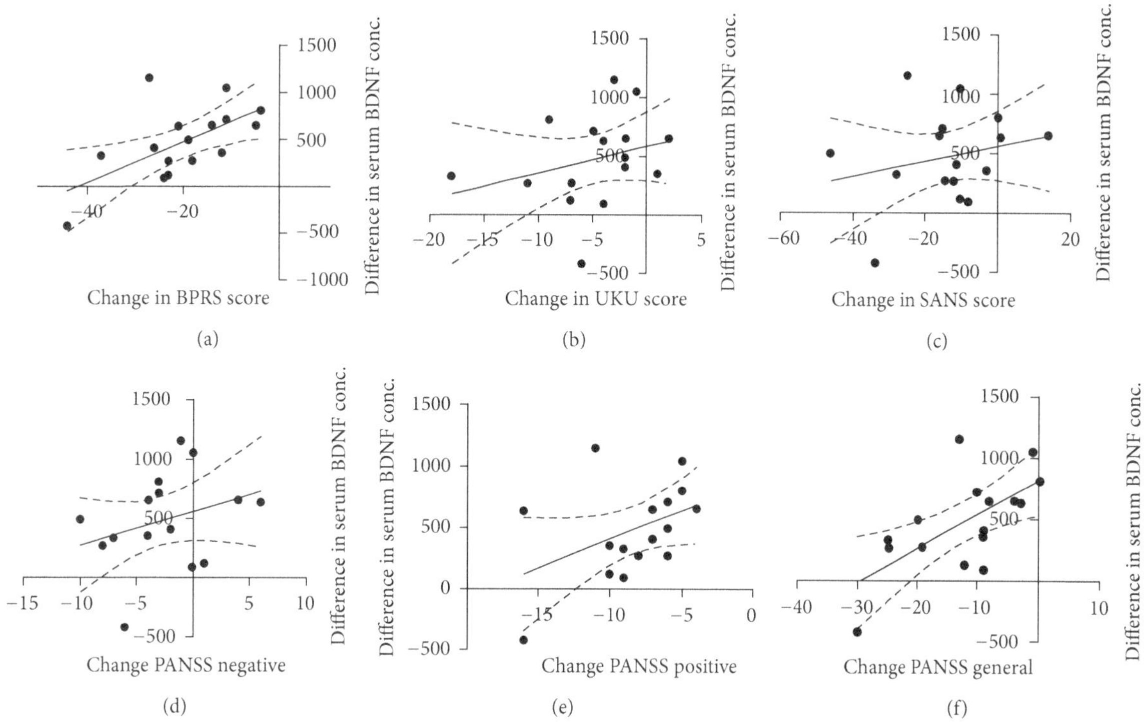

FIGURE 2: Relationship between changes in serum BDNF concentrations with changes in outcome measures. There were significant positive correlations between serum BDNF levels and improved scores on the BPRS (a) and PANNS general (f). There were no significant correlations for changes in scores of UKU (b), SANS (c), PANSS negative (d), and PANSS positive (e) with the difference in BDNF levels across both time points.

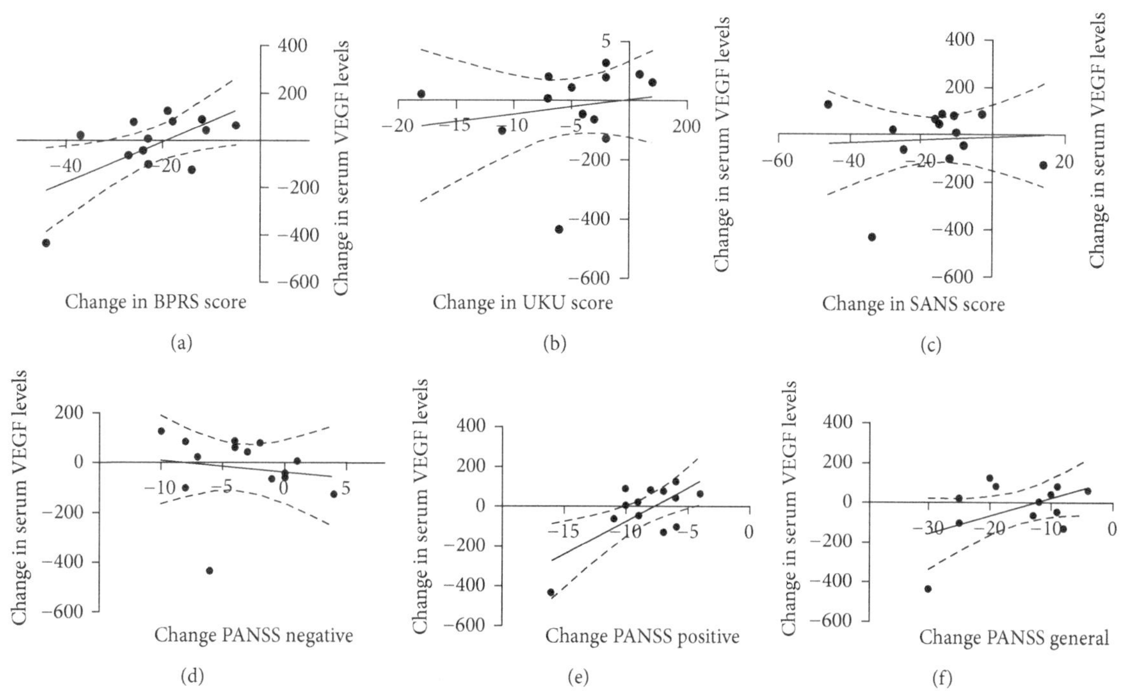

FIGURE 3: Relationship between changes in serum VEGF concentrations with changes in outcome measures. There were significant positive correlations between serum VEGF levels and improved scores on the BPRS (a) and PANNS positive (d). There were no significant correlations for changes in scores of UKU (b), SANS (c), PANSS negative (d), and PANSS general (f) with the difference in VEGF levels across both time points.

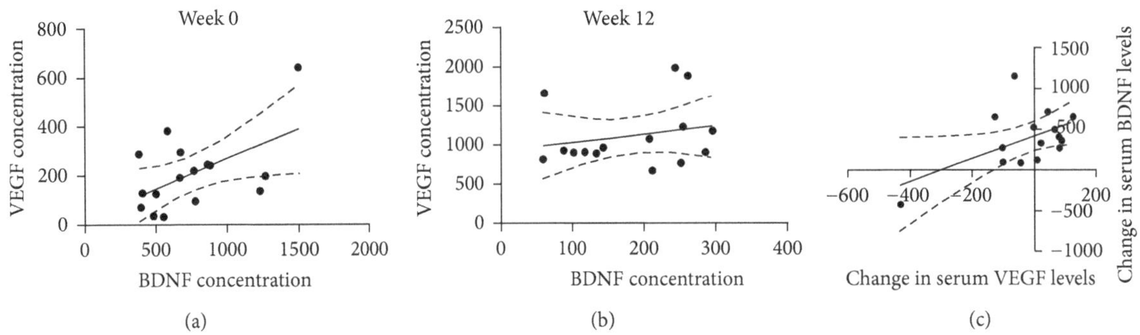

FIGURE 4: Relationship between BDNF and VEGF levels. Correlation analysis of serum BDNF and VEGF levels at separate time points reveals a significant relationship at week 0 (a) but not at week 12 (b). Further analysis found a significant correlation between the differences in BDNF and VEGF levels (c).

4. Discussion

This study has uncovered a correlative relationship between serum BDNF and VEGF levels in a drug-naive FEP sample. Each was differentially altered by twelve weeks of quetiapine treatment and was associated with specific measures of psychopathology. We believe this is the first study reporting on serum VEGF levels in first episode psychosis. The inverse relationship of serum BDNF levels with BPRS and PANSS general scores raises the possibility of its use in gauging effective antipsychotic treatment for patients in the absence of psychiatric evaluation. The study was limited by the relatively small number of enrolled subjects who had provided both baseline and Week 12 blood samples; however, a high attrition rate and loss to followup are widely acknowledged as two significant challenges facing studies of this nature. Week 12 blood samples from the healthy control group were unavailable so we cannot definitively conclude that our observations are solely attributable to quetiapine treatment. There was also an imbalance in the male/female numbers so we were unable to further examine the trend for males receiving the higher dose of quetiapine to have higher BDNF levels. Finally, full interpretation of our findings is hindered by the lack of knowledge regarding the function of BDNF and VEGF in peripheral circulation.

We found significantly raised BDNF levels following three months of treatment with quetiapine. Furthermore, no significant difference was found between Week 12 levels and controls suggesting that BDNF levels normalise with treatment. While there was no correlation between the absolute serum concentration and outcome measures at baseline or week 12, we found that the change in serum BDNF levels was positively correlated with specific reductions in BPRS and PANSS general psychopathology scores. No association was found with PANNS positive, negative, SANS, or UKU scores. It is known that negative symptoms take longer to respond to treatment so it is possible that with extended treatment beyond 12 weeks, changes in the other outcome measures could display a relationship with BDNF levels. This could be the focus of follow-up studies.

The few other studies that have attempted to correlate serum BDNF levels with outcome measures in FEP have had mixed results. In a study of 15 FEP subjects, a negative correlation between baseline BDNF levels and positive symptom scores was found but not with negative symptoms scores or any cognitive or motor function scores [42]. In two separate studies, Rizos et al., found negative correlations between baseline BDNF levels and both positive and negative symptom scores in 14 FEP subjects [48] and to the duration of untreated psychosis in 37 drug-naive FEP subjects [47]. Only one other published FEP study has correlated serum BDNF levels with outcome scores *after* treatment with antipsychotics. González-Pinto et al. (2010) found that serum BDNF levels were correlated to functional outcome and improved positive symptoms, though not to negative symptoms or general psychopathology in 11 olanzapine treated FEP subjects [44]. That study reported raised serum BDNF levels following treatment with antipsychotics, as have three other FEP studies (unspecified treatment [46]; aripiprazole [46]; risperidone, olanzapine, and aripiprazole [53]) which are consistent with the findings of this study. Amongst chronic cohorts, risperidone [47, 53], amisulpride [47], and haloperidol [47] did not raise BDNF levels, whilst clozapine [32, 68] and olanzapine [47] did. Collectively, there is some evidence that outcome measures are associated with serum BDNF levels, regardless of whether that relationship is direct or indirect; however, further studies involving larger cohorts of subjects and incorporating multiple antipsychotic drugs will be required before a more definitive conclusion can be reached.

Besides outcome measures, serum BDNF levels have been positively correlated with right hippocampal volumes in 20 drug-naive FEP subjects, with subjects having smaller hippocampi than controls [69]. There has been extensive research over the past decade examining the influence of the val66met single nucleotide polymorphism (SNP) of the BDNF gene [70] and its association with psychiatric conditions including schizophrenia, anorexia nervosa [71], and obsessive-compulsive disorder [72]. While young healthy carriers of the val66met polymorphism have smaller hippocampi, older healthy carriers do not, although this disparity could be due to an age-by-allele interaction since both BDNF expression and hippocampal volumes decrease with age [73]. Studies in schizophrenic subjects have reported mixed findings, one study finding smaller volumes with the met polymorphism [74], another smaller volumes with val homozygotes [75], and three finding no association [76–78]. A recent study in first-episode psychosis (FEP) patients found no difference in hippocampal volumes between healthy met controls and FEP met carriers but reduced volumes for FEP val homozygotes compared to healthy val controls. It would be interesting to probe our dataset for associations between BDNF, VEGF, and hippocampal volumes.

Beyond the hippocampus, others have found a relationship between the met polymorphism, temporal, and occipital lobe volume reductions and cognitive impairment [79], as well as reduced frontal lobe volumes in FEP met carriers compared to val homozygotes [80]. While the SNP has not been shown to influence response to treatment [81], it has been associated with an earlier age of onset of symptoms [82] and the development of tardive dyskinesia [3, 83]; though there have been negative findings [84, 85], the positive reports complementing the findings of lower serum BDNF levels amongst those with tardive dyskniesia [86, 87].

Though there was a trend for males on 400 mg of quetiapine to have higher BDNF levels at T12, no correlation was found between dose of quetiapine and BDNF levels. While this may have been due to low sample size or the fact that the doses were too similar (and doses in both groups were increased from week 4 to 12 according to clinical need), the only other FEP study to correlate antipsychotic dose with serum BDNF found no correlation with aripiprazole dose [49]. This accords with the aforementioned meta-analysis [54], though clozapine dose does correlate with serum BDNF in chronic schizophrenia [32, 68].

To our knowledge this is the first report that serum BDNF levels are increased by treatment with quetiapine in subjects with psychosis and complements the other positive findings of raised BDNF with atypical antipsychotic treatment and improvement in outcome scores following treatment. It also suggests a direct neurotrophic role for quetiapine via raising BDNF. Quetiapine has been shown to decrease the stress-induced reduction in BDNF expression in rat hippocampus [5], increase BDNF mRNA expression in rat hippocampus [88], and reverse the stress-induced suppression of rat hippocampal neurogenesis [89]. Taken together with our findings, these results suggest that quetiapine has a direct neurotrophic effect in schizophrenia, promoting neuroplasticity via the up-regulation of BDNF.

We also found that VEGF levels at baseline were significantly associated with BDNF levels, though this relationship was lost by Week 12. Nevertheless, the change in serum BDNF levels from Week 0 to Week 12 was associated with a change in serum VEGF levels. Furthermore, as with BDNF, the increase in serum VEGF positively correlated with a reduction in both BPRS and PANSS positive symptom scores. This is the first study to measure serum VEGF levels in psychosis and the findings are extremely novel. The correlation between increases in VEGF and BDNF and their similar impact on BPRS and general psychopathology scores suggests a direct neurotrophic role for VEGF, independent of secondary neurogenesis via brain angiogenesis. The findings also suggest that any direct neurotrophic effect quetiapine possesses maybe via several pathways including promoting BDNF and VEGF expression. Finally, it raises the possibility of gauging improvement of psychotic symptoms based by measuring changes in serum levels of BDNF and VEGF.

5. Conclusion

Our study investigated the peripheral levels of two key neurotrophic factors and report on their differential regulation by quetiapine treatment. Our results revealed an intriguing prospect that increases of serum BDNF levels might reflect the positive behavioural effects of antipsychotic treatment. Further research will be required to validate this as well as to examine if other antipsychotic agents similarly moderate VEGF levels.

Conflict of Interests

Drs. Terence Y. Pang, Anthony J. Hannan, Gregor E. Berger, and Colin O'Donnell and Mss. Tina-Marie Proffitt, Mirabel McConchie, Melissa Kerr, and Connie Markulev report no additional financial or other relationships relevant to the subject of this paper. There are no other conflict of interests.

Acknowledgments

This research was conducted with support from the Investigator-Sponsored Study Program of AstraZeneca. Dr. Brendan P. Murphy has received grant support from Sanofi and AstraZeneca and has received honoraria from AstraZeneca Janssen-Cilag, and Bristol-Myers Squibb. Dr. Patrick D. McGorry has been a consultant for and has received grant support from AstraZeneca, and has been a member of the advisory boards for AstraZeneca, Janssen, Pfizer, Eli Lilly, and Sanofi. This research was conducted with support from the Investigator-Sponsored Study Program of AstraZeneca. AstraZeneca reviewed the paper prior to publication, made no changes to the paper, and put no restrictions on any of our findings (study code 196691).

References

[1] K. H. Choi, B. W. Higgs, S. Weis et al., "Effects of typical and atypical antipsychotic drugs on gene expression profiles in the liver of schizophrenia subjects," *BMC Psychiatry*, vol. 9, artcile 57, 2009.

[2] M. W. Jann, "Implications for atypical antipsychotics in the treatment of schizophrenia: neurocognition effects and a neuroprotective hypothesis," *Pharmacotherapy*, vol. 24, no. 12 I, pp. 1759–1783, 2004.

[3] S. W. Park, J. G. Lee, B. G. Kong et al., "Genetic association of BDNF val66met and GSK-3β-50T/C polymorphisms with tardive dyskinesia: regular article," *Psychiatry and Clinical Neurosciences*, vol. 63, no. 4, pp. 433–439, 2009.

[4] M. D. Hammonds and S. S. Shim, "Effects of 4-week treatment with lithium and olanzapine on levels of brain-derived neurotrophic factor, B-Cell CLL/Lymphoma 2 and phosphorylated cyclic adenosine monophosphate response element-binding

protein in the sub-regions of the hippocampus," *Basic & Clinical Pharmacology & Toxicology*, vol. 105, no. 2, pp. 113–119, 2009.

[5] H. Xu, H. Qing, W. Lu et al., "Quetiapine attenuates the immobilization stress-induced decrease of brain-derived neurotrophic factor expression in rat hippocampus," *Neuroscience Letters*, vol. 321, no. 1-2, pp. 65–68, 2002.

[6] G. Favalli, J. Li, P. Belmonte-de-Abreu, A. H. C. Wong, and Z. J. Daskalakis, "The role of BDNF in the pathophysiology and treatment of schizophrenia," *Journal of Psychiatric Research*, vol. 46, no. 1, pp. 1–11, 2012.

[7] F. I. Tarazi, K. Zhang, and R. J. Baldessarini, "Long-term effects of olanzapine, risperidone, and quetiapine on dopamine receptor types in regions of rat brain: implications for antipsychotic drug treatment," *The Journal of Pharmacology and Experimental Therapeutics*, vol. 297, no. 2, pp. 711–717, 2001.

[8] A. Gonzalez-Pinto, E. Vieta, C. Reed et al., "Effectiveness of olanzapine monotherapy and olanzapine combination treatment in the long term following acute mania—results of a two year observational study in bipolar disorder (EMBLEM)," *Journal of Affective Disorders*, vol. 131, no. 1–3, pp. 320–329, 2011.

[9] M. Bibel and Y.-A. Barde, "Neurotrophins: key regulators of cell fate and cell shape in the vertebrate nervous system," *Genes & Development*, vol. 14, no. 23, pp. 2919–2937, 2000.

[10] L. Pezawas, B. A. Verchinski, V. S. Mattay et al., "The brain-derived neurotrophic factor val66met polymorphism and variation in human cortical morphology," *The Journal of Neuroscience*, vol. 24, no. 45, pp. 10099–10102, 2004.

[11] H. Thoenen, "Neurotrophins and activity-dependent plasticity," *Progress in Brain Research*, vol. 128, pp. 183–191, 2000.

[12] G. R. Lewin and Y.-A. Barde, "Physiology of the neurotrophins," *Annual Review of Neuroscience*, vol. 19, pp. 289–317, 1996.

[13] P. T. Pang, H. K. Teng, E. Zaitsev et al., "Cleavage of proBDNF by tPA/plasmin is essential for long-term hippocampal plasticity," *Science*, vol. 306, no. 5695, pp. 487–491, 2004.

[14] P. C. Ashe, M. D. Berry, and A. A. Boulton, "Schizophrenia, a neurodegenerative disorder with neurodevelopmental antecedents," *Progress in Neuro-Psychopharmacology & Biological Psychiatry*, vol. 25, no. 4, pp. 691–707, 2001.

[15] M. Malcangio and V. Lessmann, "A common thread for pain and memory synapses? Brain-derived neurotrophic factor and trkB receptors," *Trends in Pharmacological Sciences*, vol. 24, no. 3, pp. 116–121, 2003.

[16] J.-S. Mu, W.-P. Li, Z.-B. Yao, and X.-F. Zhou, "Deprivation of endogenous brain-derived neurotrophic factor results in impairment of spatial learning and memory in adult rats," *Brain Research*, vol. 835, no. 2, pp. 259–265, 1999.

[17] P. F. Buckley, S. Mahadik, A. Pillai, and A. Terry Jr., "Neurotrophins and schizophrenia," *Schizophrenia Research*, vol. 94, no. 1–3, pp. 1–11, 2007.

[18] R. S. Duman, G. R. Heninger, and E. J. Nestler, "A molecular and cellular theory of depression," *Archives of General Psychiatry*, vol. 54, no. 7, pp. 597–606, 1997.

[19] R. S. Duman, "Synaptic plasticity and mood disorders," *Molecular Psychiatry*, vol. 7, supplement 1, pp. S29–S34, 2002.

[20] G. Shoval and A. Weizman, "The possible role of neurotrophins in the pathogenesis and therapy of schizophrenia," *European Neuropsychopharmacology*, vol. 15, no. 3, pp. 319–329, 2005.

[21] O. Guillin, J. Diaz, P. Carroll, N. Griffon, J.-C. Schwartz, and P. Sokoloff, "BDNF controls dopamine D3 receptor expression and triggers behavioural sensitization," *Nature*, vol. 411, no. 6833, pp. 86–89, 2001.

[22] C. Anthony Altar, N. Cai, T. Bliven et al., "Anterograde transport of brain-derived neurotrophic factor and its role in the brain," *Nature*, vol. 389, no. 6653, pp. 856–860, 1997.

[23] T. Hashimoto, S. E. Bergen, Q. L. Nguyen et al., "Relationship of brain-derived neurotrophic factor and its receptor TrkB to altered inhibitory prefrontal circuitry in schizophrenia," *The Journal of Neuroscience*, vol. 25, no. 2, pp. 372–383, 2005.

[24] C. S. Weickert, T. M. Hyde, B. K. Lipska, M. M. Herman, D. R. Weinberger, and J. E. Kleinman, "Reduced brain-derived neurotrophic factor in prefrontal cortex of patients with schizophrenia," *Molecular Psychiatry*, vol. 8, no. 6, pp. 592–610, 2003.

[25] C. S. Weickert, D. L. Ligons, T. Romanczyk et al., "Reductions in neurotrophin receptor mRNAs in the prefrontal cortex of patients with schizophrenia," *Molecular Psychiatry*, vol. 10, no. 7, pp. 637–650, 2005.

[26] N. Durany, T. Michel, R. Zöchling et al., "Brain-derived neurotrophic factor and neurotrophin 3 in schizophrenic psychoses," *Schizophrenia Research*, vol. 52, no. 1-2, pp. 79–86, 2001.

[27] S. Iritani, K. Niizato, H. Nawa, K. Ikeda, and P. C. Emson, "Immunohistochemical study of brain-derived neurotrophic factor and its receptor, TrkB, in the hippocampal formation of schizophrenic brains," *Progress in Neuro-Psychopharmacology & Biological Psychiatry*, vol. 27, no. 5, pp. 801–807, 2003.

[28] M. Takahashi, O. Shirakawa, K. Toyooka et al., "Abnormal expression of brain-derived neurotrophic factor and its receptor in the corticolimbic system of schizophrenic patients," *Molecular Psychiatry*, vol. 5, no. 3, pp. 293–300, 2000.

[29] M. T. Ray, C. S. Weickert, E. Wyatt, and M. J. Webster, "Decreased BDNF, trkB-TK+ and GAD67 mRNA expression in the hippocampus of individuals with schizophrenia and mood disorders," *Journal of Psychiatry & Neuroscience*, vol. 36, no. 3, pp. 195–203, 2011.

[30] W. Pan, W. A. Banks, M. B. Fasold, J. Bluth, and A. J. Kastin, "Transport of brain-derived neurotrophic factor across the blood-brain barrier," *Neuropharmacology*, vol. 37, no. 12, pp. 1553–1561, 1998.

[31] F. Karege, M. Schwald, and M. Cisse, "Postnatal developmental profile of brain-derived neurotrophic factor in rat brain and platelets," *Neuroscience Letters*, vol. 328, no. 3, pp. 261–264, 2002.

[32] R. W. Grillo, G. L. Ottoni, R. Leke, D. O. Souza, L. V. Portela, and D. R. Lara, "Reduced serum BDNF levels in schizophrenic patients on clozapine or typical antipsychotics," *Journal of Psychiatric Research*, vol. 41, no. 1-2, pp. 31–35, 2007.

[33] Y. Ikeda, N. Yahata, I. Ito et al., "Low serum levels of brain-derived neurotrophic factor and epidermal growth factor in patients with chronic schizophrenia," *Schizophrenia Research*, vol. 101, no. 1–3, pp. 58–66, 2008.

[34] E. N. Rizos, A. Papadopoulou, E. Laskos et al., "Reduced serum BDNF levels in patients with chronic schizophrenic disorder in relapse, who were treated with typical or atypical antipsychotics," *World Journal of Biological Psychiatry*, vol. 11, no. 2, part 2, pp. 251–255, 2010.

[35] Y. L. Tan, D. F. Zhou, L. Y. Cao, Y. Z. Zou, and X. Y. Zhang, "Decreased BDNF in serum of patients with chronic schizophrenia on long-term treatment with antipsychotics," *Neuroscience Letters*, vol. 382, no. 1-2, pp. 27–32, 2005.

[36] K. Toyooka, K. Asama, Y. Watanabe et al., "Decreased levels of brain-derived neurotrophic factor in serum of chronic schizophrenic patients," *Psychiatry Research*, vol. 110, no. 3, pp. 249–257, 2002.

[37] M. H. Xiu, L. Hui, Y. F. Dang et al., "Decreased serum BDNF levels in chronic institutionalized schizophrenia on long-term treatment with typical and atypical antipsychotics," *Progress in Neuro-Psychopharmacology & Biological Psychiatry*, vol. 33, no. 8, pp. 1508–1512, 2009.

[38] X. Y. Zhang, Y. L. Tan, D. F. Zhou et al., "Serum BDNF levels and weight gain in schizophrenic patients on long-term treatment with antipsychotics," *Journal of Psychiatric Research*, vol. 41, no. 12, pp. 997–1004, 2007.

[39] C. S. Gama, A. C. Andreazza, M. Kunz, M. Berk, P. S. Belmonte-de-Abreu, and F. Kapczinski, "Serum levels of brain-derived neurotrophic factor in patients with schizophrenia and bipolar disorder," *Neuroscience Letters*, vol. 420, no. 1, pp. 45–48, 2007.

[40] Ş. Pirildar, A. S. Gönül, F. Taneli, and F. Akdeniz, "Low serum levels of brain-derived neurotrophic factor in patients with schizophrenia do not elevate after antipsychotic treatment," *Progress in Neuro-Psychopharmacology & Biological Psychiatry*, vol. 28, no. 4, pp. 709–713, 2004.

[41] H. J. Reis, R. Nicolato, I. G. Barbosa, P. H. T. D. Prado, M. A. Romano-Silva, and A. L. Teixeira, "Increased serum levels of brain-derived neurotrophic factor in chronic institutionalized patients with schizophrenia," *Neuroscience Letters*, vol. 439, no. 2, pp. 157–159, 2008.

[42] P. F. Buckley, A. Pillai, D. Evans, E. Stirewalt, and S. Mahadik, "Brain derived neurotropic factor in first-episode psychosis," *Schizophrenia Research*, vol. 91, no. 1–3, pp. 1–5, 2007.

[43] D. C. Chen, J. Wang, B. Wang et al., "Decreased levels of serum brain-derived neurotrophic factor in drug-naïve first-episode schizophrenia: relationship to clinical phenotypes," *Psychopharmacology*, vol. 207, no. 3, pp. 375–380, 2009.

[44] A. González-Pinto, F. Mosquera, A. Palomino et al., "Increase in brain-derived neurotrophic factor in first episode psychotic patients after treatment with atypical antipsychotics," *International Clinical Psychopharmacology*, vol. 25, no. 4, pp. 241–245, 2010.

[45] R. D. Jindal, A. K. Pillai, S. P. Mahadik, K. Eklund, D. M. Montrose, and M. S. Keshavan, "Decreased BDNF in patients with antipsychotic naïve first episode schizophrenia," *Schizophrenia Research*, vol. 119, no. 1–3, pp. 47–51, 2010.

[46] A. Palomino, A. Vallejo-Illarramendi, A. González-Pinto et al., "Decreased levels of plasma BDNF in first-episode schizophrenia and bipolar disorder patients," *Schizophrenia Research*, vol. 86, no. 1–3, pp. 321–322, 2006.

[47] E. N. Rizos, P. G. Michalopoulou, N. Siafakas et al., "Association of serum brain-derived neurotrophic factor and duration of untreated psychosis in first-episode patients with schizophrenia," *Neuropsychobiology*, vol. 62, no. 2, pp. 87–90, 2010.

[48] E. N. Rizos, I. Rontos, E. Laskos et al., "Investigation of serum BDNF levels in drug-naive patients with schizophrenia," *Progress in Neuro-Psychopharmacology & Biological Psychiatry*, vol. 32, no. 5, pp. 1308–1311, 2008.

[49] R. Yoshimura, H. Hori, A. Ikenouchi-Sugita et al., "Aripiprazole altered plasma levels of brain-derived neurotrophic factor and catecholamine metabolites in first-episode untreated Japanese schizophrenia patients," *Human Psychopharmacology*, vol. 27, no. 1, pp. 33–38, 2012.

[50] N. Goto, R. Yoshimura, S. Kakeda et al., "Comparison of brain N-acetylaspartate levels and serum brain-derived neurotrophic factor (BDNF) levels between patients with first-episode schizophrenia psychosis and healthy controls," *European Psychiatry*, vol. 26, no. 1, pp. 57–63, 2011.

[51] T.-L. Huang and C.-T. Lee, "Associations between serum brain-derived neurotrophic factor levels and clinical phenotypes in schizophrenia patients," *Journal of Psychiatric Research*, vol. 40, no. 7, pp. 664–668, 2006.

[52] E. Shimizu, K. Hashimoto, H. Watanabe et al., "Serum brain-derived neurotrophic factor (BDNF) levels in schizophrenia are indistinguishable from controls," *Neuroscience Letters*, vol. 351, no. 2, pp. 111–114, 2003.

[53] R. Yoshimura, H. Hori, A. Sugita et al., "Treatment with risperidone for 4 weeks increased plasma 3-methoxy-4-hydroxy-pnenylglycol (MHPG) levels, but did not alter plasma brain-derived neurotrophic factor (BDNF) levels in schizophrenic patients," *Progress in Neuro-Psychopharmacology & Biological Psychiatry*, vol. 31, no. 5, pp. 1072–1077, 2007.

[54] M. J. Green, S. L. Matheson, A. Shepherd, C. S. Weickert, and V. J. Carr, "Brain-derived neurotrophic factor levels in schizophrenia: a systematic review with meta-analysis," *Molecular Psychiatry*, vol. 16, no. 9, pp. 960–972, 2011.

[55] J. M. Rosenstein, J. M. Krum, and C. Ruhrberg, "VEGF in the nervous system," *Organogenesis*, vol. 6, no. 2, pp. 107–114, 2010.

[56] H. P. Blumberg, F. Wang, L. G. Chepenik et al., "Influence of vascular endothelial growth factor variation on human hippocampus morphology," *Biological Psychiatry*, vol. 64, no. 10, pp. 901–903, 2008.

[57] N. M. Fournier and R. S. Duman, "Role of vascular endothelial growth factor in adult hippocampal neurogenesis: implications for the pathophysiology and treatment of depression," *Behavioural Brain Research*, vol. 227, no. 2, pp. 440–449, 2012.

[58] S. Fulzele and A. Pillai, "Decreased VEGF mRNA expression in the dorsolateral prefrontal cortex of schizophrenia subjects," *Schizophrenia Research*, vol. 115, no. 2-3, pp. 372–373, 2009.

[59] A. Pillai and S. P. Mahadik, "Differential effects of haloperidol and olanzapine on levels of vascular endothelial growth factor and angiogenesis in rat hippocampus," *Schizophrenia Research*, vol. 87, no. 1–3, pp. 48–59, 2006.

[60] B. Misztal-Dethloff, H. Stepień, and J. Komorowski, "Effect of diazepam and chlorpromazine on proliferative activity and vascular endothelial growth factor (VEGF) secretion from cultured endothelial HECa10 cells in vitro," *Pharmacological Reports*, vol. 57, no. 5, pp. 670–674, 2005.

[61] M. Takebayashi, R. Hashimoto, K. Hisaoka, M. Tsuchioka, and H. Kunugi, "Plasma levels of vascular endothelial growth factor and fibroblast growth factor 2 in patients with major depressive disorders," *Journal of Neural Transmission*, vol. 117, no. 9, pp. 1119–1122, 2010.

[62] B.-H. Lee and Y.-K. Kim, "Increased plasma VEGF levels in major depressive or manic episodes in patients with mood disorders," *Journal of Affective Disorders*, vol. 136, no. 1-2, pp. 181–184, 2012.

[63] M. Ventriglia, R. Zanardini, L. Pedrini et al., "VEGF serum levels in depressed patients during SSRI antidepressant treatment," *Progress in Neuro-Psychopharmacology & Biological Psychiatry*, vol. 33, no. 1, pp. 146–149, 2009.

[64] A. Minelli, R. Zanardini, M. Abate, M. Bortolomasi, M. Gennarelli, and L. Bocchio-Chiavetto, "Vascular endothelial growth factor (VEGF) serum concentration during electroconvulsive therapy (ECT) in treatment resistant depressed patients," *Progress in Neuro-Psychopharmacology & Biological Psychiatry*, vol. 35, no. 5, pp. 1322–1325, 2011.

[65] G. E. Berger, T.-M. Proffitt, M. McConchie et al., "Dosing quetiapine in drug-naive first-episode psychosis: a controlled,

double-blind, randomized, single-center study investigating efficacy, tolerability, and safety of 200 mg/day vs. 400 mg/day of quetiapine fumarate in 141 patients aged 15 to 25 years," *The Journal of Clinical Psychiatry*, vol. 69, no. 11, pp. 1702–1714, 2008.

[66] E. Ozan, H. Okur, Ç. Eker, Ö. D. Eker, A. S. Gönül, and N. Akarsu, "The effect of depression, BDNF gene val66met polymorphism and gender on serum BDNF levels," *Brain Research Bulletin*, vol. 81, no. 1, pp. 61–65, 2010.

[67] P. D. McGorry, J. Edwards, C. Mihalopoulos, S. M. Harrigan, and H. J. Jackson, "EPPIC: an evolving system of early detection and optimal management," *Schizophrenia Bulletin*, vol. 22, no. 2, pp. 305–326, 1996.

[68] M. Pedrini, I. Chendo, I. Grande et al., "Serum brain-derived neurotrophic factor and clozapine daily dose in patients with schizophrenia: a positive correlation," *Neuroscience Letters*, vol. 491, no. 3, pp. 207–210, 2011.

[69] E. N. Rizos, M. Papathanasiou, P. G. Michalopoulou et al., "Association of serum BDNF levels with hippocampal volumes in first psychotic episode drug-naive schizophrenic patients," *Schizophrenia Research*, vol. 129, no. 2-3, pp. 201–204, 2011.

[70] M. Neves-Pereira, E. Mundo, P. Muglia, N. King, F. Macciardi, and J. L. Kennedy, "The brain-derived neurotrophic factor gene confers susceptibility to bipolar disorder: evidence from a family-based association study," *The American Journal of Human Genetics*, vol. 71, no. 3, pp. 651–655, 2002.

[71] M. Gratacòs, J. R. González, J. M. Mercader, R. de Cid, M. Urretavizcaya, and X. Estivill, "Brain-derived neurotrophic factor val66met and psychiatric disorders: meta-analysis of case-control studies confirm association to substance-related disorders, eating disorders, and schizophrenia," *Biological Psychiatry*, vol. 61, no. 7, pp. 911–922, 2007.

[72] D. Hall, A. Dhilla, A. Charalambous, J. A. Gogos, and M. Karayiorgou, "Sequence variants of the brain-derived neurotrophic factor (BDNF) gene are strongly associated with obsessive-compulsive disorder," *The American Journal of Human Genetics*, vol. 73, no. 2, pp. 370–376, 2003.

[73] G. N. Smith, A. E. Thornton, D. J. Lang et al., "Hippocampal volume and the brain-derived neurotrophic factor val66met polymorphism in first episode psychosis," *Schizophrenia Research*, vol. 134, no. 2-3, pp. 253–259, 2012.

[74] P. R. Szeszko, R. Lipsky, C. Mentschel et al., "Brain-derived neurotrophic factor val66met polymorphism and volume of the hippocampal formation," *Molecular Psychiatry*, vol. 10, no. 7, pp. 631–636, 2005.

[75] P. C. M. P. Koolschijn, N. E. M. van Haren, S. C. Bakker, M. L. C. Hoogendoorn, H. E. Hulshoff Pol, and R. S. Kahn, "Effects of brain-derived neurotrophic factor val66met polymorphism on hippocampal volume change in schizophrenia," *Hippocampus*, vol. 20, no. 9, pp. 1010–1017, 2010.

[76] I. Agartz, G. C. Sedvall, L. Terenius et al., "BDNF gene variants and brain morphology in schizophrenia," *The American Journal of Medical Genetics B*, vol. 141, no. 5, pp. 513–523, 2006.

[77] A. Dutt, C. McDonald, E. Dempster et al., "The effect of COMT, BDNF, 5-HTT, NRG1 and DTNBP1 genes on hippocampal and lateral ventricular volume in psychosis," *Psychological Medicine*, vol. 39, no. 11, pp. 1783–1797, 2009.

[78] T. Takahashi, M. Suzuki, M. Tsunoda et al., "Association between the brain-derived neurotrophic factor val66met polymorphism and brain morphology in a Japanese sample of schizophrenia and healthy comparisons," *Neuroscience Letters*, vol. 435, no. 1, pp. 34–39, 2008.

[79] B.-C. Ho, P. Milev, D. S. O'Leary, A. Librant, N. C. Andreasen, and T. H. Wassink, "Cognitive and magnetic resonance imaging brain morphometric correlates of brain-derived neurotrophic factor val66met gene polymorphism in patients with schizophrenia and healthy volunteers," *Archives of General Psychiatry*, vol. 63, no. 7, pp. 731–740, 2006.

[80] B.-C. Ho, N. C. Andreasen, J. D. Dawson, and T. H. Wassink, "Association between brain-derived neurotrophic factor val66met gene polymorphism and progressive brain volume changes in schizophrenia," *The American Journal of Psychiatry*, vol. 164, no. 12, pp. 1890–1899, 2007.

[81] S. Anttila, A. Illi, O. Kampman, K. M. Mattila, T. Lehtimäki, and E. Leinonen, "Lack of association between two polymorphisms of brain-derived neurotrophic factor and response to typical neuroleptics," *Journal of Neural Transmission*, vol. 112, no. 7, pp. 885–890, 2005.

[82] H. M. Chao, H.-T. Kao, and B. Porton, "BDNF val66met variant and age of onset in schizophrenia," *The American Journal of Medical Genetics B*, vol. 147, no. 4, pp. 505–506, 2008.

[83] Y.-J. Liou, D.-L. Liao, J.-Y. Chen et al., "Association analysis of the dopamine D3 receptor gene ser9gly and brain-derived neurotrophic factor gene val66met polymorphisms with antipsychotic-induced persistent tardive dyskinesia and clinical expression in Chinese schizophrenic patients," *NeuroMolecular Medicine*, vol. 5, no. 3, pp. 243–251, 2004.

[84] S.-G. Kang, J.-E. Choi, H. An et al., "No association between the brain-derived neurotrophic factor gene val66met polymorphism and tardive dyskinesia in schizophrenic patients," *Progress in Neuro-Psychopharmacology & Biological Psychiatry*, vol. 32, no. 6, pp. 1545–1548, 2008.

[85] Y. Wang, J. D. Wang, H. R. Wu et al., "The val66met polymorphism of the brain-derived neurotrophic factor gene is not associated with risk for schizophrenia and tardive dyskinesia in Han Chinese population," *Schizophrenia Research*, vol. 120, no. 1-3, pp. 240–242, 2010.

[86] Y. L. Tan, D. F. Zhou, and X. Y. Zhang, "Decreased plasma brain-derived neurotrophic factor levels in schizophrenic patients with tardive dyskinesia: association with dyskinetic movements," *Schizophrenia Research*, vol. 74, no. 2-3, pp. 263–270, 2005.

[87] Y. Q. Yang, S. Sun, Y. Q. Yu et al., "Decreased serum brain-derived neurotrophic factor levels in schizophrenic patients with tardive dyskinesia," *Neuroscience Letters*, vol. 502, no. 1, pp. 37–40, 2011.

[88] F. Fumagalli, R. Molteni, F. Bedogni et al., "Quetiapine regulates FGF-2 and BDNF expression in the hippocampus of animals treated with MK-801," *NeuroReport*, vol. 15, no. 13, pp. 2109–2112, 2004.

[89] C. Luo, H. Xu, and X.-M. Li, "Quetiapine reverses the suppression of hippocampal neurogenesis caused by repeated restraint stress," *Brain Research*, vol. 1063, no. 1, pp. 32–39, 2005.

7

The Impact of Childhood Adversity on the Clinical Features of Schizophrenia

Ravi Philip Rajkumar

Department of Psychiatry, Jawaharlal Institute of Postgraduate Medical Education and Research (JIPMER), Pondicherry 605 006, India

Correspondence should be addressed to Ravi Philip Rajkumar; ravi.psych@gmail.com

Academic Editor: Brian Kirkpatrick

Introduction. Recent research has drawn attention to the link between childhood maltreatment and schizophrenia. Child abuse and neglect may have an impact on symptoms and physical health in these patients. This association has not been studied to date in India. *Materials and Methods.* Clinically stable patients with schizophrenia ($n = 62$) were assessed for childhood adversity using the Childhood Trauma Questionnaire. The association of specific forms of adversity with symptomatology and associated variables was examined. *Results.* Emotional abuse was reported by 56.5% patients and physical abuse by 33.9%; scores for childhood neglect were also high. Persecutory delusions were linked to physical abuse, while anxiety was linked to emotional neglect and depression to emotional abuse and childhood neglect. Physical abuse was linked to elevated systolic blood pressure, while emotional abuse and neglect in women were linked to being overweight. *Conclusions.* Childhood adversity is common in schizophrenia and appears to be associated with a specific symptom profile. Certain components of the metabolic syndrome also appear to be related to childhood adversity. These results are subject to certain limitations as they are derived from remitted patients, and no control group was used for measures of childhood adversity.

1. Introduction

In the past two decades, a growing body of research has called attention to the association between childhood adversity and psychotic disorders, particularly schizophrenia [1]. Patients with psychotic disorders have high rates of self-reported childhood abuse and neglect, ranging from 30% to over 75% [2–4]. This has led some authors to speculate that, in at least some cases of schizophrenia, childhood traumatic events play a causal role by affecting brain development, a "traumagenic neurodevelopmental model" [5]. Other researchers have focused on the role of specific types of childhood trauma, such as physical, emotional, or sexual abuse, in the development of specific symptoms such as auditory hallucinations [6–8] or delusions [8–10]. Along similar lines, preliminary evidence suggests that childhood abuse may be associated with positive psychotic symptoms, while neglect correlates more strongly with negative symptoms [11]. In addition to its effect on psychotic symptoms, childhood adversity may also be associated with components of the metabolic syndrome, such as dyslipidemia and elevated blood pressure, in patients with schizophrenia [12].

Despite the above evidence, the relationship between childhood adversity and schizophrenia is neither simple nor linear. Childhood adversity is neither necessary nor sufficient to cause schizophrenia [13], and a critical review of the association between childhood trauma and psychosis found only tentative evidence of a positive relationship, largely due to methodological problems with individual studies [14]. Moreover, childhood adversity is common both in other psychiatric disorders [15, 16] and in the general population [17], ruling out a one-to-one causal relationship. It is likely that childhood adversity may be associated with particular groups of symptoms, rather than with a categorical diagnosis such as schizophrenia [16], and that the association between childhood adversity and psychosis may be mediated by several factors. These include genetic variants [18, 19], the abuse of substances such as cannabis [20], ethnicity [21], gender [22], stressful life events in adulthood [23], and other environmental risk factors, such as urbanicity [24].

Most of the evidence linking childhood trauma and schizophrenia has been derived from studies in Western cultures. The impact of adversities during childhood in Eastern cultures, where parenting practices and social structures differ significantly from the West, may be different; however, there is preliminary evidence that rates of childhood trauma are elevated in Turkish [25] and Korean [26] patients with schizophrenia. To date, no study has examined the relationship between specific forms of childhood adversity and symptoms or symptom dimensions in schizophrenia in such a cultural setting.

In the current study, we examine the impact of different forms of childhood adversity—both abuse and neglect—on the clinical presentation of adult South Indian patients with a diagnosis of schizophrenia.

2. Materials and Methods

We screened all consecutive patients with a DSM-IV-TR diagnosis of schizophrenia who were being followed up at the out-patient unit of a general hospital psychiatry service in Pondicherry, South India. Of these patients, only those who had been stable on antipsychotic medication for the past six months, with no recent exacerbation of symptoms and with no psychiatric comorbidity, were included. Of the 139 patients screened, 62 fulfilled these criteria. Of the 77 patients excluded, seventy-four had experienced a psychotic episode in the six months prior to assessment. Further three were excluded due to a comorbid Axis I diagnosis, obsessive-compulsive disorder in two patients and social anxiety disorder in one. All patients provided written informed consent.

Information about the onset, duration, diagnostic subtype, symptom profile, and number of episodes of illness, as well as any medical or substance use comorbidity, was obtained from patients' medical records and was confirmed by interviewing patients and their accompanying caregivers. Systolic and diastolic blood pressure and height and weight were recorded during the interview, and the Body Mass Index (BMI) was calculated from this information.

Patients were assessed for the presence of various forms of childhood adversity using the Childhood Trauma Questionnaire (CTQ), a 28-item self-report instrument [27] which has been widely used to assess childhood trauma in patients with psychosis [4, 7, 8] and for which a Tamil adaptation is available [28]. Each item on the CTQ is scored from 1 to 5, and besides a total score, the instrument provides specific subscores for physical, emotional, and sexual abuse and for physical and emotional neglect.

Residual psychopathology was assessed using the Positive and Negative Syndrome Scale for Schizophrenia (PANSS) [28], and current depressive symptoms were assessed using the Calgary Depression Scale for Schizophrenia (CDSS) [29]. Patients' current level of functioning in various domains was assessed using the Functioning Assessment Short Test (FAST) [30] and the DSM-IV Global Assessment of Functioning (GAF) Scale [31].

Associations between the presence or absence of particular symptoms or illness variables and the CTQ total and subscores were assessed using the independent samples t-test or the Mann-Whitney U test, depending on the distribution of data. Correlations between the CTQ total and subscale scores and measures of psychopathology and functioning were examined using Pearson's r or Spearman's *rho*, again depending on the data distribution. All tests were two-tailed, and a value of $p < 0.05$ was considered significant.

3. Results

3.1. General Description of the Study Sample. The sample consisted of 62 patients, 31 men and 31 women. The mean age of the study subjects was 35.3 ± 8.5 years (range 19–54 years) and did not vary significantly by sex. 27 patients were single, 24 were currently married, 10 were divorced or separated from their spouses, and one was widowed; male patients were significantly more likely than women to be single ($\chi^2 = 10.57$, $p = 0.014$). Patients had received an average of 9.9 ± 4.3 years of formal education (range 0–18 years), with no significant gender difference. Seventeen patients were unemployed, fourteen (all women) were homemakers, and the remainder were employed as skilled or unskilled labourers or farmers.

Description of the sample's clinical characteristics is provided in Table 1. Male and female patients were comparable in terms of PANSS symptom scores, CDSS-rated depression, and current levels of functioning and impairment. Male patients had higher rates of comorbid substance dependence, particularly nicotine ($\chi^2 = 4.77$, $p = 0.029$), while female patients had a higher mean Body Mass Index ($t = 2.184$, $p = 0.033$).

3.2. Childhood Adversities Reported by Patients. The mean CTQ total and subscale scores are presented in Table 1. The highest scores were noted on the subscales for emotional neglect, followed by physical neglect and emotional abuse; scores on the physical and sexual abuse subscale scores were low. Overall, emotional abuse was reported by 35 (56.5%) patients, physical abuse by 21 (33.9%) patients, and sexual abuse by two (3.2%). Neither these categorical rates nor any of the CTQ subscores were significantly different across the sexes. We did not attempt a similar description of emotional or physical neglect, as almost all patients endorsed at least one item pertaining to these categories; besides, unlike sexual or physical abuse, neglect is difficult to categorize as a yes/no phenomenon. CTQ total and subscale scores did not differ according to place of childhood residence (rural or urban) or marital status and were not significantly correlated with total years of education.

3.3. Relationship between CTQ Scores and Clinical Course and Outcome. There was no difference in CTQ scores between patients with an acute onset of schizophrenia and those with an insidious onset; however, the CTQ Physical Abuse subscore was significantly higher in those patients ($n = 53$) whose illness was not triggered by a life event or stressor (Mann-Whitney $U = 144.0$, $p = 0.025$). Age at onset, total duration of illness, illness course, and duration of untreated psychosis were not correlated with any of the CTQ

TABLE 1: Clinical description of the sample by gender.

Variable	Male patients (n = 31)	Female patients (n = 31)	Total
Age at onset, years	24.9 ± 7.4	26.6 ± 7.9	25.8 ± 7.6
Duration of illness, years	10.8 ± 8.6	8.3 ± 7.2	9.6 ± 7.9
Duration of untreated illness, years	1.4 ± 1.8	1.5 ± 1.5	1.5 ± 1.7
Diagnostic subtype			
Paranoid	22	22	44
Undifferentiated	7	5	12
Catatonic	2	2	4
Disorganized	—	2	2
Body mass index, kg/m^2	23.2 ± 4.2	25.9 ± 5.4	24.5 ± 4.9*
Blood pressure, mmHg			
Systolic	118.3 ± 10.3	115.1 ± 12.4	116.7 ± 11.4
Diastolic	80.9 ± 10.2	77.5 ± 10.2	79.2 ± 10.2
Lifetime substance use disorder			
Total	10	3	13*
Nicotine dependence	10	3	13*
Alcohol abuse/dependence	2	0	2
Lifetime suicide attempt	9	8	17
Lifetime violent suicide attempt	5	4	9
CTQ scores			
Emotional abuse	7.9 ± 3.9	8.0 ± 3.3	8.0 ± 3.6
Physical abuse	6.4 ± 2.9	5.7 ± 1.9	6.1 ± 2.4
Sexual abuse	5.0 ± 0.2	5.1 ± 0.4	5.0 ± 0.3
Emotional neglect	11.6 ± 3.5	11.5 ± 3.3	11.5 ± 3.4
Physical neglect	9.3 ± 2.7	9.6 ± 3.3	9.5 ± 3.0
Total	40.4 ± 10.4	39.9 ± 10.1	40.1 ± 10.2
PANSS scores			
Positive	8.9 ± 2.2	8.9 ± 2.1	8.9 ± 2.2
Negative	15.4 ± 6.4	15.5 ± 6.3	15.5 ± 6.3
General psychopathology	24.5 ± 6.6	26.6 ± 7.5	25.6 ± 7.1
Total	48.8 ± 13.7	51.0 ± 14.4	49.9 ± 14.0
CDSS score, total	1.3 ± 2.3	1.5 ± 2.7	1.4 ± 2.5
FAST score			
Autonomy	2.9 ± 2.6	3.8 ± 2.8	3.4 ± 2.7
Occupational activity	7.2 ± 4.8	7.7 ± 4.6	7.4 ± 4.7
Cognitive functioning	4.6 ± 3.0	5.2 ± 3.0	4.9 ± 3.0
Finances	1.8 ± 1.6	1.9 ± 1.8	1.9 ± 1.7
Interpersonal relationships	7.0 ± 4.9	8.6 ± 5.5	7.8 ± 5.2
Leisure	1.9 ± 1.6	2.5 ± 1.7	2.2 ± 1.6
Total	25.4 ± 16.7	29.6 ± 17.4	27.5 ± 17.0
GAF score	61.7 ± 11.5	58.9 ± 11.6	60.2 ± 11.5

PANSS: Positive and Negative Symptom Scale for Schizophrenia; CDSS: Calgary Depression Scale for Schizophrenia; CTQ: Childhood Trauma Questionnaire; FAST: Functional Assessment Short Test; GAF: Global Assessment of Functioning.
*Difference is significant at $p < 0.05$.

scores. CTQ scores did not differ according to the course of the illness (episodic versus continuous), and CTQ scores in remitted patients did not differ from those who had significant residual symptoms; these findings held true for both men and women. There was no significant relationship between the GAF or FAST scores and any of the CTQ scores, and this remained true even after controlling for sex.

3.4. Relationship between CTQ Scores and Symptomatology. The PANSS positive, negative, general psychopathology, and total scores did not correlate significantly with the CTQ total or subscale scores; this association remained negative in both men and women. When the presence or absence of individual symptoms was used as a grouping variables, the CTQ Physical Abuse subscore was significantly associated with lifetime delusions ($t = 2.89$, $p < 0.01$), and more specifically with delusions having a persecutory theme ($t = 2.81$, $p < 0.01$). The presence of auditory hallucinations, disorganization, catatonic symptoms, and first-rank schizophrenic symptoms was not associated with a significant difference in any CTQ scores. Similarly, the presence or absence of individual negative symptoms—affective flattening, asociality, alogia, attentional impairment, and anhedonia—was not associated with CTQ abuse, neglect, or total scores. However, when we examined only the 31 patients with significant negative symptoms and a diagnosis of residual schizophrenia, the CTQ Physical Neglect subscore was positively correlated with the PANSS negative symptom score (Pearson's $r = 0.364$, $p = 0.048$). When categorical definitions of physical, emotional, and sexual abuse were used in the analysis, no specific psychotic symptom or PANSS score was specifically associated with any individual form of abuse.

3.5. Relationship between CTQ Scores and Other Illness Variables. The total CTQ score was associated with lifetime suicide attempts in male patients, but not in women ($t = 2.11$, $p = 0.043$); similarly, the CTQ Physical Neglect score was associated with violent suicide attempts, but only in men ($t = 2.47$, $p = 0.02$). Lifetime substance use disorders were not associated with elevated CTQ scores irrespective of gender.

The PANSS anxiety scale score was significantly correlated with the CTQ Emotional Neglect subscore (Spearman's $\rho = 0.253$, $p = 0.049$), and this remained significant even after correcting for gender. The PANSS depression score was positively correlated with the CTQ Emotional Neglect ($\rho = 0.278$, $p = 0.03$), Physical Neglect ($\rho = 0.271$, $p = 0.035$), and total ($\rho = 0.27$, $p = 0.036$) scores. Similarly, the CDSS total score was positively correlated with the CTQ Emotional Abuse, Emotional Neglect, Physical Neglect, and total scores ($p < 0.01$ for all correlations except Physical Neglect, $p = 0.022$), and mean CDSS scores were significantly higher in those with lifetime emotional abuse ($t = -2.44$, $p = 0.018$).

Systolic and diastolic blood pressures were not correlated with CTQ scores in either men or women. However, the CTQ Emotional Abuse subscore was positively correlated with patients' Body Mass Index (BMI) (Pearson's $r = 0.335$, $p < 0.01$). When using a cut-off value of 25 kg/m^2 for the BMI, patients whose BMI was above 25 had significantly higher total CTQ scores ($t = 2.84$, $p < 0.01$) and higher subscores for emotional abuse ($t = 3.15$, $p < 0.01$), emotional neglect ($t = 2.53$, $p = 0.014$), and physical neglect ($t = 2.23$, $p = 0.03$); an analysis of covariance revealed that this association was not mediated by exposure to atypical antipsychotics ($F = 0.05$, $p =$ NS); however, there was a significant effect of gender, with differences remaining significant in female, but not in male patients. Mean systolic blood pressure was higher in those reporting lifetime physical abuse (mean 120.86 mmHg versus 114.53 mmHg in those without physical abuse; $t = 2.12$, $p = 0.038$).

4. Discussion

The rates of physical and emotional abuse reported by our patients are comparable to those reported in the literature [2, 3]; however, rates of reported sexual abuse are much lower. While this may represent a genuine difference, it is far more likely to reflect underreporting on the part of patients. This is probably due to the cultural taboos and stigma that surround child sexual abuse in the Indian context [32], as a survey conducted by the Government of India suggested that up to 42% of a sample of 2211 children had experienced some form of sexual abuse [33]; moreover, higher rates of childhood sexual abuse in patients with psychosis are well-documented in other settings [34, 35]. Measures of the different types of abuse and neglect did not differ according to gender; this is in accordance with a recent meta-analysis which found that the various forms of childhood maltreatment, except for sexual abuse, were equally common in male and female patients with schizophrenia [2].

The onset of schizophrenia was slightly more likely to be spontaneous, that is, to occur in the absence of an obvious proximal stressor, in those with higher scores on the Physical Abuse subscale. This is consistent with the hypothesis that childhood physical abuse represents a form of "social defeat" which can itself predispose to psychosis, by causing cognitive changes and/or altered dopamine transmission [36]. The latter alteration may involve a gene/environment ($G \times E$) interaction in which genetic variants which affect frontal dopamine levels interact with physical abuse to increase the likelihood of developing psychotic symptoms [18]. Though we did not find a relationship between outcome measures and childhood adversity in our sample, this result is unlikely to be significant as our patients were already selected for relative clinical and functional stability.

Among the different types of psychotic symptoms reported by patients, only delusions—particularly those with a persecutory theme—were significantly associated with physical abuse. This result is consistent with work indicating that child victims of physical abuse are likely to experience impaired reality testing [37] and that physical abuse can lead to the development of paranoid ideation [38] or a paranoid personality [39]. Similarly, a study of patients with schizophrenia has also reported an association between physical abuse and positive psychotic symptoms such as delusions [10]. Variables that may mediate this association include variants of the catechol-O-methyltransferase gene [18], anxiety [38], and negative beliefs about the self or others [38, 40]. We could not replicate the often-reported association between childhood sexual abuse and auditory hallucinations [6–8, 21], most probably because of the under-reporting of sexual abuse in our sample. We found some evidence of an association between negative symptoms and physical neglect, as suggested by earlier literature [11], but this result must be interpreted with caution as it was derived from a subgroup analysis.

Besides delusions, childhood adversity was associated with a range of other nonpsychotic symptomatology, depression, anxiety, and suicidal behavior. The latter association was more marked in men, while the others remained true irrespective of gender. Further, similar associations were obtained regardless of which depression measure—the ordinal PANSS depression score or continuous CDSS total score—was used. In other words, there was good concurrent validity for the association between depression and childhood adversity—particularly childhood neglect—in patients with schizophrenia. This is consistent with the results of the Genetic Risk and Outcome of Psychosis (GROUP) investigators, who suggest that childhood trauma is linked to a cluster of symptoms—depression, anxiety, and positive psychotic symptoms—which transcends existing diagnostic categories or groups [16, 41]. An association between childhood abuse and suicide risk in schizophrenia has been reported in earlier studies [3, 10], though our finding that male gender may mediate this association requires further exploration.

Finally, we found evidence of an association between specific forms of abuse and components of the metabolic syndrome. First, physical abuse was linked to elevated systolic blood pressure. The latter relationship has already been observed in patients with schizophrenia [12] and is unlikely to be an artefact of the interview conditions, as blood pressure was measured before any enquiries were made about childhood trauma. Second, female patients who were overweight reported significantly more emotional abuse and neglect during childhood. A link between childhood maltreatment and obesity has been demonstrated in the general population [42] and in patients with mood disorders [43] and has been shown to be mediated by gender [44]. However, this association has not been examined so far in schizophrenia. In our patients, this finding could not be explained by antipsychotic exposure and is likely to involve both biological and psychological mechanisms [45, 46].

Our results are subject to certain limitations. First, the sample size was small compared to similar work in other populations. Second, we relied on a single self-report measure of childhood adversity, which may have resulted in an underreporting of the scope of this problem. Third, owing to the small number of patients in each group, we may have underestimated the associations between specific psychotic symptoms and childhood adversity. Fourth, as some of the information was collected retrospectively, it is subject to recall bias. Fifth, our sample included only clinically stable patients. While this might have led to a loss of information, it was necessitated by the strictures of the institute's Ethics Committee against administering the potentially stressful CTQ to acutely ill, unstable patients. Sixth, we excluded a small number of patients with comorbid diagnoses, in order to clearly delineate the relationship between childhood adversity and schizophrenia alone; however, these patients did not differ significantly from the rest of the sample in terms of CTQ scores. Finally, due to the preliminary and exploratory nature of our work, our study lacked a control group, and we are therefore unable to comment on whether the patients in our sample experienced higher levels of abuse and neglect than appropriately matched controls from the same population. It is hoped that the latter deficit, which is admittedly the greatest shortcoming of our study, will be addressed by a continuation of our work which is currently in progress and involves the recruitment of a control sample.

5. Conclusion

In spite of these shortcomings, our results replicate many of the positive findings in the schizophrenia literature on the impact of childhood adversity. They are consistent with the view that childhood maltreatment, despite not being necessary to cause schizophrenia, can have a significant impact on symptomatology. To our knowledge, this report is the first study from India to explore the association between childhood adversity and schizophrenia. From a clinical perspective, our findings highlight the need to actively enquire about childhood maltreatment in patients with schizophrenia, particularly those who are overweight or who present with symptoms of anxiety or depression even after improvement in positive psychotic symptoms.

Conflict of Interests

The author declares that there is no conflict of interests regarding the publication of this paper.

References

[1] J. Read, J. van Os, A. P. Morrison, and C. A. Ross, "Childhood trauma, psychosis and schizophrenia: a literature review with theoretical and clinical implications," *Acta Psychiatrica Scandinavica*, vol. 112, no. 5, pp. 330–350, 2005.

[2] I. Bonoldi, E. Simeone, M. Rocchetti et al., "Prevalence of self-reported childhood abuse in psychosis: a meta-analysis of retrospective studies," *Psychiatry Research*, vol. 210, no. 1, pp. 8–15, 2013.

[3] S. Shah, A. Mackinnon, C. Galletly et al., "Prevalence and impact of childhood abuse in people with a psychotic illness. Data from the second Australian national survey of psychosis," *Schizophrenia Research*, vol. 159, no. 1, pp. 20–26, 2014.

[4] M. Duhing, S. Patterson, M. Connell et al., "The prevalence and correlates of childhood trauma in patients with early psychosis," *Australian & New Zealand Journal of Psychiatry*, vol. 49, no. 7, pp. 651–659, 2015.

[5] J. Read, B. D. Perry, A. Moskowitz, and J. Connolly, "The contribution of early traumatic events to schizophrenia in some patients: a traumagenic neurodevelopmental model," *Psychiatry*, vol. 64, no. 4, pp. 319–345, 2001.

[6] K. Daalman, K. M. J. Diederen, E. M. Derks, R. van Lutterveld, R. S. Kahn, and I. E. C. Sommer, "Childhood trauma and auditory verbal hallucinations," *Psychological Medicine*, vol. 42, no. 12, pp. 2475–2484, 2012.

[7] J. M. Sheffield, L. E. Williams, J. U. Blackford, and S. Heckers, "Childhood sexual abuse increases risk of auditory hallucinations in psychotic disorders," *Comprehensive Psychiatry*, vol. 54, no. 7, pp. 1098–1104, 2013.

[8] A. Üçok and S. Bikmaz, "The effects of childhood trauma in patients with first-episode schizophrenia," *Acta Psychiatrica Scandinavica*, vol. 116, no. 5, pp. 371–377, 2007.

[9] J. Read, K. Agar, N. Argyle, and V. Aderhold, "Sexual and physical abuse during childhood and adulthood as predictors of hallucinations, delusions and thought disorder," *Psychology and Psychotherapy: Theory, Research and Practice*, vol. 76, no. 1, pp. 1–22, 2003.

[10] L. S. Schenkel, W. D. Spaulding, D. DiLillo, and S. M. Silverstein, "Histories of childhood maltreatment in schizophrenia: relationships with premorbid functioning, symptomatology, and cognitive deficits," *Schizophrenia Research*, vol. 76, no. 2-3, pp. 273–286, 2005.

[11] B. J. Gallagher III and B. J. Jones, "Childhood stressors and symptoms of schizophrenia," *Clinical Schizophrenia and Related Psychoses*, vol. 7, no. 3, pp. 124–130, 2013.

[12] B. Misiak, A. Kiejna, and D. Frydecka, "The history of childhood trauma is associated with lipid disturbances and blood pressure in adult first-episode schizophrenia patients," *General Hospital Psychiatry*, vol. 37, no. 4, pp. 365–367, 2015.

[13] L. Sideli, A. Mulé, D. La Barbera, and R. M. Murray, "Do child abuse and maltreatment increase risk of schizophrenia?" *Psychiatry Investigation*, vol. 9, no. 2, pp. 87–99, 2012.

[14] S. Bendall, H. J. Jackson, C. A. Hulbert, and P. D. McGorry, "Childhood trauma and psychotic disorders: a systematic, critical review of the evidence," *Schizophrenia Bulletin*, vol. 34, no. 3, pp. 568–579, 2008.

[15] I. A. Rubino, R. C. Nanni, D. M. Pozzi, and A. Siracusano, "Early adverse experiences in schizophrenia and unipolar depression," *Journal of Nervous and Mental Disease*, vol. 197, no. 1, pp. 65–68, 2009.

[16] M. van Nierop, W. Viechtbauer, N. Gunther et al., "Childhood trauma is associated with a specific admixture of affective, anxiety, and psychosis symptoms cutting across traditional diagnostic boundaries," *Psychological Medicine*, vol. 45, no. 6, pp. 1277–1288, 2015.

[17] G. R. Chiu, K. E. Lutfey, H. J. Litman, C. L. Link, S. A. Hall, and J. B. McKinlay, "Prevalence and overlap of childhood and adult physical, sexual, and emotional abuse: a descriptive analysis of results from the boston area community health (BACH) survey," *Violence and Victims*, vol. 28, no. 3, pp. 381–402, 2013.

[18] M. J. Green, T.-Y. Chia, M. J. Cairns et al., "Catechol-O-methyltransferase (COMT) genotype moderates the effects of childhood trauma on cognition and symptoms in schizophrenia," *Journal of Psychiatric Research*, vol. 49, no. 1, pp. 43–50, 2014.

[19] M. Aas, U. K. Haukvik, S. Djurovic et al., "BDNF val66met modulates the association between childhood trauma, cognitive and brain abnormalities in psychoses," *Progress in Neuro-Psychopharmacology and Biological Psychiatry*, vol. 46, pp. 181–188, 2013.

[20] S. Alemany, B. Arias, M. Fatjó-Vilas et al., "Psychosis-inducing effects of cannabis are related to both childhood abuse and COMT genotypes," *Acta Psychiatrica Scandinavica*, vol. 129, no. 1, pp. 54–62, 2014.

[21] A. O. Berg, M. Aas, S. Larsson et al., "Childhood trauma mediates the association between ethnic minority status and more severe hallucinations in psychotic disorder," *Psychological Medicine*, vol. 45, no. 1, pp. 133–142, 2015.

[22] H. Fisher, C. Morgan, P. Dazzan et al., "Gender differences in the association between childhood abuse and psychosis," *British Journal of Psychiatry*, vol. 194, no. 4, pp. 319–325, 2009.

[23] R. van Winkel, N. C. Stefanis, and I. Myin-Germeys, "Psychosocial stress and psychosis. A review of the neurobiological mechanisms and the evidence for gene-stress interaction," *Schizophrenia Bulletin*, vol. 34, no. 6, pp. 1095–1105, 2008.

[24] A. Frissen, R. Lieverse, M. Drukker et al., "Childhood trauma and childhood urbanicity in relation to psychotic disorder," *Social Psychiatry and Psychiatric Epidemiology*, 2015.

[25] S. Şahin, Ç. Yüksel, J. Güler et al., "The history of childhood trauma among individuals with ultra high risk for psychosis is as common as among patients with first-episode schizophrenia," *Early Intervention in Psychiatry*, vol. 7, no. 4, pp. 414–420, 2013.

[26] D. Kim, H. Bae, C. Han, H. Y. Oh, and K. MacDonald, "Psychometric properties of the Childhood Trauma Questionnaire-Short Form (CTQ-SF) in Korean patients with schizophrenia," *Schizophrenia Research*, vol. 144, no. 1–3, pp. 93–98, 2013.

[27] D. P. Bernstein, L. Fink, L. Handelsman et al., "Initial reliability and validity of a new retrospective measure of child abuse and neglect," *The American Journal of Psychiatry*, vol. 151, no. 8, pp. 1132–1136, 1994.

[28] S. R. Kay, A. Fiszbein, and L. A. Opler, "The positive and negative syndrome scale (PANSS) for schizophrenia," *Schizophrenia Bulletin*, vol. 13, no. 2, pp. 261–276, 1987.

[29] D. Addington, J. Addington, and E. Maticka-Tyndale, "Assessing depression in schizophrenia: the Calgary depression scale," *British Journal of Psychiatry*, vol. 163, no. 22, pp. S39–S44, 1993.

[30] A. R. Rosa, J. Sánchez-Moreno, A. Martínez-Aran et al., "Validity and reliability of the Functioning Assessment Short Test (FAST) in bipolar disorder," *Clinical Practice and Epidemiology in Mental Health*, vol. 3, article 5, 2007.

[31] American Psychiatric Association, *Diagnostic and Statistical Manual of Mental Disorders*, American Psychiatric Association, Washington, DC, USA, 4th edition, 1994.

[32] R. K. J. Karthiga and R. Ravikumar, "Child sexual abuse in Madurai, India: a literary review and empirical study," *Journal of Child Sexual Abuse*, vol. 23, no. 6, pp. 727–744, 2014.

[33] L. Kacker, S. Varadan, and P. Kumar, *Study on Child Abuse: India*, Ministry of Women and Child Development, Government of India, New Delhi, India, 2007.

[34] P. Bebbington, S. Jonas, E. Kuipers et al., "Childhood sexual abuse and psychosis: data from a cross-sectional national psychiatric survey in England," *The British Journal of Psychiatry*, vol. 199, no. 1, pp. 29–37, 2011.

[35] P. Bebbington, "Unravelling psychosis: psychosocial epidemiology, mechanism, and meaning," *Shanghai Archives of Psychiatry*, vol. 27, pp. 70–81, 2015.

[36] J.-P. Selten, E. van der ven, B. P. F. Rutten, and E. Cantor-Graae, "The social defeat hypothesis of schizophrenia: an update," *Schizophrenia Bulletin*, vol. 39, no. 6, pp. 1180–1186, 2013.

[37] M. G. Haviland, J. L. Sonne, and L. R. Woods, "Beyond posttraumatic stress disorder: object relations and reality testing disturbances in physically and sexually abused adolescents," *Journal of the American Academy of Child and Adolescent Psychiatry*, vol. 34, no. 8, pp. 1054–1059, 1995.

[38] H. L. Fisher, E. Appiah-Kusi, and C. Grant, "Anxiety and negative self-schemas mediate the association between childhood maltreatment and paranoia," *Psychiatry Research*, vol. 196, no. 2-3, pp. 323–324, 2012.

[39] L. M. Bierer, R. Yehuda, J. Schmeidler et al., "Abuse and neglect in childhood: relationship to personality disorder diagnosis," *CNS Spectrums*, vol. 8, no. 10, pp. 737–749, 2003.

[40] C. Bortolon, D. Capdevielle, J.-P. Boulenger, M.-C. Gely-Nargeot, and S. Raffard, "Early maladaptive schemas predict positive symptomatology in schizophrenia: a cross-sectional study," *Psychiatry Research*, vol. 209, no. 3, pp. 361–366, 2013.

[41] E. Ruby, K. Rothman, C. Corcoran, R. R. Goetz, and D. Malaspina, "Influence of early trauma on features of schizophrenia," *Early Intervention in Psychiatry*, 2015.

[42] K. Peltzer, S. Pengpid, T. A. Samuels et al., "Prevalence of overweight/obesity and its associated factors among university students from 22 countries," *International Journal of Environmental Research and Public Health*, vol. 11, no. 7, pp. 7425–7441, 2014.

[43] R. S. McIntyre, J. K. Soczynska, S. S. Liauw et al., "The association between childhood adversity and components of metabolic syndrome in adults with mood disorders: results from the international mood disorders collaborative project," *International Journal of Psychiatry in Medicine*, vol. 43, no. 2, pp. 165–177, 2012.

[44] E. Fuller-Thomson, D. A. Sinclair, and S. Brennenstuhl, "Carrying the pain of abuse: gender-specific findings on the relationship between childhood physical abuse and obesity in adulthood," *Obesity Facts*, vol. 6, no. 4, pp. 325–336, 2013.

[45] M. O. Min, S. Minnes, H. Kim, and L. T. Singer, "Pathways linking childhood maltreatment and adult physical health," *Child Abuse and Neglect*, vol. 37, no. 6, pp. 361–373, 2013.

[46] B. R. Keeshin, P. F. Cronholm, and J. R. Strawn, "Physiologic changes associated with violence and abuse exposure: an examination of related medical conditions," *Trauma, Violence, and Abuse*, vol. 13, no. 1, pp. 41–56, 2012.

8

Twenty Years of Schizophrenia Research in the Northern Finland Birth Cohort 1966: A Systematic Review

Erika Jääskeläinen,[1,2,3] Marianne Haapea,[2,3,4] Nina Rautio,[1,2,5] Pauliina Juola,[2,3,4] Matti Penttilä,[2,3,4] Tanja Nordström,[1,2] Ina Rissanen,[1,2,3] Anja Husa,[2,3,4] Emmi Keskinen,[1,2,3] Riikka Marttila,[1,2,3] Svetlana Filatova,[1,2,3,4] Tiina-Mari Paaso,[1,2] Jenni Koivukangas,[3,6] Kristiina Moilanen,[2,3,4] Matti Isohanni,[3,4] and Jouko Miettunen[1,2,3,4]

[1] *Center for Life Course Epidemiology and Systems Medicine, University of Oulu, P.O. Box 5000, 90014 Oulu, Finland*
[2] *Medical Research Center Oulu, Oulu University Hospital and University of Oulu, P.O. Box 5000, 90014 Oulu, Finland*
[3] *Department of Psychiatry, Center for Clinical Neurosciences, University of Oulu, P.O. Box 5000, 90014 Oulu, Finland*
[4] *Department of Psychiatry, Oulu University Hospital, P.O. Box 26, 90029 Oulu, Finland*
[5] *Unit of Primary Health Care, Oulu University Hospital, P.O. Box 10, 90029 Oulu, Finland*
[6] *Aurora Doctoral Programme, Thule Institute, University of Oulu, P.O. Box 7300, Oulu, Finland*

Correspondence should be addressed to Erika Jääskeläinen; erika.jaaskelainen@oulu.fi

Academic Editor: Hugo Schnack

Birth cohort designs are useful in studying adult disease trajectories and outcomes, such as schizophrenia. We review the schizophrenia research performed in the Northern Finland Birth Cohort 1966 (NFBC 1966), which includes 10,934 individuals living in Finland at 16 years of age who have been monitored since each mother's mid-pregnancy. By the age of 44, 150 (1.4%) had developed schizophrenia. There are 77 original papers on schizophrenia published from the NFBC 1966. The early studies have found various risk factors for schizophrenia, especially related to pregnancy and perinatal phase. Psychiatric and somatic outcomes were heterogeneous, but relatively poor. Mortality in schizophrenia is high, especially due to suicides. Several early predictors of outcomes have also been found. Individuals with schizophrenia have alterations in brain morphometry and neurocognition, and our latest studies have found that the use of high lifetime doses of antipsychotics associated with these changes. The schizophrenia research in the NFBC 1966 has been especially active for 20 years, the prospective study design and long follow-up enabling several clinically and epidemiologically important findings. When compared to other birth cohorts, the research in the NFBC 1966 has offered also unique findings on course and outcome of schizophrenia.

1. Introduction

Birth cohort studies were originally designed to study early health outcomes, but as the earliest birth cohorts started in the 1940s to the 1960s have matured, adult outcomes have also been studied [1]. Welham and colleagues [1] reviewed birth cohort studies on antecedents of schizophrenia, finding 11 birth cohorts from seven countries. The authors concluded that birth cohort studies have provided important insights into how the premorbid developmental trajectory of individuals who develop schizophrenia differs from their peers.

The Northern Finland Birth Cohort 1966 (NFBC 1966) is a birth cohort which has been studied extensively with almost 1000 peer-review publications in various fields of medicine (http://www.oulu.fi/nfbc). The NFBC 1966 was collected during the mid-1960s by paediatrician and Professor of Public Health Paula Rantakallio, the first aim being to analyze perinatal health [2]. In the 1980s, adolescent health and, in the 1990s, adult somatic and psychiatric disorders emerged as the main foci. Schizophrenia research in the NFBC 1966 has been especially active, with the first studies performed in the mid-1990s. The first studies focused on early risk factors, but later on clinical and social outcomes, neurocognition, brain morphometry, somatic illnesses, and genetics have also been studied.

In this paper, we systematically review the schizophrenia research performed in the NFBC 1966.

2. Methods

2.1. Literature Search. The literature search was completed in PubMed in September 2014. The keywords included "Northern Finland Birth Cohort" and words related to schizophrenia (including schizotypy and psychotic disorders). Additionally, we manually searched for articles from the extensive publication list maintained by the NFBC 1966 (http://www.oulu.fi/nfbc). We found 77 original articles related to schizophrenia. In addition, previous reviews from the NFBC 1966 were utilized in this review.

2.2. Sample. The sample was drawn from the NFBC 1966, which is based on 12,068 pregnant women and their 12,058 live-born babies in two northernmost Finnish provinces (Oulu and Lapland), with an expected date of birth during 1966 [2]. The live-births in this study represent 96% of all births in the region. The information has been collected during pregnancy, delivery, childhood, and the follow-up periods at adulthood. The schizophrenia studies are based on 10,934 cohort members who lived in Finland in 1982. The original articles of this literature review are largely based on three data collections: the 31-year follow-up of the cohort members alive in 1997, and two smaller psychiatric follow-up studies. Register data and earlier collected data of the NFBC 1966 have also been utilized in the studies. The overall study design has been approved and is under the review of the Ethical Committee of the Northern Ostrobothnia Hospital District.

The 31-year follow-up of the whole cohort was conducted in 1997. Comprehensive data on somatic and mental health and the use of health services and medications as well as socioeconomic status were collected using a postal questionnaire ($N = 8{,}297$). A clinical examination of the cohort members living in Northern Finland or Helsinki area included, for instance, a blood sample draw, which has been utilized in genetic studies ($N = 5{,}960$). Additional questionnaires including, for example, schizotypal traits, were also filled in ($N = 5{,}084$) [41].

The 34-year follow-up for psychoses was conducted in 1999–2001. Cohort members with a psychotic episode by the end of the year 1997 (cases) were detected using the Finnish Hospital Discharge Register (FHDR), currently known as Care Register for Health Care. The control subjects were selected randomly from the cohort members without a psychotic episode, living in the region of Oulu. The 34-year follow-up consisted of structural magnetic resonance imaging (MRI) of the brain (GE Signa 1.5T scanner), measures of cognitive functioning, psychiatric interviews, and questions related to, for example, the use of antipsychotic medication, social background, and substance use. In the 34-year follow-up, 91 cases with a psychotic disorder (61 with schizophrenia) and 104 controls participated and provided written informed consent [42, 43].

The 43-year follow-up for psychoses was conducted in 2008–2010. In addition to those with regard to whom a psychosis had been detected during the 34-year follow-up, those who had developed a psychosis between the years 1998 and 2008 according to the nationwide registers or self-report were invited to participate. The new control subjects were selected randomly from all the cohort members. The procedure was extended from the 34-year follow-up with functional MRI and more measures of cognitive functioning. Out of the eligible subjects, 107 cases with a psychotic disorder (54 with schizophrenia) and 194 controls participated and provided written informed consent. Of the participants, 54 cases with a psychotic disorder (40 with schizophrenia) and 76 controls participated, both at ages 34 and 43 [44].

2.3. Diagnostics. The diagnoses of the participants of the 34-year follow-up were validated in accordance with DSM-III-R [45, 46]. New cases with schizophrenia and other psychoses have been included in the later studies: these cases are detected continuously from several nationwide registers. Due to the more comprehensive set of registers, the later studies include more outpatients than the previous studies.

3. Risk Factors

The first schizophrenia studies in the NFBC 1966 focused on risk factors. The main results of the studies are presented in Table 1. Twenty original studies and also some reviews (e.g., [47]) concerning the various risk factors of schizophrenia have been published. These risk factors can be divided into risks during pregnancy and birth, childhood, and adolescence and later premorbid factors.

The most essential risk factors identified in the latest NFBC 1966 review [47] were male gender, parental psychosis, unwanted pregnancy, perinatal brain damage, low birth weight, late age at learning to stand and walk, not being potty-trained by the age of one, central nervous system infections by the age of 14 years, and not attending normal school grade.

Later, other risk factors have also been found, such as severe injuries [19] and both high and low birth length and weight [5, 10]. New aspects of the studies were to link parental psychosis and known risk factors [5, 22, 24] and to study their interactions. It has been found, for instance, that the presence of early biological risk factors increased the risk of schizophrenia only among those with parental psychosis [5] and that low birth weight and length increased the risk only among those without parental psychosis, whereas high birth weight and length did so only among those with parental psychosis [5].

In each stage of human development, there are risk factors influencing the occurrence of schizophrenia. It is important to identify the risk and create awareness among health professionals and decision makers to develop and implement preventive strategies, though it should be noted that most of the effect sizes detected are small or medium level. In schizophrenia risk studies in general, the risk factors with highest quality evidence have shown medium effect sizes [48].

TABLE 1: Risk factors of schizophrenia in the Northern Finland Birth Cohort 1966.

Risk factors	Risk estimates
	Pregnancy and birth
Male gender	Risk of schizophrenia OR 1.8 (95% CI 1.1–3.0) [3, 4]
Parental psychosis	Risk of schizophrenia HR 2.8 (95% CI 1.7–4.5) [5]
Maternal antenatal depression	Nonsignificant risk of schizophrenia RR 1.5 (95% CI 0.9–2.4) [6]
Unwantedness of a pregnancy	Risk of schizophrenia OR 2.4 (95% CI 1.2–4.8) [7]
High paternal social class at birth (females)	Risk of schizophrenia RR 2.4 (95% CI 1.2–4.9) [8]
Perinatal brain damage	Risk of schizophrenia OR 4.6 (95% CI 1.7–12.1) [3, 9]
Deviant intrauterine growth	Increased risk of schizophrenia for both low (OR 2.5; 95% CI 1.2–5.1) and high (OR 2.4; 95% CI 1.1–4.9) birth weight and for both low (OR 2.6; 95% CI 1.1–5.9) and high (OR 1.8; 95% CI 1.0–3.5) birth length [5, 9, 10]
Birth order	Risk of schizophrenia among male first-borns (observed-expected ratio 1.5; 95% CI 1.0–2.2) and nonsignificant risk among female last-borns (1.3; 95% CI 0.9–1.9) [11]
Grand multiparity, six or more	Nonsignificant risk of schizophrenia OR 1.1 (95% CI 0.6–2.1), significant risk of other psychosis OR 2.3 (95% CI 1.2–4.7) [12]
	Childhood and adolescence
Use of vitamin D supplementation, at least 2000 IU	Decreased risk of schizophrenia RR range: 0.08–0.23 [13]
Markers of development in childhood	Risk of schizophrenia, later age of learning to stand (RR 1.5; 95% CI 1.0–2.2) and walk (RR 1.3; 95% CI 1.0–1.6) [14]
Family type (single-parent versus two-parent) at birth to 14 years	No significant differences [15]
Viral central nervous system infection before age 14	Risk of schizophrenia OR 4.8 (95% CI 1.6–14.0) [3, 16]
Intelligence Quotient (IQ) <85 up to the age of 14 years	Risk of schizophrenia OR 4.8 (95% CI 2.2–10.3) [3]
Excellent school performance age 16 years (males)	Risk of schizophrenia OR 3.8 (95% CI 1.6–9.3) [17]
Lower school marks and below normal class age 16 years	Lower school marks associated with risk for nonpsychotic disorders, but not for schizophrenia or other psychoses. Below normal class associated with schizophrenia risk in boys OR 2.8 (95% CI 1.5–5.7) [18].
	Other premorbid factors
Severe injuries (e.g., fractures) before onset of psychosis	Risk of psychotic disorder, having a fracture HR 2.9 (95% CI 1.4–6.0) [19]
Seasonality	Rate of first admission for schizophrenia lower in spring compared to other seasons [20]
Paternal age	No significant risk by paternal age categories [21]
	Interaction studies
Parental psychosis and maternal antenatal depression	Risk of schizophrenia highest in the offspring with both maternal depressed mood during pregnancy and parental psychosis (OR 9.4; 95% CI 4.2–20.9) [22]
Parental psychosis and early risk factors	Risk for schizophrenia highest among those with parental psychosis and biological risk factor: parental psychosis and high birth weight HR 7.9 (95% CI 1.8–34.8), parental psychosis and high birth length HR 4.3 (95% CI 1.1–16.2), parental psychosis and any biological risk HR 3.6 (95% CI 1.3–10.3), and parental psychosis and high maternal education HR 0.2 (95% CI 0.1–0.9) [5]

TABLE 1: Continued.

Risk factors	Risk estimates
	Associations between risk factors
Motor performance at age 1 and school performance at age 16	Age of learning to stand associated with school mark of physical education in schizophrenia but not in controls [23]
Parental psychosis and advanced paternal age	Maternal schizophrenia associated with higher advanced paternal age [24]

OR = odds ratio, CI = confidence interval, HR = hazard ratio, RR = risk ratio, and IU = international unit.

TABLE 2: Predictors of poor outcomes in schizophrenia in the Northern Finland Birth Cohort 1966.

Definition of poor outcome	Predictor of poor outcome
	Poor clinical outcomes
(i) More hospitalizations, rehospitalization after first episode [25–30]	Family history of psychosis Sociodemographic factors: father's high social class Childhood development: earlier age of learning to stand or walk Illness-related factors: insidious mode of illness onset, suicidal ideations at first episode, short first hospitalization, long DUP in short-term, and short DUP in long-term Brain morphology: reduced density of the left limbic area
(ii) More symptoms, lack of remission [27, 29, 31, 32]	Adolescence factors: smoking at age 14 years, poorer school performance at high school Illness-related factors: earlier age at onset, poor work adjustment at illness onset, single at illness onset, psychosocial stressor before illness onset, and more symptoms at first episode Temperament traits: lower reward dependence and persistence Brain morphology: decreased white matter volume
(iii) Treatment resistance [33]	Higher birth length and weight
	Poor social outcomes
(i) Poor occupational functioning (ii) Disability pension (iii) Low score on SOFAS [25, 29, 32, 34, 35]	Childhood and adolescence factors: lack of friends at childhood, poorer school performance at high school Illness-related factors: earlier age of illness onset, single at illness onset Temperament traits: lower persistence and higher harm avoidance Brain morphology: reduced density of the grey matter in left frontal lobe and left limbic area

DUP = duration of untreated psychosis, SOFAS = Social and Occupational Functioning Assessment Scale.

4. Course of Illness and Outcomes

4.1. Course of Illness and Outcomes. In the NFBC 1966 on average of ten years from the onset of illness, the outcomes were heterogeneous, but relatively poor [25, 49]. A total of 81% of subjects with schizophrenic psychoses needed rehospitalization [26]. Adult educational level was significantly lower in subjects with schizophrenia, compared to the controls [50].

At the age of 34, outcomes were heterogeneous and varied largely, depending on the measures of outcomes. More than half (56%) of the individuals with schizophrenia were on disability pension [34], whereas 21% were in symptomatic remission, with only 3.4% having recovered [25, 49]. These numbers are somewhat smaller than the average rate of recovery (13.5%) worldwide, based on a meta-analysis [51].

4.2. Predictors of Outcomes. There are several relevant predictors of outcomes, but especially factors related to illness onset are significant to course of illness. Statistically significant predictors of poor outcomes are presented in Table 2. Many of these factors are not modifiable, but some could possibly be affected by means of early interventions, for example, duration of untreated psychosis (DUP) [52]. One of the most important factors associated with poor outcome in schizophrenia is the early age of illness onset [27], and in the future it is necessary to further study ways to delay the onset of psychosis [53].

Clinical and functional course of illness associates also with biological markers: earlier motor development at age one [28] and morphological abnormalities in several brain areas at age 34 [29] associated with poor outcomes. The difference in early development and brain morphology in good and poor outcomes may reflect separable aetiologies and developmental trajectories in schizophrenia.

5. Brain Morphometry

5.1. Differences between Individuals with Schizophrenia and Controls. Differences between subjects with schizophrenia and controls in brain volumes and densities in several brain regions were found at the 34-year follow-up. Subjects with schizophrenia showed 2-3% lower whole brain, grey matter (GM), and white matter (WM) volumes and 7% higher cerebrospinal fluid volume when compared to controls [54]. Subjects with schizophrenia showed reduced density of GM in several brain regions, for example, frontal, temporal, parietal, and occipital regions at the 34-year follow-up. WM deficits in inter- and intrahemispheric tracts were also found in these lobes. Increased GM density was found, for example, in basal ganglia [55].

The volume of hippocampus was reduced in individuals with schizophrenia or any psychosis when compared to the controls, but the difference was explained by the total brain volume reduction. In the amygdala, significant volume differences between individuals with schizophrenia and controls were not found [56].

5.2. Predictors of Brain Morphometry. At age 34, associations between GM and WM densities and earlier onset age (i.e., longer duration of illness) were found [55]. One study also detected that longer DUP associated with lower GM density of the right limbic area [57]. Earlier infant motor development associated with greater density of GM in, for example, premotor cortex and WM in frontal and parietal lobes in control group, but these associations were not significant in schizophrenia [58].

Between 34 and 43 years of age, Veijola et al. [37] found the rate of annual brain volume reduction to be greater in the schizophrenia group (0.69%) than in the controls (0.49%). The greatest volume loss in schizophrenia occurred in the temporal lobe and periventricular area. The high amount of antipsychotic medication predicted excessive brain volume loss.

6. Cognition

Neurocognitive performance, longitudinal change in cognition, and their associations with infant motor developmental markers, brain volume change, and antipsychotic medication have all been studied in the NFBC 1966 in schizophrenia in comparison with nonpsychotic controls.

6.1. Developmental Markers and Cognition. Delayed infant motor development was associated with poorer adult cognition in schizophrenia at the age of 34 years in executive functions, verbal learning, and visuospatial working memory, but not in visual learning [59]. Earlier motor development, better adult executive functions, and higher grey matter density in frontocerebellar systems were associated with each other in controls, but there was a disruption of these normative associations in schizophrenia at 34 years [58].

Age of learning to stand in infancy significantly inversely predicted later deterioration of executive functions with memory in adult schizophrenia between 34 and 43 years of age [60]. This connection between delayed infant development and greater cognitive decline in adulthood may possibly suggest a link between abnormal neurodevelopmental and neurodegenerative processes in schizophrenia [60].

6.2. Longitudinal Change of Cognitive Performance. Global cognitive functioning as well as performance in domains of executive functions, working memory, and visual and verbal memory were lower in subjects with schizophrenia in comparison to control subjects cross-sectionally, both at the age of 34 [37, 38, 58–60] and 43 [37, 38, 60]. No significantly greater decrease in overall cognition [37] or in verbal learning [61], visual learning, or executive functions without memory component [60] was observed during midlife in schizophrenia, compared to the controls. All in all, change of cognition in schizophrenia followed mostly normative age-related decline [61]. The only exception for this pattern was the significant deterioration of executive functions with the memory component in cases compared to controls [60]. The results of mostly no deterioration extend the findings of other studies that have shown no decline in cognition around illness onset and first episode [62] also to later stages of illness in schizophrenia.

6.3. Antipsychotic Medication and Cognition. Higher lifetime antipsychotic medication exposure was associated with poorer verbal learning and memory performance at the age of 34 and greater decline in verbal learning and memory between the ages of 34 and 43 years [38]. Although antipsychotic exposure also predicted brain volume reduction in schizophrenia during that time, this volume reduction was not associated with a decrease in overall cognition or specific cognitive processes [37], so the associations between antipsychotic medication, cognition, and longitudinal brain changes seem complex in schizophrenia.

7. Somatic Illnesses, Mortality, and Criminality

7.1. Smoking and Somatic Illnesses. In the NFBC 1966, the proportion of smokers was about 50% among people with schizophrenia and the initiation of regular smoking was closely associated with the onset of the disorder [63]. Riala et al. [64] found poor premorbid school performance to associate with later cigarette smoking among schizophrenia patients. People with psychotic disorders have increased weight gain [65] and individuals with schizophrenia had almost a 4-fold risk of metabolic syndrome by the age of 31 [66]. The prevalence of metabolic syndrome among individuals with schizophrenia varied between 19 and 29%, depending on the measurement criteria [66, 67], and 45% had insulin resistance [68]. Total cholesterol and triglyceride levels were higher in schizophrenia compared to the controls [69], especially among those who used antipsychotic medication [40]. Also, higher triglyceride levels have been found among people with early-onset (less than 20 years of age) of schizophrenia [70]. These results imply that regular monitoring and active treatment of metabolic abnormalities are important already at a relatively young age in schizophrenia.

In addition, in the NFBC 1966, schizophrenia has been associated strongly with epilepsy by the age of 28 years, neurological diseases in general, and inflammatory bowel diseases [71], but rheumatoid arthritis and appendicitis were not more common than in the general population [72].

7.2. Mortality and Suicidality. In the NFBC 1966, the overall mortality rate among subjects with schizophrenia was 14%

TABLE 3: Factors associated with the use of antipsychotic medication in the Northern Finland Birth Cohort 1966.

Factors	Effect of higher use of antipsychotic medication
Sex	Females used more often medication [36]
Age at onset of psychosis	No association [36]
Psychiatric hospital treatment	Increased need of hospital treatment [36]
Clinical measures (PANSS, CGI, SOFAS, and remission)	Poorer clinical and social outcome [36]
Occupational functioning	Higher rate of disability pensions and lower rate of employment [36]
Brain volume loss	Increased brain loss [37]
Change of cognition	Decline of verbal learning and memory [38]
Suicidal ideation	No association when symptoms of depression and anxiety were controlled for [39]
Hyperlipidemia	Increased risk of hyperlipidemia [40]

PANSS = Positive and Negative Syndrome Scale, CGI = Clinical Global Impression, and SOFAS = Social and Occupational Functioning Assessment Scale.

before the age of 27 years, with half of the deaths being suicides [73]. The suicide rate among people with schizophrenia before the age of 39 was 7% with 71% of suicides occurring during the first three years after the onset of illness [74]. Good school performance at the age of 16 years increased the risk of suicide in schizophrenia and other psychoses but decreased risk of suicide in the healthy controls [75]. A history of attempted and committed suicides associated with specific genetic traits among schizophrenic males [76], and the use of antipsychotic medication increased the risk of suicidal ideation among people with schizophrenia, but this association disappeared when adjusted for the severity of depression and anxiety symptoms [39].

7.3. Criminality and Violent Behavior. Those with psychotic disorders exhibited higher risks of criminal behavior [77], and increased risk for violent behavior was associated with schizophrenia and coexisting alcohol abuse [78] or with alcohol-induced psychoses [77]. Men with schizophrenia with comorbid alcohol abuse were also more likely to repeat the violent crimes [78]. However, also men with schizophrenia without alcohol abuse were more likely to commit violent crimes, but none of the women with schizophrenia had committed any crimes in the NFBC 1966 by the age of 26 [78].

8. Antipsychotic Medication

8.1. Use of Antipsychotic Medication. In the NFBC 1966, the associations between the use of antipsychotic medication and related factors have been extensively studied [36–40]. The predictors and consequences of the use of antipsychotic medication in schizophrenia are described in detail in Table 3. Of the predictors studied, only female gender was found to be a significant predictor of the use of antipsychotic medication.

8.2. Antipsychotic Medication and Outcome. The use of antipsychotic medication predicted an overall poorer outcome; for example, subjects using antipsychotics needed more hospital treatment, had poorer clinical and social outcomes, and were more often unemployed or on disability pension [36]. The subjects using antipsychotic medication had increased risk of hyperlipidemia compared to subjects not using antipsychotics [40]. Use of antipsychotic medication associated with increased suicidal ideation and symptoms of depression and anxiety [39].

8.3. Antipsychotic Medication, Brain Morphometry, and Cognition. Higher cumulative antipsychotic medication exposure (chlorpromazine equivalent dose-years) over the 9-year follow-up between the two brain scans was associated with brain volume reduction [37] and higher cumulative lifetime antipsychotic medication exposure associated with poorer performance and decline in verbal learning and memory in midlife in schizophrenia [38]. These associations remained statistically significant even after controlling for illness severity. Schizophrenia subjects with high antipsychotic doses declined more than the controls in some verbal learning and memory measures, whereas cognitive change in subjects with low doses did not differ from the controls [38]. The annual reduction in brain volume was significantly predicted by exposure to atypical antipsychotics but not typical antipsychotics [37], but higher exposure to both typical and atypical antipsychotics by the age of 34 associated with poorer verbal learning and memory [38].

9. Schizotypal Traits and Genetic Research

9.1. Schizotypal Traits as a Marker of Schizophrenia Risk. Schizophrenia is a highly heritable disease. Recently, the Schizophrenia Working Group of the Psychiatric Genomics Consortium [79] identified 128 independent associations spanning 108 conservatively defined loci that met genome-wide significance. The consortium also included data from the NFBC 1966. The genetic studies utilizing only the NFBC 1966 data have focused on schizotypal traits as an indication of schizophrenia risk. The schizotypal traits in the NFBC 1966 were assessed in a large (almost 5,000 individuals) follow-up at the age of 31, with the Wisconsin schizotypy scales (Social Anhedonia Scale, Physical Anhedonia Scale, and Perceptual Aberration Scale) and the Hypomanic Personality Scale.

The cohort studies have focused on psychometric properties on these scales and differences in the traits by gender and education [80]. Men reported higher anhedonia, whereas women had higher scores in hypomanic personality and perceptual aberration. Participants with a lower level of education scored higher in all scales [80]. Of the various traits, perceptual aberration and hypomanic personality associated most strongly with psychosis diagnoses in the 11-year follow-up [81], whereas physical anhedonia separated depression from other psychiatric disorders [82]. Many of the early-life risk factors linked to schizophrenia also associated with schizotypal traits, including, for instance, lower birth weight and gestational age [83].

9.2. Genes Associated with Schizophrenia and Schizotypal Traits. The genetic studies in the NFBC 1966 have focused especially on DISC1 (disrupted-in-schizophrenia 1), finding associations between DISC1 and social anhedonia [84]. The authors later reanalyzed the genome-wide association data and found several genes with biological relevance to mental illnesses through loci displaying suggestive evidence for association [85]. Bader et al. [86] found CRMP1 (collapsin-response mediator protein 1) locus to associate with social and physical anhedonia, suggesting the potential role of CRMP1 expression as a blood-based diagnostic marker. The NFBC 1966 data have also been used in a study that found a positive correlation between neuropeptide precursor VGF single-nucleotide polymorphisms and social anhedonia [87]. It has also been investigated as to whether large copy number variant deletions [88] or Chromosome 22q deletions [89] associate with various neurodevelopmental phenotypes. In these studies, no associations were found with regard to psychotic disorders.

10. Discussion

10.1. Main Results. The NFBC 1966 has been especially active for 20 years. The prospective study design and long follow-up have enabled several clinically and epidemiologically important findings. The early studies in the NFBC 1966 focused on risk factors for schizophrenia. Various risk factors have been found, related to, for example, family history of psychosis, adverse events during pregnancy and delivery, and delays in early developmental milestones. Psychiatric course of illness and outcomes are heterogeneous and unfortunately relatively poor. There are several predictors for outcomes, one of the most important being early age of illness onset. Some of the predictors of outcomes may be modified, such as substance use and duration of untreated psychosis.

There are differences between subjects with schizophrenia and controls in brain volume and densities in several brain areas. Global cognitive functioning and performance in various cognitive domains were worse in schizophrenia than in the controls cross-sectionally, but longitudinally cognition mostly followed the normal course of aging in midlife. High doses of antipsychotics associated with both brain volume loss and decline in cognition, and also more severe illness in terms of symptomatology, the need of hospitalization, and functional outcomes. Additionally, the use of antipsychotics was related to hyperlipidemia. Physical diseases, such as metabolic syndrome and epilepsy, are common in schizophrenia, and mortality is high, especially due to suicides.

10.2. Significance and Novelty of the NFBC 1966 Findings. The NFBC 1966 has provided important knowledge on epidemiology and etiology of schizophrenia. In particular, the possibility of prospectively and reliably analyzing the very early risk factors of schizophrenia is unique. Additionally, the results from the last ten years have brought information that can be utilized in developing clinical practice as well. For example, results on psychiatric and somatic outcomes, mortality, and predictors of outcomes are important with regard to the health promotion and clinical care in schizophrenia. The results also indicate that suicide prevention, early detection and intervention, monitoring somatic health, and active treatment of metabolic abnormalities are highly important. The sample is naturalistic, describing the real-life situation, so the results are generalizable to other settings. The NFBC 1966 studies have analysed also methodological questions, such as diagnostic validity [45, 46] and attrition [41–43]. The studies have been basis also for theoretical, holistic longitudinal models in schizophrenia [47].

The especially interesting and novel findings of the NFBC 1966 are those concerning potentially harmful effects of high doses of antipsychotics on changes in brain morphometry and cognitive functioning [37, 38]. These results support some earlier studies [90, 91], now detecting similar findings in unselected, nonclinical schizophrenia population. The finding of the higher cumulative lifetime dose of antipsychotics and decrease of cognition is new. Earlier studies investigating the association between antipsychotic medication and cognition in schizophrenia have been conducted most commonly in clinical trials with relatively short follow-up, in which two or more antipsychotic drugs are compared with each other. Additionally, high doses of antipsychotics were associated with increased suicidal thoughts among persons without diagnosis of psychosis (i.e., off-label use), even when depression and anxiety symptoms were controlled for [39]. Together with earlier studies [91], these results do not support the view that antipsychotics in general prevent cognitive decline or promote cognitive recovery in schizophrenia and highlight the importance of careful assessment of risks and benefits of dosage and duration of antipsychotic treatment.

10.3. Comparison to Other Birth Cohort Studies. The NFBC 1966 is not the only birth cohort that has studied schizophrenia. Welham et al. [1] have identified 11 birth cohort studies focusing on premorbid developmental trajectories of schizophrenia. Most consistent risk factors identified were behavioral disturbances and psychopathology, intellectual and language deficits, and early motor delays [1]. The NFBC 1966 studies have contributed to conclusions of the review, and especially results regarding early motor developmental delays are comparable to other birth cohort studies and ours. Recently, a register-based Danish National Birth Cohort study has shown that maternal HSV-2 antibodies increase the risk of schizophrenia in offspring [92]. The Prenatal Determinants of Schizophrenia (PDS) study based on the Child Health and Development Study cohort assembled in 1959–1967 in USA has identified various prenatal infection, nutrition, and toxic exposure for schizophrenia; these studies have been reviewed by Bresnahan et al. [93].

Studies on cognition on other birth cohorts have focused mostly on premorbid cognition. MacCabe [94] concluded in his review that children and adolescents with poor cognitive abilities in childhood are at increased risk of schizophrenia. Regarding adulthood cognition, patients exposed to maternal genital/reproductive infection performed more poorly on verbal memory, fine-motor coordination, and working memory in a US birth cohort (Child Health and Development Study) [95]. Also low birth weight has been linked with cognitive impairment in schizophrenia [96]. In the Dunedin cohort, including cognitive tests both before and after onset of schizophrenia disease specific decline in IQ and various mental functions in schizophrenia was found [97]. Later age of learning to stand in infancy predicted deterioration of executive functions with memory in schizophrenia between 34 and 43 years of age in the NFBC 1966 [60]. These above-mentioned studies support the idea of neurodevelopmental but also neurodegenerative processes in schizophrenia.

To our knowledge only one other birth cohort study has focused on brain MRI, showing structural alterations of the cerebral cortex, particularly in the frontal and temporal lobes, and ventricular enlargement in schizophrenia [98], as in our sample.

Somatic comorbidities have been studied in the Helsinki Birth Cohort Study, where individuals with schizophrenia had a higher risk of hospitalization and mortality for coronary heart disease; however, patients with schizophrenia used less lipid-lowering and antihypertensive drug treatment [99]. These and the results of our study highlight the importance of both detecting and treating the somatic illness in schizophrenia early and efficiently. As in our study, violence and criminality have been studied, for example, in the Dunedin Birth Cohort, where the researchers found that those with schizophrenia were 2.5 times more likely to be violent than control subjects [100].

The register-based Danish national birth cohort has been utilized when studying family history and variation in single-nucleotide polymorphisms to risk of schizophrenia. Agerbo et al. [101] found that offspring schizophrenia risk was elevated in those whose mother, father, or siblings had been diagnosed with schizophrenia or related psychosis, bipolar affective disorder, or any other psychiatric disorder. Regarding schizotypal symptoms, in the Australian Mater-University of Queensland Study of Pregnancy, high childhood psychopathology predicted high levels of delusional-like experiences at the age of 21 [102].

There is also younger birth cohort based on the same geographical area than the NFBC 1966; the studies relating to schizophrenia in the Northern Finland Birth Cohort 1986 have so far studied mainly those with clinical or familial risk for psychosis or schizophrenia [103].

In all, many of the risk factor findings from the NFBC 1966 have been replicated in other birth cohorts. To our knowledge, other birth cohort studies have not analyzed clinical and occupational course of illness and their determinants after onset of schizophrenia, though these kind of clinically relevant studies would be especially important in epidemiologically sound samples like birth cohorts. There is a lack of birth cohort studies with straight clinical implications, including postmorbid data, and this should be corrected in the future as birth cohorts get older.

10.4. Strengths and Limitations. The strengths of the birth cohort samples in general and also of the NFBC 1966 include the prospective design and large number of unselected matched controls. This design provides unique possibilities of analyzing causal relationships, for example, between risk factors during pregnancy and delivery and later risk of illness. The major benefit in the NFBC 1966 is also the ability to utilize large nationwide health registers [104]. Linking the cohort data to register data enables researchers to study relatively easily and with low attrition various outcomes, such as hospital treatments, employment, use of social benefits, and mortality. The NFBC 1966 studies utilizing cognitive and brain imaging data differ from most of the other studies on these topics, as in those studies cases are often from clinical samples, collected from one treatment setting, and controls are not included or are selected volunteers.

The NFBC 1966 and other birth cohort studies have various limitations. Participants are not randomly assigned to exposure; thus, any observed associations may be confounded by unmeasured factors. For example, very sick individuals get more antipsychotics than persons with minimal symptomatology. Also, naturally, birth cohort studies include only case and outcome data until the point of data collection used in each study. In the birth cohort studies, the number of cases is often relatively small and power to detect even moderate signal may be low. Additionally, originally birth cohort was not planned for schizophrenia studies specifically: this means that all relevant data regarding schizophrenia research has not been collected (e.g., childhood behaviour and symptoms or treatment aspects, especially regarding psychosocial treatments).

11. Conclusions

Schizophrenia research has been conducted for over 20 years in the NFBC 1966. Several interesting and unique findings regarding risk factors, somatic and psychiatric outcomes, brain morphology and cognition, antipsychotics use, and genetics have been reported. In the future, with the cohort members aging, somatic health, consequences of the use of antipsychotics, and the long-term psychiatric and functional outcomes will be important to explore.

Disclosure

The funders had no role in the design or conduct of the study.

Conflict of Interests

The authors declare that there is no conflict of interests regarding the publication of this paper.

Acknowledgments

This study has been funded by the Academy of Finland (no. 132071, no. 268336, and no. 278286), Brain and Behavior Research Foundation, Jalmari and Rauha Ahokas Foundation, Sigrid Jusélius Foundation, and Northern Finland

Health Care Support Foundation. The authors would like to acknowledge all the participants in this study and researchers collecting the data.

References

[1] J. Welham, M. Isohanni, P. Jones, and J. McGrath, "The antecedents of Schizophrenia: a review of birth cohort studies," *Schizophrenia Bulletin*, vol. 35, no. 3, pp. 603–623, 2009.

[2] P. Rantakallio, "Groups at risk in low birth weight infants and perinatal mortality," *Acta Paediatrica Scandinavica*, vol. 193, supplement 193, pp. 1–71, 1969.

[3] P. Rantakallio, P. Jones, J. Moring, and L. von Wendt, "Association between central nervous system infections during childhood and adult onset schizophrenia and other psychoses: a 28-year follow-up," *International Journal of Epidemiology*, vol. 26, no. 4, pp. 837–843, 1997.

[4] S. Räsänen, J. Veijola, H. Hakko, M. Joukamaa, and M. Isohanni, "Gender differences in incidence and age at onset of DSM-III-R schizophrenia. Preliminary results of the Northern Finland 1966 birth cohort study," *Schizophrenia Research*, vol. 37, no. 2, pp. 197–198, 1999.

[5] E. Keskinen, J. Miettunen, H. Koivumaa-Honkanen, P. Mäki, M. Isohanni, and E. Jääskeläinen, "Interaction between parental psychosis and risk factors during pregnancy and birth for schizophrenia—the Northern Finland 1966 Birth Cohort study," *Schizophrenia Research*, vol. 145, no. 1–3, pp. 56–62, 2013.

[6] P. Mäki, J. Veijola, P. Rantakallio, J. Jokelainen, P. B. Jones, and M. Isohanni, "Schizophrenia in the offspring of antenatally depressed mothers: a 31-year follow-up of the Northern Finland 1966 Birth Cohort," *Schizophrenia Research*, vol. 66, no. 1, pp. 79–81, 2004.

[7] A. Myhrman, P. Rantakallio, M. Isohanni, P. Jones, and U. Rartanen, "Unwantedness of a pregnancy and schizophrenia in the child," *British Journal of Psychiatry*, vol. 169, no. 5, pp. 637–640, 1996.

[8] T. Mäkikyrö, M. Isohanni, J. Moring et al., "Is a child's risk of early onset schizophrenia increased in the highest social class?" *Schizophrenia Research*, vol. 23, no. 3, pp. 245–252, 1997.

[9] P. B. Jones, P. Rantakallio, A.-L. Hartikainen, M. Isohanni, and P. Sipila, "Schizophrenia as a long-term outcome of pregnancy, delivery, and perinatal complications: a 28-year follow-up of the 1966 North Finland general population birth cohort," *The American Journal of Psychiatry*, vol. 155, no. 3, pp. 355–364, 1998.

[10] K. Moilanen, J. Jokelainen, P. B. Jones, A.-L. Hartikainen, M.-R. Järvelin, and M. Isohanni, "Deviant intrauterine growth and risk of schizophrenia: a 34-year follow-up of the Northern Finland 1966 Birth Cohort," *Schizophrenia Research*, vol. 124, no. 1–3, pp. 223–230, 2010.

[11] L. Kemppainen, J. Veijola, J. Jokelainen et al., "Birth order and risk for schizophrenia: a 31-year follow-up of the Northern Finland 1966 Birth Cohort," *Acta Psychiatrica Scandinavica*, vol. 104, no. 2, pp. 148–152, 2001.

[12] L. Kemppainen, T. Mäkikyrö, J. Jokelainen, P. Nieminen, M.-R. Järvelin, and M. Isohanni, "Is grand multiparity associated with offsprings' hospital-treated mental disorders? A 28-year follow-up of the North Finland 1966 birth cohort," *Social Psychiatry and Psychiatric Epidemiology*, vol. 35, no. 3, pp. 104–108, 2000.

[13] J. McGrath, K. Saari, H. Hakko et al., "Vitamin D supplementation during the first year of life and risk of schizophrenia: a Finnish birth cohort study," *Schizophrenia Research*, vol. 67, no. 2-3, pp. 237–245, 2004.

[14] M. Isohanni, P. B. Jones, K. Moilanen et al., "Early developmental milestones in adult schizophrenia and other psychoses. A 31-year follow-up of the Northern Finland 1966 Birth Cohort," *Schizophrenia Research*, vol. 52, no. 1-2, pp. 1–19, 2001.

[15] T. Mäkikyrö, A. Sauvola, J. Moring et al., "Hospital-treated psychiatric disorders in adults with a single-parent and two-parent family background: a 28-year follow-up of the 1966 Northern Finland Birth Cohort," *Family Process*, vol. 37, no. 3, pp. 335–344, 1998.

[16] H. Koponen, P. Rantakallio, J. Veijola, P. Jones, J. Jokelainen, and M. Isohanni, "Childhood central nervous system infections and risk for schizophrenia," *European Archives of Psychiatry and Clinical Neuroscience*, vol. 254, no. 1, pp. 9–13, 2004.

[17] I. Isohanni, M.-R. Järvelin, P. Jones, J. Jokelainen, and M. Isohanni, "Can excellent school performance be a precursor of schizophrenia? A 28-year follow-up in the Northern Finland 1966 birth cohort," *Acta Psychiatrica Scandinavica*, vol. 100, no. 1, pp. 17–26, 1999.

[18] I. Isohanni, M.-R. Järvelin, P. Nieminen et al., "School performance as a predictor of psychiatric hospitalization in adult life. A 28-year follow-up in the Northern Finland 1966 Birth Cohort," *Psychological Medicine*, vol. 28, no. 4, pp. 967–974, 1998.

[19] S. Luoma, H. Hakko, M. Marttunen, A. Taanila, and S. Lindeman, "Severe injuries in adolescence predict psychosis: a nested case control study of the Northern Finland 1966 Birth Cohort," *Schizophrenia Research*, vol. 118, no. 1–3, pp. 48–53, 2010.

[20] P. Rasanen, H. Hakko, M.-R. Jarvelin, M. Isohanni, and J. Tiihonen, "Schizophrenia and seasonality of admissions: the Northern Finland 1966 birth cohort study," *Schizophrenia Research*, vol. 35, no. 2, pp. 183–185, 1999.

[21] B. Miller, E. Messias, J. Miettunen et al., "Meta-analysis of paternal age and schizophrenia risk in male versus female offspring," *Schizophrenia Bulletin*, vol. 37, no. 5, pp. 1039–1047, 2011.

[22] P. Mäki, T. Riekki, J. Miettunen et al., "Schizophrenia in the offspring of antenatally depressed mothers in the Northern Finland 1966 birth cohort: Relationship to family history of psychosis," *The American Journal of Psychiatry*, vol. 167, no. 1, pp. 70–77, 2010.

[23] M. Isohanni, G. K. Murray, J. Jokelainen, T. Croudace, and P. B. Jones, "The persistence of developmental markers in childhood and adolescence and risk for schizophrenic psychoses in adult life. A 34-year follow-up of the Northern Finland 1966 birth cohort," *Schizophrenia Research*, vol. 71, no. 2-3, pp. 213–225, 2004.

[24] B. Miller, J. Suvisaari, J. Miettunen et al., "Advanced paternal age and parental history of schizophrenia," *Schizophrenia Research*, vol. 133, no. 1–3, pp. 125–132, 2011.

[25] E. Lauronen, J. Miettunen, J. Veijola, M. Karhu, P. B. Jones, and M. Isohanni, "Outcome and its predictors in schizophrenia within the Northern Finland 1966 Birth Cohort," *European Psychiatry*, vol. 22, no. 2, pp. 129–136, 2007.

[26] J. Miettunen, E. Lauronen, J. Veijola, H. Koponen, O. Saarento, and M. Isohanni, "Patterns of psychiatric hospitalizations in schizophrenic psychoses within the Northern Finland 1966 birth cohort," *Nordic Journal of Psychiatry*, vol. 60, no. 4, pp. 286–293, 2006.

[27] P. Juola, J. Miettunen, J. Veijola, M. Isohanni, and E. Jääskeläinen, "Predictors of short-and long-term clinical outcome in schizophrenic psychosis-the Northern Finland

1966 Birth Cohort study," *European Psychiatry*, vol. 28, no. 5, pp. 263–268, 2013.

[28] E. Jääskeläinen, J. Miettunen, J. Veijola et al., "Associations between early development and outcome in schizophrenia—a 35-year follow-up of the Northern Finland 1966 Birth Cohort," *Schizophrenia Research*, vol. 99, no. 1–3, pp. 29–37, 2008.

[29] E. Jääskeläinen, P. Juola, J. Kurtti et al., "Associations between brain morphology and outcome in schizophrenia in a general population sample," *European Psychiatry*, vol. 29, no. 7, pp. 456–462, 2014.

[30] M. Penttilä, J. Miettunen, H. Koponen et al., "Association between the duration of untreated psychosis and short- and long-term outcome in schizophrenia within the Northern Finland 1966 Birth Cohort," *Schizophrenia Research*, vol. 143, no. 1, pp. 3–10, 2013.

[31] J. Mäkinen, J. Miettunen, E. Jääskeläinen, J. Veijola, M. Isohanni, and H. Koponen, "Negative symptoms and their predictors in schizophrenia within the Northern Finland 1966 Birth Cohort," *Psychiatry Research*, vol. 178, no. 1, pp. 121–125, 2010.

[32] L. Poustka, G. K. Murray, E. Jääskeläinen et al., "The influence of temperament on symptoms and functional outcome in people with psychosis in the Northern Finland 1966 Birth Cohort," *European Psychiatry*, vol. 25, no. 1, pp. 26–32, 2010.

[33] T. Mäkikyrö, E. Leinonen, H. Koponen et al., "Early developmental differences between DSM-III-R schizophrenics treated with clozapine and typical neuroleptics," *Journal of Psychiatric Research*, vol. 32, no. 2, pp. 105–110, 1998.

[34] J. Miettunen, E. Lauronen, J. Veijola et al., "Socio-demographic and clinical predictors of occupational status in schizophrenic psychoses-follow-up within the Northern Finland 1966 Birth Cohort," *Psychiatry Research*, vol. 150, no. 3, pp. 217–225, 2007.

[35] S. Luoma, H. Hakko, T. Ollinen, M.-R. Järvelin, and S. Lindeman, "Association between age at onset and clinical features of schizophrenia: the Northern Finland 1966 birth cohort study," *European Psychiatry*, vol. 23, no. 5, pp. 331–335, 2008.

[36] J. Moilanen, M. Haapea, J. Miettunen et al., "Characteristics of subjects with schizophrenia spectrum disorder with and without antipsychotic medication—a 10-year follow-up of the Northern Finland 1966 Birth Cohort study," *European Psychiatry*, vol. 28, no. 1, pp. 53–58, 2013.

[37] J. Veijola, J. Y. Guo, J. S. Moilanen et al., "Longitudinal changes in total brain volume in schizophrenia: relation to symptom severity, cognition and antipsychotic medication," *PLoS ONE*, vol. 9, no. 7, Article ID e101689, 2014.

[38] A. P. Husa, I. Rannikko, J. Moilanen et al., "Lifetime use of antipsychotic medication and its relation to change of verbal learning and memory in midlife schizophrenia—an observational 9-year follow-up study," *Schizophrenia Research*, vol. 158, no. 1–3, pp. 134–141, 2014.

[39] I. Rissanen, E. Jääskeläinen, M. Isohanni et al., "Use of antipsychotic medication and suicidality—the Northern Finland Birth Cohort 1966," *Human Psychopharmacology*, vol. 27, no. 5, pp. 476–485, 2012.

[40] K. Saari, H. Koponen, J. Laitinen et al., "Hyperlipidemia in persons using antipsychotic medication: a general population-based birth cohort study," *The Journal of Clinical Psychiatry*, vol. 65, no. 4, pp. 547–550, 2004.

[41] M. Haapea, J. Miettunen, E. Läärä et al., "Non-participation in a field survey with respect to psychiatric disorders," *Scandinavian Journal of Public Health*, vol. 36, no. 7, pp. 728–736, 2008.

[42] M. Haapea, J. Miettunen, J. Veijola, E. Lauronen, P. Tanskanen, and M. Isohanni, "Non-participation may bias the results of a psychiatric survey. An analysis from the survey including magnetic resonance imaging within the Northern Finland 1966 Birth Cohort," *Social Psychiatry and Psychiatric Epidemiology*, vol. 42, no. 5, pp. 403–409, 2007.

[43] M. Haapea, J. Veijola, P. Tanskanen, E. Jääskeläinen, M. Isohanni, and J. Miettunen, "Use of inverse probability weighting to adjust for non-participation in estimating brain volumes in schizophrenia patients," *Psychiatry Research*, vol. 194, no. 3, pp. 326–332, 2011.

[44] M. Haapea, M. Isohanni, E. Jääskeläinen, J. Veijola, and J. Miettunen, "Using home recruitment to increase representativeness of schizophrenia research," *European Psychiatry*, vol. 28, supplement 1, meeting abstract 1725, 2013.

[45] M. Isohanni, T. Mäkikyrö, J. Moring et al., "A comparison of clinical and research DSM-III-R diagnoses of schizophrenia in a Finnish national birth cohort. Clinical and research diagnoses of schizophrenia," *Social Psychiatry and Psychiatric Epidemiology*, vol. 32, no. 5, pp. 303–308, 1997.

[46] K. Moilanen, J. Veijola, K. Läksy et al., "Reasons for the diagnostic discordance between clinicians and researchers in schizophrenia in Northern Finland 1966 Birth Cohort," *Social Psychiatry and Psychiatric Epidemiology*, vol. 38, no. 6, pp. 305–310, 2003.

[47] M. Isohanni, J. Miettunen, P. Mäki et al., "Risk factors for schizophrenia. Follow-up data from the Northern Finland 1966 Birth Cohort Study," *World Psychiatry*, vol. 5, no. 3, pp. 168–171, 2006.

[48] S. L. Matheson, A. M. Shepherd, K. R. Laurens, and V. J. Carr, "A systematic meta-review grading the evidence for non-genetic risk factors and putative antecedents of schizophrenia," *Schizophrenia Research*, vol. 133, no. 1–3, pp. 133–142, 2011.

[49] E. Lauronen, J. Koskinen, J. Veijola et al., "Recovery from schizophrenic psychoses within the northern Finland 1966 birth cohort," *Journal of Clinical Psychiatry*, vol. 66, no. 3, pp. 375–383, 2005.

[50] I. Isohanni, P. B. Jones, M.-R. Järvelin et al., "Educational consequences of mental disorders treated in hospital. A 31-year follow-up of the Northern Finland 1966 Birth Cohort," *Psychological Medicine*, vol. 31, no. 2, pp. 339–349, 2001.

[51] E. Jääskeläinen, P. Juola, N. Hirvonen et al., "A systematic review and meta-analysis of recovery in schizophrenia," *Schizophrenia Bulletin*, vol. 39, no. 6, pp. 1296–1306, 2013.

[52] M. Penttilä, E. Jääskeläinen, N. Hirvonen, M. Isohanni, and J. Miettunen, "Duration of untreated psychosis as predictor of long-term outcome in schizophrenia: systematic review and meta-analysis," *The British Journal of Psychiatry*, vol. 205, no. 2, pp. 88–94, 2014.

[53] P. Fusar-Poli, S. Borgwardt, A. Bechdolf et al., "The psychosis high-risk state: a comprehensive state-of-the-art review," *Archives of General Psychiatry*, vol. 70, no. 1, pp. 107–120, 2013.

[54] P. Tanskanen, M. Haapea, J. Veijola et al., "Volumes of brain, grey and white matter and cerebrospinal fluid in schizophrenia in the Northern Finland 1966 Birth Cohort: an epidemiological approach to analysis," *Psychiatry Research*, vol. 174, no. 2, pp. 116–120, 2009.

[55] P. Tanskanen, K. Ridler, M. Haapea et al., "Morphometric brain abnormalities in schizophrenia in a population-based sample: relationship to duration of illness," *Schizophrenia Bulletin*, vol. 36, no. 4, pp. 766–777, 2010.

[56] P. Tanskanen, J. M. Veijola, U. K. Piippo et al., "Hippocampus and amygdala volumes in schizophrenia and other psychoses

in the Northern Finland 1966 birth cohort," *Schizophrenia Research*, vol. 75, no. 2-3, pp. 283–294, 2005.

[57] M. Penttilä, E. Jääskeläinen, M. Haapea et al., "Association between duration of untreated psychosis and brain morphology in schizophrenia within the Northern Finland 1966 Birth Cohort," *Schizophrenia Research*, vol. 123, no. 2-3, pp. 145–152, 2010.

[58] K. Ridler, J. M. Veijola, P. Tanskanen et al., "Fronto-cerebellar systems are associated with infant motor and adult executive functions in healthy adults but not in schizophrenia," *Proceedings of the National Academy of Sciences of the United States of America*, vol. 103, no. 42, pp. 15651–15656, 2006.

[59] G. K. Murray, P. B. Jones, K. Moilanen et al., "Infant motor development and adult cognitive functions in schizophrenia," *Schizophrenia Research*, vol. 81, no. 1, pp. 65–74, 2006.

[60] H. Kobayashi, M. Isohanni, E. Jääskeläinen et al., "Linking the developmental and degenerative theories of schizophrenia: association between infant development and adult cognitive decline," *Schizophrenia Bulletin*, vol. 40, no. 6, pp. 1319–1327, 2014.

[61] I. Rannikko, M. Haapea, J. Miettunen et al., "Longitudinal change in verbal learning and memory in schizophrenia and controls: a nine-year study in the Northern Finland Birth Cohort 1966," *European Psychiatry*, vol. 28, supplement 1, meeting abstract 1913, 2013.

[62] E. Bora and R. M. Murray, "Meta-analysis of cognitive deficits in ultra-high risk to psychosis and first-episode psychosis: do the cognitive deficits progress over, or after, the onset of psychosis?" *Schizophrenia Bulletin*, vol. 40, no. 4, pp. 744–755, 2014.

[63] K. Riala, H. Hakko, M. Isohanni, A. Pouta, and P. Räsänen, "Is initiation of smoking associated with the prodromal phase of schizophrenia?" *Journal of Psychiatry and Neuroscience*, vol. 30, no. 1, pp. 26–32, 2005.

[64] K. Riala, H. Hakko, M. Isohanni, J. Jokelainen, M. Weiser, and P. Räsänen, "Poor premorbid school performance is associated with later cigarette smoking among schizophrenia patients," *Psychiatry Research*, vol. 137, no. 1-2, pp. 137–141, 2005.

[65] H. Hakko, M. T. Komulainen, H. Koponen et al., "Are females at special risk of obesity if they become psychotic? The longitudinal Northern Finland 1966 Birth Cohort Study," *Schizophrenia Research*, vol. 84, no. 1, pp. 15–19, 2006.

[66] K. M. Saari, S. M. Lindeman, K. M. Viilo et al., "A 4-fold risk of metabolic syndrome in patients with schizophrenia: the Northern Finland 1966 birth cohort study," *Journal of Clinical Psychiatry*, vol. 66, no. 5, pp. 559–563, 2005.

[67] H. J. Koponen, H. H. Hakko, K. M. Saari et al., "The prevalence and predictive value of individual criteria for metabolic syndrome in schizophrenia: a Northern Finland 1966 Birth Cohort Study," *World Journal of Biological Psychiatry*, vol. 11, no. 2, part 2, pp. 262–267, 2010.

[68] M. J. Timonen, K. M. Saari, J. J. Jokelainen, V. B. Meyer-Rochow, P. K. Räsänen, and H. J. Koponen, "Insulin resistance and schizophrenia: results from the Northern Finland 1966 Birth Cohort," *Schizophrenia Research*, vol. 113, no. 1, pp. 107–108, 2009.

[69] K. Saari, J. Jokelainen, J. Veijola et al., "Serum lipids in schizophrenia and other functional psychoses: a general population northern Finland 1966 birth cohort survey," *Acta Psychiatrica Scandinavica*, vol. 110, no. 4, pp. 279–285, 2004.

[70] K. Saari, S. Lindeman, H. Koponen, J. Jokelainen, and M. Isohanni, "Higher serum triglyceride levels in early-onset schizophrenia," *The American Journal of Psychiatry*, vol. 161, no. 1, p. 176, 2004.

[71] T. Mäkikyrö, J. T. Karvonen, H. Hakko et al., "Comorbidity of hospital-treated psychiatric and physical disorders with special reference to schizophrenia: a 28 year follow-up of the 1966 northern Finland general population birth cohort," *Public Health*, vol. 112, no. 4, pp. 221–228, 1998.

[72] H. Lauerma, V. Lehtinen, M. Joukamaa, M.-R. Järvelin, H. Helenius, and M. Isohanni, "Schizophrenia among patients treated for rheumatoid arthritis and appendicitis," *Schizophrenia Research*, vol. 29, no. 3, pp. 255–261, 1998.

[73] P. Räsänen, J. Tiihonen, M. Isohanni, J. Moring, and M. Koiranen, "Juvenile mortality, mental disturbances and criminality: a prospective study of the Northern Finland 1966 birth cohort," *Acta Psychiatrica Scandinavica*, vol. 97, no. 1, pp. 5–9, 1998.

[74] A. Alaräisänen, J. Miettunen, P. Räsänen, W. Fenton, H.-T. J. Koivumaa-Honkanen, and M. Isohanni, "Suicide rate in schizophrenia in the Northern Finland 1966 Birth Cohort," *Social Psychiatry and Psychiatric Epidemiology*, vol. 44, no. 12, pp. 1107–1110, 2009.

[75] A. Alaräisänen, J. Miettunen, E. Lauronen, P. Räsänen, and M. Isohanni, "Good school performance is a risk factor of suicide in psychoses: a 35-year follow up of the Northern Finland 1966 Birth Cohort," *Acta Psychiatrica Scandinavica*, vol. 114, no. 5, pp. 357–362, 2006.

[76] K. A. Nolan, J. Volavka, P. Czobor et al., "Suicidal behavior in patients with schizophrenia is related to COMT polymorphism," *Psychiatric Genetics*, vol. 10, no. 3, pp. 117–124, 2000.

[77] J. Tiihonen, M. Isohanni, P. Räsänen, M. Koiranen, and J. Moring, "Specific major mental disorders and criminality: a 26-year prospective study of the 1966 Northern Finland birth cohort," *The American Journal of Psychiatry*, vol. 154, no. 6, pp. 840–845, 1997.

[78] P. Rasanen, J. Tiihonen, M. Isohanni, P. Rantakallio, J. Lehtonen, and J. Moring, "Schizophrenia, alcohol abuse, and violent behavior: a 26-year followup study of an unselected birth cohort," *Schizophrenia Bulletin*, vol. 24, no. 3, pp. 437–441, 1998.

[79] Schizophrenia Working Group of the Psychiatric Genomics Consortium, "Biological insights from 108 schizophrenia-associated genetic loci," *Nature*, vol. 511, no. 7510, pp. 421–427, 2014.

[80] J. Miettunen, J. Veijola, N. Freimer et al., "Data on schizotypy and affective scales are gender and education dependent—study in the Northern Finland 1966 Birth Cohort," *Psychiatry Research*, vol. 178, no. 2, pp. 408–413, 2010.

[81] J. Miettunen, J. Veijola, M. Isohanni et al., "Identifying schizophrenia and other psychoses with psychological scales in the general population," *Journal of Nervous and Mental Disease*, vol. 199, no. 4, pp. 230–238, 2011.

[82] J. Miettunen, M. Isohanni, T. Paunio et al., "Predicting depression with psychopathology and temperament traits—the Northern Finland 1966 birth cohort," *Depression Research and Treatment*, vol. 2012, Article ID 160905, 9 pages, 2012.

[83] J. Lahti, K. Räikkönen, U. Sovio et al., "Early-life origins of schizotypal traits in adulthood," *British Journal of Psychiatry*, vol. 195, no. 2, pp. 132–137, 2009.

[84] L. Tomppo, W. Hennah, J. Miettunen et al., "Association of variants in DISC1 with psychosis-related traits in a large population cohort," *Archives of General Psychiatry*, vol. 66, no. 2, pp. 134–141, 2009.

[85] L. Tomppo, J. Ekelund, D. Lichtermann, J. Veijola, M.-R. Järvelin, and W. Hennah, "DISC1 conditioned GWAS for

psychosis proneness in a large Finnish birth cohort," *PLoS ONE*, vol. 7, no. 2, Article ID e30643, 2012.

[86] V. Bader, L. Tomppo, S. V. Trossbach et al., "Proteomic, genomic and translational approaches identify CRMP1 for a role in schizophrenia and its underlying traits," *Human Molecular Genetics*, vol. 21, no. 20, Article ID dds273, pp. 4406–4418, 2012.

[87] A. Ramos, C. Rodríguez-Seoane, I. Rosa et al., "Neuropeptide precursor VGF is genetically associated with social anhedonia and underrepresented in the brain of major mental illness: its downregulation by DISC1," *Human Molecular Genetics*, vol. 23, no. 22, pp. 5859–5865, 2014.

[88] O. P. H. Pietiläinen, K. Rehnström, E. Jakkula et al., "Phenotype mining in CNV carriers from a population cohort," *Human Molecular Genetics*, vol. 20, no. 13, pp. 2686–2695, 2011.

[89] G. Stoll, O. P. H. Pietiläinen, B. Linder et al., "Deletion of TOP3β, a component of FMRP-containing mRNPs, contributes to neurodevelopmental disorders," *Nature Neuroscience*, vol. 16, no. 9, pp. 1228–1237, 2013.

[90] B.-C. Ho, N. C. Andreasen, S. Ziebell, R. Pierson, and V. Magnotta, "Long-term antipsychotic treatment and brain volumes: a longitudinal study of first-episode schizophrenia," *Archives of General Psychiatry*, vol. 68, no. 2, pp. 128–137, 2011.

[91] P. Fusar-Poli, R. Smieskova, M. J. Kempton, B. C. Ho, N. C. Andreasen, and S. Borgwardt, "Progressive brain changes in schizophrenia related to antipsychotic treatment? A meta-analysis of longitudinal MRI studies," *Neuroscience & Biobehavioral Reviews*, vol. 37, no. 8, pp. 1680–1691, 2013.

[92] P. B. Mortensen, C. B. Pedersen, D. M. Hougaard et al., "A Danish National Birth Cohort study of maternal HSV-2 antibodies as a risk factor for schizophrenia in their offspring," *Schizophrenia Research*, vol. 122, no. 1–3, pp. 257–263, 2010.

[93] M. Bresnahan, C. A. Schaefer, A. S. Brown, and E. S. Susser, "Prenatal determinants of schizophrenia: what we have learned thus far?" *Epidemiologia e Psichiatria Sociale*, vol. 14, no. 4, pp. 194–197, 2005.

[94] J. H. MacCabe, "Population-based cohort studies on premorbid cognitive function in schizophrenia," *Epidemiologic Reviews*, vol. 30, no. 1, pp. 77–83, 2008.

[95] A. S. Brown, S. Vinogradov, W. S. Kremen et al., "Association of maternal genital and reproductive infections with verbal memory and motor deficits in adult schizophrenia," *Psychiatry Research*, vol. 188, no. 2, pp. 179–186, 2011.

[96] D. Freedman, Y. Bao, W. S. Kremen, S. Vinogradov, I. W. McKeague, and A. S. Brown, "Birth weight and neurocognition in schizophrenia spectrum disorders," *Schizophrenia Bulletin*, vol. 39, no. 3, pp. 592–600, 2013.

[97] M. H. Meier, A. Caspi, A. Reichenberg et al., "Neuropsychological decline in schizophrenia from the premorbid to the postonset period: evidence from a population-representative longitudinal study," *The American Journal of Psychiatry*, vol. 171, no. 1, pp. 91–101, 2014.

[98] T. D. Cannon, T. G. M. van Erp, M. Huttunen et al., "Regional gray matter, white matter, and cerebrospinal fluid distributions in schizophrenic patients, their siblings, and controls," *Archives of General Psychiatry*, vol. 55, no. 12, pp. 1084–1091, 1998.

[99] M. Lahti, J. Tiihonen, H. Wildgust et al., "Cardiovascular morbidity, mortality and pharmacotherapy in patients with schizophrenia," *Psychological Medicine*, vol. 42, no. 11, pp. 2275–2285, 2012.

[100] L. Arseneault, T. E. Moffitt, A. Caspi, P. J. Taylor, and P. A. Silva, "Mental disorders and violence in a total birth cohort: results from the Dunedin study," *Archives of General Psychiatry*, vol. 57, no. 10, pp. 979–986, 2000.

[101] E. Agerbo, P. B. Mortensen, C. Wiuf et al., "Modelling the contribution of family history and variation in single nucleotide polymorphisms to risk of schizophrenia: a Danish national birth cohort-based study," *Schizophrenia Research*, vol. 134, no. 2-3, pp. 246–252, 2012.

[102] J. Scott, G. Martin, J. Welham et al., "Psychopathology during childhood and adolescence predicts delusional-like experiences in adults: a 21-year birth cohort study," *American Journal of Psychiatry*, vol. 166, no. 5, pp. 567–574, 2009.

[103] J. Veijola, P. Mäki, E. Jääskeläinen et al., "Young people at risk for psychosis: case finding and sample characteristics of the Oulu Brain and Mind Study," *Early Intervention in Psychiatry*, vol. 7, no. 2, pp. 146–154, 2013.

[104] J. Miettunen, J. Suvisaari, J. Haukka, and M. Isohanni, "Use of register data for psychiatric epidemiology in the Nordic countries," in *Textbook in Psychiatric Epidemiology*, M. Tsuang, M. Tohen, and P. Jones, Eds., pp. 117–131, Wiley-Blackwell, Singapore, 3rd edition, 2011.

9

Residual Negative Symptoms Differentiate Cognitive Performance in Clinically Stable Patients with Schizophrenia and Bipolar Disorder

Rajeev Krishnadas,[1] Seethalakshmi Ramanathan,[2] Eugene Wong,[3] Ajita Nayak,[4] and Brian Moore[5]

[1] *Sackler Institute of Psychobiological Research, Southern General Hospital, Room 25, University Corridor, Ground Floor, Neurology Building, Glasgow G51 4TF, UK*
[2] *Hutchings Psychiatric Center, NYS Office of Mental Health, Syracuse, NY 13210, USA*
[3] *Gartnavel Royal Hospital, Glasgow G12 0XH, UK*
[4] *Department of Psychiatry, KEM Hospital, Mumbai 400012, India*
[5] *Newcastle General Hospital, 1st Floor, Building 15, Westgate Road, Newcastle upon Tyne NE4 6BE, UK*

Correspondence should be addressed to Rajeev Krishnadas; rajeev.krishnadas@glasgow.ac.uk

Academic Editor: Luis San

Cognitive deficits in various domains have been shown in patients with bipolar disorder and schizophrenia. The purpose of the present study was to examine if residual psychopathology explained the difference in cognitive function between clinically stable patients with schizophrenia and bipolar disorder. We compared the performance on tests of attention, visual and verbal memory, and executive function of 25 patients with schizophrenia in remission and 25 euthymic bipolar disorder patients with that of 25 healthy controls. Mediation analysis was used to see if residual psychopathology could explain the difference in cognitive function between the patient groups. Both patient groups performed significantly worse than healthy controls on most cognitive tests. Patients with bipolar disorder displayed cognitive deficits that were milder but qualitatively similar to those of patients with schizophrenia. Residual negative symptoms mediated the difference in performance on cognitive tests between the two groups. Neither residual general psychotic symptoms nor greater antipsychotic doses explained this relationship. The shared variance explained by the residual negative and cognitive deficits that the difference between patient groups may be explained by greater frontal cortical neurophysiological deficits in patients with schizophrenia, compared to bipolar disorder. Further longitudinal work may provide insight into pathophysiological mechanisms that underlie these deficits.

1. Introduction

Cognitive deficits represent stable traits in both schizophrenia and bipolar disorder [1]. Studies that have directly compared the two groups show qualitatively similar deficits, but quantitatively, milder deficits in bipolar disorder [2–4]. More recently, it has been postulated that this quantitative difference may depend on the presence or severity of psychotic symptoms [5, 6]. For example, Simonsen et al. found that as compared to those without psychosis, subjects with a history of psychosis, irrespective of the diagnosis, showed poorer performance on neurocognitive measures [5]. Additionally, depressive and negative symptoms have also been associated with cognitive deficits [7, 8]. However, very few studies have tried to address these issues during symptomatic remission. It is not clear if residual/subthreshold psychopathology during periods of remission would explain the trait difference between the two groups. In other words, do patients with schizophrenia perform poorer on cognitive tests than patients with bipolar disorder, due to the presence of residual/subthreshold psychotic/negative symptoms?

In this study, we aimed to compare cognitive function in patients with euthymic bipolar disorder with those with schizophrenia in remission. Our second aim was to examine if differences in residual symptoms (psychotic/negative symptoms) between the patient groups could explain (mediate) the difference in cognitive dysfunction between the groups. In other words, the question we are attempting to answer is whether the presence of residual symptoms, including psychotic and specifically negative symptoms, in schizophrenia explains the poorer cognitive performance in schizophrenia? We hypothesise that the difference in cognitive performance could be explained by the presence of residual symptoms.

2. Materials and Methods

The study received ethical approval from the institutional ethics review board, and all subjects gave written informed consent. Twenty-five 18–60 year-old subjects were recruited into each group. Both the patient groups were recruited from the outpatients' clinics of BYL Nair Hospital. Those in the bipolar disorder group (BD), fulfilled the DSM IV criteria for bipolar I disorder—most recent episode manic—severe without psychotic features (with no life-time history of a psychotic episode confirmed using MINI 5.0). Those in the schizophrenia group (SZ), fulfilled the DSM IV criteria for schizophrenia [10, 11]. Euthymia was ascertained using a cut-off score of less than 8 on Hamilton Depression Rating Scale (HRSD) and Young Mania Rating Scale (YMRS) [12, 13]. Remission in schizophrenia was confirmed using a cut-off score of 8 with a score of less than 2 on individual items on the Brief Psychiatric Rating Scale (BPRS) and Scale for the Assessment of Negative Symptoms (SANS) [9, 14, 15]. Antipsychotic doses were measured using the defined daily dose (DDD) method described by WHO [16]. The control group consisted of 25 healthy subjects who had no past or family history of major psychiatric illness in a first-degree relative. Subjects with comorbid Axis I (including substance use disorder—except nicotine use based on MINI 5.0 screening) and Axis II diagnoses, those with medical comorbidity, and those who had received ECT in the last 6 months were excluded.

2.1. Cognitive Assessment

2.1.1. Verbal and Visual Memory. Memory was assessed using Postgraduate Institute Memory Scale (PGIMS), an Indian adaptation of Wechsler memory scale and Boston memory scale that takes into account the language, educational level, and norms standardized for the Indian population [17]. Dysfunction scores adjusted for education level are scored 0, 2, or 3, with higher scores suggesting greater dysfunction. We used the total dysfunction score as well as the raw scores on digit span tests. The Rey-Osterrieth complex figure test with copy component (ROCFT1) and a 30-minute recall component (ROCFT2) was used to evaluate visual attention (copy component), visuoconstructional ability, and delayed visual memory [18].

2.1.2. Trail-Making Test (TMT). TMT A and B have been commonly used and validated in the Indian population [19].

2.1.3. Verbal Fluency. Based on previous studies of verbal fluency, one Hindi phoneme (denoted in English as /*p*/["pa:"]) was used in this task and participants were asked to generate words that started with the sounds associated with these letters in the 60 s time limit. The total number of words in the trial, after excluding proper nouns, numbers, and multiple forms of the same root word, was taken as the verbal fluency score [20].

2.1.4. Go-No Go Task. Sensitivity to interference and inhibitory control was tested using a two-step go-no go task, as described in the frontal assessment battery [21]. In the first task, the subject was asked to provide an opposite response to the examiner's alternating signal. Thus, the subject should obey the initial verbal command and refrain following what they see. On the second task, the subject must inhibit a response that was previously given to the same stimulus. A total of the correct responses on the two tests were taken as the total score.

3. Statistical Analysis

Firstly, we examined zero-order correlation between demographic/clinical variables and cognition (b path on mediation). To address our first aim, we compared cognitive function between groups using MANCOVA, with cognitive functions as dependent variable, diagnosis as the fixed factor, and those variables that correlated with cognitive function (dependent variable), but not diagnostic group (independent variable), as covariates [22]. We correlated the effect sizes of cognitive deficits between the two diagnostic groups to look at the similarity of cognitive deficits, as previously done by Schretlen et al. [3].

Finally, to address our second aim, we conducted a mediation analysis to see if variables, SANS, BPRS, and DDD (mediators), that differed significantly between diagnostic groups mediated the relationship between group membership (independent variable: IV) and cognitive function (dependent variable: DV) in each domain. The analysis tests the hypothesis that the diagnostic category (IV) accounts for variance in the mediator and in turn, this variance in the mediator accounts for a proportion of the variance of the cognitive deficits (DV) (Figure 1). "The adjustable parameters of the model represent the unidirectional influence between pairs of variable in the model. The best fitting values of the parameters are estimated by using the General Linear Model to solve the linear equations that describe the relationships within the model. This analysis differs from multiple regression which estimates the proportion of variance in the dependent variable accounted for by each of several independent predictor variables while allowing for the variance accounted for by the other predictors in the model. In other words, the mediation analysis partitions the variance explained by the predictor into a part that is independent of the mediating variable and a part that is accounted for via the mediating variable" [23]. In classic mediation analysis, causal models are tested using longitudinal data; such an assumption was not made here. The purpose of this analysis was to

TABLE 1: Demographic and illness characteristics.

	BP	SZ	HC	Test statistic	P	BP versus SZ
Female, n (%)	7 (28)	9 (36)	7 (28)	Chi square = 0.502	0.778	
Age, years : mean (s.d.)	35.44 (11.18)	40.16 (8.153)	35.48 (5.49)	$F = 2.49^b$	0.09	
Years in education	10.08 (2.08)	9.08 (1.47)	9.92 (1.03)	$F = 2.86^b$	0.064	
Unemployed	3	6	0	$2.7E-09^a$	<0.001	NS
YMRS, mean (s.d.)	2.28 (1.1)	2.04 (1.02)	0	$F = 52.32^b$	<0.001	NS
HRSD, mean (s.d.)	1.52 (0.58)	1.36 (0.95)	0	$F = 41.85^b$	<0.001	NS
BPRS, mean (s.d.)	0.56 (0.65)	3.68 (1.24)	0	$F = 148.67^b$	<0.001	$t = -11.07$; $P < 0.001$
SANS, mean (s.d.)	0.32 (0.55)	2.68 (0.69)	0	$F = 204.2^b$	<0.001	$t = -13.3$; $P < 0.001$
IDEAS, mean (s.d.)	1.52 (2.00)	2.16 (2.26)	—	$F = 1.12^b$	0.295	
Number of manic episodes, mean (s.d.)	2.88 (1.45)	—	—			
Number of depressive episodes, mean (s.d.)	1.08 (1.57)	—	—			
Duration of illness, mean (s.d.)	8.48 (6.61)	11.32 (5.81)	—	$F = 2.6^b$	0.113	
Medication						
DDD	0.72 (0.50)	1.68 (0.62)		$t = -5.94$;	<0.001	
Lithium, n (%)	7 (28)	—	—			
Valproate, n (%)	6 (24)	—	—			
Carbamazepine, n (%)	6 (24)	—	—			
Lithium + carbamazepine, n (%)	6 (24)	—	—			
Antipsychotics, n (%)	18 (72)	25 (100)	—			
Benzodiazepine, n (%)	5 (20)	8 (32)	—			
Anticholinergics, n (%)	8 (32)	24 (96)	—			
Antidepressant, n (%)	3 (12)	3 (12)	—			

[a]Fisher's exact test for rXc tables; [b]ANOVA IDEAS: Indian Disability Evaluation and Assessment Scale; DDD: defined daily dose of antipsychotics; BP: bipolar disorder; SZ: schizophrenia; HC: healthy control; BPRS: Brief Psychiatric Rating Scale (measured on a scale of 0–6 as in [9]); HDRS: Hamilton Depression Rating Scale; YMRS: Young Mania Rating Scale; SANS: Scale for the Assessment of Negative Symptoms.

identify overlapping variance in cognitive function, explained by the diagnostic groups and mediator variables. This type of approach has been taken previously to examine the contribution of MRI surface based measures to volume-based measures measured using VBM [19]. We used the bootstrap method of Preacher and Hayes to estimate the indirect effect and bias-corrected 95% confidence interval (CI) for each mediator based on 20,000 bootstrap samples using an SPSS macro [24]. This analysis requires no assumption regarding the underlying distributions since the statistical significance level is determined nonparametrically.

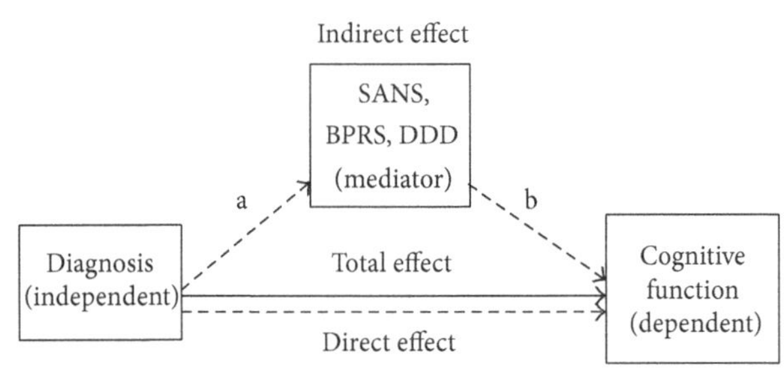

FIGURE 1: Mediation analysis. The figure depicts the relationship between the independent, mediator, and dependent variables. The mediation analysis partitions the total variance (total effect) explained by the predictor into a part that is independent of the mediating variable (direct effect) and a part that is accounted for via the mediating variable (indirect effect). a represents the "a" path and b represents the "b" path.

4. Results

Demographic and illness variables are shown in Table 1. The two patient groups did not differ on most of the variables. Notably, BPRS, SANS scores, and defined daily dose (DDD) of antipsychotics were greater in the schizophrenia group compared to the bipolar group.

The results of the correlation are shown in Table 2. Age showed a significant association with performance on trail-making test. HDRS scores were associated with memory dysfunction. DDD of medication was associated with poorer performance on digit forward trail-making test B and ROCFT. There was also a significant association between BPRS and SANS across a number of domains.

Mean effect size of cognitive deficits was $\eta_p^2 = -0.56$ in bipolar disorder and $\eta_p^2 = -0.72$ in schizophrenia. Figure 2 shows the relationship between the effect sizes of cognitive function in both groups. As can be seen, patients performed worse than controls on all tests, after controlling for gender, age, and number of years in education. Performing a Pearson's correlation of effect sizes between groups tested the similarity of cognitive deficits. This was found to be $r = 0.88$.

TABLE 2: Spearman's correlation between clinical and demographic variables and performance on cognitive tests.

	Digit forward	Digit backward	Trail making A	Trail making B	Verbal fluency	Go-no go	ROCFT1	ROCFT2	PGIMS
Age	−0.164	−0.032	−0.313*	0.263	−0.247	−0.183	0.075	−0.187	0.191
Number of years in education	0.119	0.069	−0.045	−0.156	0.235	0.031	0.127	0.268	0.066
Duration of illness in years	−0.082	0.256	−0.079	0.096	−0.122	−0.132	0.123	−0.215	0.047
DDD	−0.362**	−0.186	0.146	0.433**	−0.245	−0.160	−0.016	−0.500**	0.483**
YMRS	0.137	0.191	−0.175	−0.151	0.154	0.169	−0.052	0.040	−0.056
HDRS	0.213	−0.010	0.244	−0.126	−0.186	−0.154	0.094	0.170	−0.300*
BPRS	−0.617**	−0.282*	0.172	0.575**	−0.478**	−0.298*	0.097	−0.589**	0.558**
SANS	−0.526**	−0.239	0.157	0.466**	−0.488**	−0.511**	0.120	−0.530**	0.526**
Total IDEAS	−0.374**	−0.416**	−0.048	0.131	−0.119	−0.331*	0.054	−0.117	0.434**

*$P < 0.05$; **$P < 0.01$; DDD: defined daily dose of antipsychotics; BPRS: Brief Psychiatric Rating Scale; HDRS: Hamilton Depression Rating Scale; YMRS: Young Mania Rating Scale; SANS: Scale for the Assessment of Negative Symptoms; IDEAS: Indian Disability Evaluation and Assessment Scale.

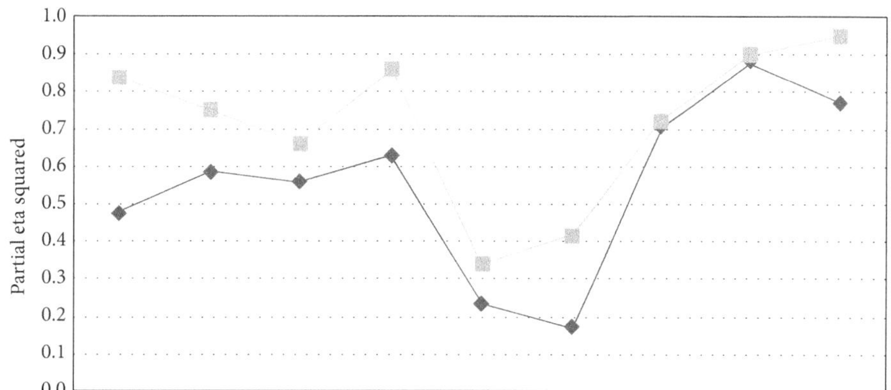

	FDS	RDS	TMT A	TMT B	Verbal fluency	Go-no go	ROCFT1	ROCFT2	Total PGIMS
Bipolar	0.477	0.588	0.561	0.629	0.233	0.171	0.709	0.879	0.772
Schizophrenia	0.837	0.749	0.661	0.863	0.339	0.419	0.725	0.900	0.951

FIGURE 2: Comparison of effect sizes of differences between cases and controls. Partial eta squared represents the size of the relationship between diagnosis and cognitive function. Greater values represent greater cognitive deficits. Covariates appearing in the model are evaluated at the following values: gender = 0.3067, number of years in education = 9.69, and age = 37.03. FDS: forward digit span; RDS: reverse digit span; TMT A: trail-making test A; TMT B: trail-making test B; ROCFT-ROCFT: Rey Osterreith Complex figure test; PGIMS: PGI memory scale.

Results of MANCOVA comparing the patient groups are shown in Table 3. Diagnosis was significantly associated with cognitive performance [Pillai's trace = 0.73; $F(9, 35) = 10.41$; $P < 0.001$; $\eta_p^2 = 0.73$]. SANS, BPRS, and DDD were not included as covariates in the above model, as they differed significantly between the patient groups. They were considered as potential mediators.

On mediation analysis, we found that SANS mediated the difference in performance between the two groups on trail-making B (Beta = −30.46; $Z = -3.07$; 95%CI = −49.67–−6.52), verbal fluency (Beta = −2.24; $Z = -2.65$; 95%CI = −4.16–−0.18), go-no go test (Beta = −1.59; $Z = -3.97$; 95%CI = −2.615–−0.61), and ROCFT2 (Beta = 2.45; $Z = 2.09$; 95%CI = 0.17–4.89). BPRS and DDD showed no mediation effects.

5. Discussion

We have shown that clinically stable patients with schizophrenia and bipolar disorder have qualitatively similar cognitive deficits. These deficits are quantitatively greater in patients with schizophrenia. This difference in performance between the patients groups was at least in part mediated by residual negative symptoms.

Recent review of meta-analyses of cognitive function in patients with remitted bipolar disorder and schizophrenia showed a weighted effect size in the range of 0.6 and 0.8–1 for letter fluency; 0.7 and 0.9 on trail-making tests; 0.7 and 0.9 on digit span backwards; 0.8 and 1.3 on verbal learning and recall, respectively [1]. Findings of our study confirm the large effect sizes observed by the aforementioned investigators

Table 3: Comparison of cognitive performance between patient groups.

	Bipolar[a]	Schizophrenia[a]	F	Sig
Total PGIMS	11.26[a]	17.94[a]	33.735	<0.001
Digit span forward	4.75[a]	3.57[a]	26.771	<0.001
Digit span backward	2.84[a]	2.32[a]	5.011	0.030
ROCFT 1	31.57[a]	31.71[a]	0.094	0.761
ROCFT 2	18.44[a]	14.55[a]	31.243	<0.001
Trail-making A	70.81[a]	78.99[a]	1.761	0.192
Trail-making B	118.99[a]	149.37[a]	24.107	<0.001
Verbal fluency test	13.06[a]	11.82[a]	5.371	0.025
Go-no go test	5.52[a]	4.84[a]	6.694	0.013

[a]Estimated marginal means; covariates appearing in the model are evaluated at the following values: age = 37.80, gender = 0.3200, number of years in education = 9.58, hdrs = 1.44, ymrs = 2.16. Adjustment for multiple comparisons: Bonferroni. ROCFT: Rey Osterreith Complex figure test; PGIMS: PGI memory scale.

in a sample from a developing country. The effect sizes of cognitive deficits in bipolar disorder and schizophrenia showed a high degree of correlation, suggesting deficits in qualitatively similar cognitive function. Schretlen et al. previously compared cognitive functioning in bipolar disorder ($d = -0.59$) with schizophrenia ($d = -0.97$) [3]. They found good correlation ($r = 0.71$) of effect sizes of cognitive tests between the two illnesses, a finding replicated in our study ($r = 0.88$). Similar results have also been shown by studies by Siedman et al. ($r = 0.81$) and Dickerson et al. ($r = 0.93$) [25, 26].

Most interestingly, using mediation analysis, we found that residual negative symptoms mediated the relationship between diagnosis and cognitive function, particularly on the executive function domain. This implies that negative symptoms and cognitive symptoms share significant common variance. In other words, poorer performance on cognitive tests by patients with schizophrenia is, at least in part, explained by the presence of residual negative symptoms in patients with schizophrenia. Neither residual BPRS scores nor greater DDD explained this relationship. This finding is in contrast to those of Simonsen et al., who found that neurocognitive dysfunction was more strongly determined by a history of psychosis [5].

Data from longitudinal studies examining the relationship between negative symptoms and cognitive dysfunction have demonstrated a temporal link between the two. Nevertheless, cognitive and negative symptoms have been shown to be sufficiently independent of each other, implying differential involvement of brain regions in these two processes [7]. More recently, Farzan et al. examined cortical inhibition of gamma band oscillations (CI_γ) in patients with schizophrenia and bipolar disorder. They found that patients with schizophrenia demonstrated selective deficits in CI_γ in the DLPFC compared to bipolar disorder and healthy subjects. They suggest that this lack of inhibition of gamma oscillations in the dorsolateral prefrontal cortex may represent a frontal neurophysiological deficit that could be responsible for the spectrum of frontal deficits in patients with schizophrenia, including executive and cognitive control deficits and negative symptoms [27, 28]. While we cannot make conclusions about the pathophysiology of these illnesses, our findings may be explained by the greater deficits in these physiological processes in patients with schizophrenia, compared to those with bipolar disorder.

While the positive aspect of our study includes the use of standardised tests in a clinical sample free of substance use and other comorbidities, the study has a number of limitations. The small sample size might have led to a type-2 error. However, the observation that negative symptoms (SANS) mediated the difference in cognitive function, despite the small sample size, suggests that the relationship is robust. It should also be noted that the bias-corrected bootstrapping method for testing the mediation is relatively robust against the effect of small sample sizes, especially when the effect sizes of the "a" path and "b" path of the mediation are large as in our sample. A possible explanation for the finding in our study is that SANS designates a number of occupational and educational performance deficits as negative symptoms that are linked with poor cognitive function [7]. It could be argued that BPRS is a general measure of psychopathology, rather than just a measure of psychosis. However, in our sample, we found that BPRS scores did not correlate significantly with any of the other psychopathology scores in patients with schizophrenia. We did not test the premorbid IQ of the patients. Previous studies have indeed shown that the difference in premorbid IQ could explain some of the differences in performance on verbal fluency and response inhibition tests [29]. Premorbid IQ has also been shown previously to link to negative symptoms. However, previous validating studies have shown that scores on PGIMS show low correlation with IQ [17]. The present study did not confirm remission prospectively. While we excluded those with a history of substance use disorder or recent substance use, this exclusion was based on self-report (and MINI screen). We did not use laboratory methods to rule out recent substance use that may have influenced performance on the cognitive tests. Finally, it is not known how generalizable the data is to the community, where symptoms might not be as controlled as in the population tested.

6. Conclusions

Persistent cognitive deficits are seen in patients with euthymic bipolar disorder and schizophrenia under remission when compared to healthy controls. The cognitive deficits are qualitatively similar but worse in patients with schizophrenia compared to patients with bipolar disorder. The worse cognitive function in patients with schizophrenia was mediated by the presence of residual negative symptoms. Further work exploring the link between negative symptoms, cognitive symptoms, and neurophysiological measures may provide insight into pathophysiological mechanisms that may underlie these deficits.

Conflict of Interests

The authors declare that there is no conflict of interests regarding the publication of this paper.

References

[1] E. Bora, M. Yücel, and C. Pantelis, "Cognitive impairment in affective psychoses: a meta-analysis," *Schizophrenia Bulletin*, vol. 36, no. 1, pp. 112–125, 2010.

[2] C. Daban, A. Martinez-Aran, C. Torrent et al., "Specificity of cognitive deficits in bipolar disorder versus schizophrenia: a systematic review," *Psychotherapy and Psychosomatics*, vol. 75, no. 2, pp. 72–84, 2006.

[3] D. J. Schretlen, N. G. Cascella, S. M. Meyer et al., "Neuropsychological functioning in bipolar disorder and schizophrenia," *Biological Psychiatry*, vol. 62, no. 2, pp. 179–186, 2007.

[4] S. K. Hill, J. L. Reilly, R. S. Keefe et al., "Neuropsychological impairments in schizophrenia and psychotic bipolar disorder: findings from the Bipolar-Schizophrenia Network on Intermediate Phenotypes (B-SNIP) study," *The American Journal of Psychiatry*, vol. 170, no. 11, pp. 1275–1284, 2013.

[5] C. Simonsen, K. Sundet, A. Vaskinn et al., "Neurocognitive dysfunction in bipolar and schizophrenia spectrum disorders depends on history of psychosis rather than diagnostic group," *Schizophrenia Bulletin*, vol. 37, no. 1, pp. 73–83, 2011.

[6] D. C. Glahn, C. E. Bearden, M. Barguil et al., "The neurocognitive signature of psychotic bipolar disorder," *Biological Psychiatry*, vol. 62, no. 8, pp. 910–916, 2007.

[7] P. D. Harvey, D. Koren, A. Reichenberg, and C. R. Bowie, "Negative symptoms and cognitive deficits: what is the nature of their relationship?" *Schizophrenia Bulletin*, vol. 32, no. 2, pp. 250–258, 2006.

[8] M. J. van der Werf-Eldering, H. Burger, E. A. E. Holthausen, A. Aleman, and W. A. Nolen, "Cognitive functioning in patients with bipolar disorder: association with depressive symptoms and alcohol use," *PLoS ONE*, vol. 5, no. 9, Article ID e13032, 2010.

[9] V. V. Sadock, B. J. Sadock, and H. I. Kaplan, "Comprehensive sex therapy training: a new approach," *American Journal of Psychiatry*, vol. 132, no. 8, pp. 858–860, 1975.

[10] AmericanPsychiatricAssociation:, *Diagnostic and Statistical Manual of Mental Disorders (DSM-IV)*, American psychiatric association, Washington, DC, USA, 1994.

[11] D. V. Sheehan, Y. Lecrubier, K. H. Sheehan et al., "The Mini-International Neuropsychiatric Interview (M.I.N.I.): the development and validation of a structured diagnostic psychiatric interview for DSM-IV and ICD-10," *Journal of Clinical Psychiatry*, vol. 59, no. 20, pp. 22–33, 1998.

[12] M. Hamilton, "A rating scale for depression," *Journal of Neurology, Neurosurgery, and Psychiatry*, vol. 23, pp. 56–62, 1960.

[13] R. C. Young, J. T. Biggs, V. E. Ziegler, and D. A. Meyer, "A rating scale for mania: reliability, validity and sensitivity," *British Journal of Psychiatry*, vol. 133, no. 11, pp. 429–435, 1978.

[14] N. C. Andreasen, "The Scale for the Assessment of Negative Symptoms (SANS): conceptual and theoretical foundations," *The British journal of psychiatry. Supplement*, no. 7, pp. 49–58, 1989.

[15] J. E. Overall and D. R. Gorham, "The brief psychiatric rating scale," *Psychological Reports*, vol. 10, no. 3, pp. 799–812, 1962.

[16] M. Nosè, M. Tansella, G. Thornicroft et al., "Is the Defined Daily Dose system a reliable tool for standardizing antipsychotic dosages?" *International Clinical Psychopharmacology*, vol. 23, no. 5, pp. 287–290, 2008.

[17] D. Pershad and S. Verma, *Handbook of PGI Battery of Brain Dysfunction (PGI-BDD)*, National psychological corporation, Agra, India, 1990.

[18] J. Hodges, *Cognitive Assessment For Clinicians*, Oxford university press, Oxford, UK, 1994.

[19] C. Mukundan, "NIMHANS neuropsychological battery: test descriptions, instructions, clinical data and interpretation," in *Proceedings of the National Workshop in Clinical Neuropsychology*, C. Mukundan, Ed., pp. 24–29, NIMHANS Publications, Bangalore, India, 1996.

[20] G. Ratcliff, M. Ganguli, V. Chandra et al., "Effects of literacy and education on measures of word fluency," *Brain and Language*, vol. 61, no. 1, pp. 115–122, 1998.

[21] B. Dubois, A. Slachevsky, I. Litvan, and B. Pillon, "The FAB: a frontal assessment battery at bedside," *Neurology*, vol. 55, no. 11, pp. 1621–1626, 2000.

[22] G. A. Miller and J. P. Chapman, "Misunderstanding analysis of covariance," *Journal of Abnormal Psychology*, vol. 110, no. 1, pp. 40–48, 2001.

[23] L. Palaniyappan and P. F. Liddle, "Differential effects of surface area, gyrification and cortical thickness on voxel based morphometric deficits in schizophrenia," *NeuroImage*, vol. 60, no. 1, pp. 693–699, 2012.

[24] K. J. Preacher and A. F. Hayes, "Asymptotic and resampling strategies for assessing and comparing indirect effects in multiple mediator models," *Behavior Research Methods*, vol. 40, no. 3, pp. 879–891, 2008.

[25] F. Dickerson, J. J. Boronow, C. Stallings, A. E. Origoni, S. K. Cole, and R. H. Yolken, "Cognitive functioning in schizophrenia and bipolar disorder: comparison of performance on the Repeatable Battery for the Assessment of Neuropsychological Status," *Psychiatry Research*, vol. 129, no. 1, pp. 45–53, 2004.

[26] L. J. Seidman, W. S. Kremen, D. Koren, S. V. Faraone, J. M. Goldstein, and M. T. Tsuang, "A comparative profile analysis of neuropsychological functioning in patients with schizophrenia and bipolar psychoses," *Schizophrenia Research*, vol. 53, no. 1-2, pp. 31–44, 2002.

[27] F. Farzan, M. S. Barr, A. J. Levinson et al., "Evidence for gamma inhibition deficits in the dorsolateral prefrontal cortex of patients with schizophrenia," *Brain*, vol. 133, no. 5, pp. 1505–1514, 2010.

[28] P. J. Uhlhaas and W. Singer, "Abnormal neural oscillations and synchrony in schizophrenia," *Nature Reviews Neuroscience*, vol. 11, no. 2, pp. 100–113, 2010.

[29] S. L. Barrett, C. C. Mulholland, S. J. Cooper, and T. M. Rushe, "Patterns of neurocognitive impairment in first-episode bipolar disorder and schizophrenia," *British Journal of Psychiatry*, vol. 195, no. 1, pp. 67–72, 2009.

10

Arousal Predisposition as a Vulnerability Indicator for Psychosis: A General Population Online Stress Induction Study

Annika Clamor, A. Malika Warmuth, and Tania M. Lincoln

Department of Clinical Psychology and Psychotherapy, University of Hamburg, Von-Melle-Park 5, 20146 Hamburg, Germany

Correspondence should be addressed to Annika Clamor; annika.clamor@uni-hamburg.de

Academic Editor: Brian Kirkpatrick

Explanatory models ascribe to arousability a central role for the development of psychotic symptoms. Thus, a disposition to hyperarousal (i.e., increased arousal predisposition (AP)) may serve as an underlying vulnerability indicator for psychosis by interacting with stressors to cause symptoms. In this case, AP, stress-response, and psychotic symptoms should be linked before the development of a diagnosable psychotic disorder. We conducted a cross-sectional online study in a population sample ($N = 104$; $M_{age} = 27.7$ years, $SD = 11.2$, range 18–70). Participants rated their AP and subclinical psychotic symptoms. Participants reported their stress-levels before and after two stress inductions including an arithmetic and a social stressor. The participants with an increased AP generally felt more stressed. However, AP was not associated with the specific stress-response. As expected, positive psychotic symptoms were significantly associated with AP, but this was not mediated by general stress-levels. Its association to subtle, nonclinical psychotic symptoms supports our assumption that AP could be a vulnerability indicator for psychosis. The trait is easily accessible via a short self-report and could facilitate the identification of people at risk and be a promising target for early stress-management. Further research is needed to clarify its predictive value for stress-responses.

1. Introduction

Psychotic symptoms such as blunted affect, hallucinations, and delusions may sometimes appear as being very distinct from usual perception and behavior. However, research indicates that "normal" personality traits such as neuroticism precede these symptoms and moderate emotional experience in psychosis [1]. As personality traits influence the perception of and coping with environmental challenges, it seems intuitive to assume that particular traits may constitute vulnerability indicators for the development of psychotic symptoms by interacting with those challenges. The mechanism as such has been postulated by vulnerability-stress-models of psychosis [2, 3], yet research on distinct vulnerability indicators and precise mechanisms is still needed. If we understand which characteristics are indicative of vulnerability, preventive approaches may be enhanced.

Both the traditional vulnerability-stress-models (e.g., [2]) and their more recent cognitive extensions [4] ascribe to the state of hyperarousal a central role in psychotic symptom formation. According to the cognitive model of persecutory delusions, vulnerability will cause individuals to respond to stressful events by a stronger increase in arousal than can be expected for nonvulnerable individuals. This arousal may be further intensified and prolonged by additive factors such as sleep-disturbances or long-term anxiety [4]. This hyperarousal of vulnerable individuals may then cause an inner-outer confusion leading to anomalous perceptual experiences such as hearing thoughts as voices. Individuals will consequently search for a meaning of their arousal and of these experiences, nurturing the threat belief [4]. In support of the role of high arousal in symptom formation, different measures of trait reactivity have been found to interact with life events to predict psychotic symptoms [5]. Also, an increased sensitivity to stressors was found not only to precede symptom exacerbations and relapse in patients with psychosis [6] but also to be characteristic of individuals at ultrahigh risk for psychosis [7, 8]. Over and above sensitivity to minor stressors, a generally elevated level of arousal is also characteristic of individuals with psychosis [9]. Thus, hyperarousal could be a promising indicator of vulnerability to psychosis.

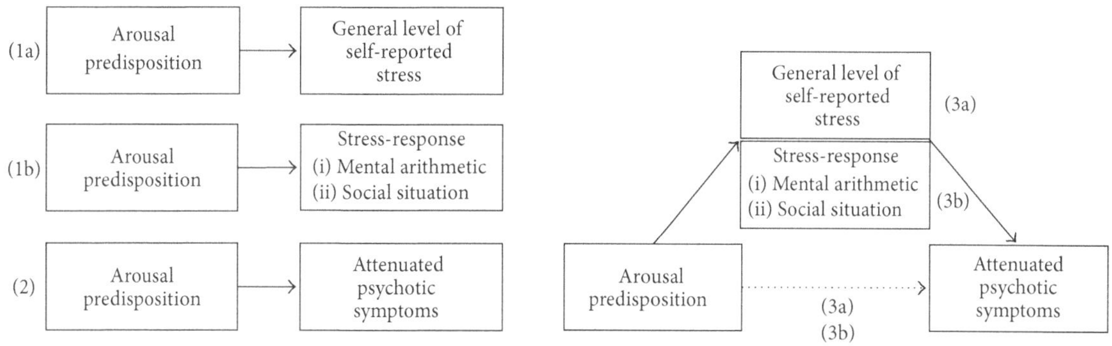

FIGURE 1: Graphical depiction of the hypotheses.

Researchers have proposed a personality trait called arousal predisposition (AP) that combines aspects of trait and stimuli processing and can readily be assessed by self-report scales [10, 11]. It is defined as the extent to which a person responds to heightened complexity, variation, and/or unexpectedness of stimuli with increased arousal [11]. Hence, it describes a person's responsiveness to the environment [10]. In line with the above definition, AP was found to be associated with larger electromyographic and electrodermal activity after the exposure to novel stimuli (e.g., white noise), thus with increased autonomic arousal responses [10]. In contrast to neuroticism, which is a more complex trait that involves characteristic unpleasant responses to situations and specific negative emotional and cognitive experiences such as guilt, AP is narrowly defined and proposed to be a possible foundation for later neuroticism (see [11, 12]). It describes the perception of immediate sensory (e.g., "I find that my heart keeps beating fast") and emotional (e.g., "I can be emotionally moved") responses rather than involving complex levels of secondary appraisals [11, 12]. Two studies found AP to be increased in participants with schizophrenia compared to healthy controls [5, 13]. The same group of researchers also reported a positive association of AP and positive and affective symptom severity [13]. Furthermore, they added support to the construct validity by demonstrating that, in the participants with schizophrenia, AP was significantly associated with the self-reported stress related to a speech stress condition [13]. The authors concluded that heightened AP increases an individual's stress-responsiveness and speculated that this could be a cause of stress-related symptom exacerbation. However, as the authors point out themselves, the increased level of AP and thus stress-responsiveness may also be a result rather than a precursor of the mental disorder [13]. Furthermore, results from later studies have been inconclusive [12] and the authors emphasized the need to examine whether and under which circumstances the association of psychotic symptoms and stress-responsiveness assigned to AP may be found. Taken together, previous findings assign AP a role in explaining psychotic symptoms but replication and further exploration are needed to corroborate the proposed assumptions and to clarify whether AP is indeed a valid indicator of vulnerability to psychosis.

Following the assumption that AP is a risk factor for the development of psychotic symptoms and that both psychotic symptoms and their risk factors occur on a continuum [14], an association between AP and symptoms should already be present before symptoms reach clinical relevance. Consequently, one would expect to find the association in any kind of population sample.

Thus, we expect individuals without a psychotic disorder but with high AP to (1a) report higher general levels of stress and (1b) show an increased response to discrete stressors (i.e., stress-response) compared to individuals with low AP. Furthermore, if AP constitutes a vulnerability factor for psychotic symptoms, we expect that (2) AP will be positively associated with the extent of subclinical psychotic symptoms. Finally, we hypothesize that the association of AP with symptoms is mediated by general levels of self-reported stress (3a) and the stress-responses (3b; see Figure 1).

2. Materials and Methods

2.1. Design and Procedure. We conducted the study within the general population as an online study and included a stress induction to measure the stress-response. Before the questionnaires and tasks, participants were told to switch off any possible source of distraction (e.g., music), to close all other browsers, and to concentrate on the participation. Then, sociodemographic data, psychotic symptoms, and AP were assessed, followed by the stress induction (see Figure 2).

Psychotic symptoms were measured with the German version of the Community Assessment of Psychic Experiences (CAPE) questionnaire [15]. Participants rated their experiences during the previous four weeks on a 4-point scale from "never" to "nearly always." The self-report scale assesses positive symptoms with 20 items, negative symptoms with 14 items, and symptoms of depression with eight items. A total score for overall psychotic symptoms is calculated from all three subscales. Good reliability and validity have been reported [16].

AP was measured with the Arousal Predisposition Scale (APS) [17]. The 12-item self-report scale incorporates a self-descriptive format, such as "I can be emotionally moved by what other people consider to be simple things," "I get excited easily," and "I am restless and fidgety." For the present study,

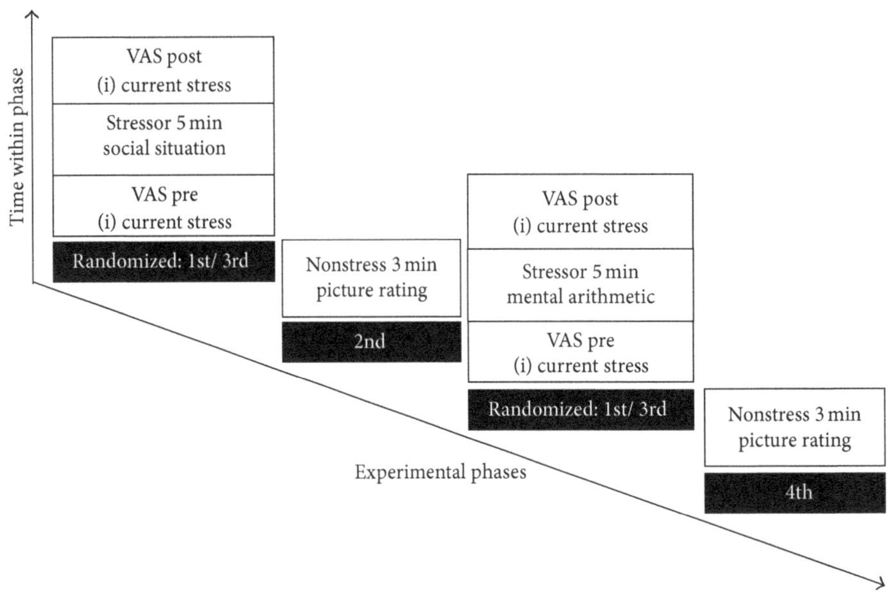

FIGURE 2: Procedure of the stress induction. VAS: Visual Analogue Scales. "1st/3rd": randomized order of the phases.

the APS was translated into German. A back translation was analyzed for concordance with the original version. All discrepancies of the new English version from the original one were due to the use of synonyms. Participants rated their consent with the statements from "1 = never" to "5 = always" and a total score was calculated. The internal consistency of the English version has been found to be acceptable or good [17, 18]. Stability, as intended by a trait index, was found by a retest correlation of .65 in a 9-month follow-up [5].

For the stress induction, participants were exposed to two different 5-minute stressors (an arithmetic stressor and a social stressor) in randomized order. This procedure was adapted from previous studies investigating stress-responses in patients with schizophrenia [13, 19]. The arithmetic stressor required mental arithmetics that were adapted from an intelligence test battery to increase the stressor's potential (e.g., $60 - 25 = A$. $A = ?$; $2/3 * 75 + 1/3 * 60 = F$. $F = ?$). Twenty-five arithmetic problems were displayed at the same time for the duration of five minutes, allowing participants to skip forward and backward. Engagement in the task was tested by reviewing the typed responses. The social stressor required the description of an everyday stressful social interaction. ("Please recall the situation and describe it in as much detail as possible. The situation should have been stressful and occurred within an everyday social context."). The participants typed in the situation within the 5-minute period, after which the next screen occurred. Similar to the arithmetic stressor, engagement in the task was considered by reviewing the typed responses. Each stress condition was followed by a 3-minute nonstress condition (18 pictures; e.g., objects and landscapes). During the nonstress conditions participants were kept committed to the experiment by rating the extent to which the pictures elicited emotions in them via Visual Analogue Scales (VAS) based on Gaab et al. [20], ranging from "not at all" to "very intensely." Before and after the stress tasks, VAS were employed to assess subjective stress with the item "I feel stressed by the situation." The stress-response was defined as the increase in stress from pre- to poststressor assessment. Furthermore, another VAS at the end of the experiment assessed the participants' subjective impression of their ability to concentrate throughout the experiment. All VAS scrollable bars had 100 invisible increments.

2.2. Participants. Participants were recruited through flyers at different universities, social networks, and Internet platforms (e.g., psychology or stress forums). Students from the authors' university were granted partial course credit after obtaining the link via an electronic credit system.

Participation was voluntary and could be stopped at any point without explanation. Anonymity of data was guaranteed as no codes, names, or residencies were assessed. In the beginning and at the end of the study, participants were given a contact address for any requests or problems that occurred before, during, or after the study. After being welcomed and thoroughly informed, participants had to explicitly give consent by clicking "continue with participation."

Previous research in clinical samples showed a medium sized correlation of AP with positive symptoms ($r = .321$) [13]. Thus, we based the power calculation on the expectation of medium effect sizes ($\rho = .30$ and $f = .25$). With $\alpha = .05$ and a power of .90, the calculations with G*Power [21] yielded a required sample size of $N = 46$ for repeated-measures within-between interaction (two groups, two measurements, correlation among measurements $r = 0.5$), of $N = 92$ for one-tailed bivariate correlations, and of $N = 88$ for a linear multiple regression analysis.

In total, 184 participants agreed to participate in the study. No adverse events were reported to the provided contact. After excluding the participants for whom a lack of engagement was evident (i.e., who did not complete the questionnaires, $n = 57$, or participate in both stressors, $n = 23$), 104 participants constituted the final sample. The reported mean age was 27.7 years ($SD = 11.2$, range 18–70). Of these participants, the majority was female ($n = 74$, 71.2%) and well educated ($n = 73$, 70.2% with 10–13 years of education and $n = 31$, 29.8% with a university degree). Furthermore, 15 participants (14.4%) reported a diagnosed mental disorder (the majority of these being depression and anxiety disorders) and 8 participants (7.7%) were in treatment at the time of participation. No participant reported having a psychotic disorder.

2.3. Data Analysis. To analyze the impact of the extent of AP for the stress-levels (hypothesis 1a) and stress-response (hypothesis 1b), we divided the sample into terciles according to the APS scores. For a better distinction from two extreme ends, the upper and lower terciles were regarded as between-subject variable and analyzed in repeated-measures ANOVA for pre- and poststress, distinctively for the two stressors. Bivariate correlations were conducted to verify the proposed association between the CAPE and the APS (hypothesis 2). After confirming the hypotheses (1a) or (1b) and (2), we planned to test the association between stress-level, stress-response (i.e., difference value post-pre), and symptoms using bivariate correlations and the mediation hypotheses (3a and 3b) using linear multiple regression models.

Prior to the analyses, the scale distributions were tested for normality with the Kolmogorov-Smirnov test and visually checked for outliers within a stem-and-leaf plot. Due to directed hypotheses, the correlations were conducted one-tailed. The level of significance was determined as $p \leq .05$. All analyses were conducted with SPSS version 20.

3. Results

3.1. Data Quality and Manipulation Check. Both the core scales of CAPE total and APS total met the requirements of normal distribution ($p \geq .61$). In the stem-and-leaf plots, three outliers ($n = 2$ for CAPE and $n = 1$ for APS) were identified and excluded in subgroup analyses (see Section 3.5). The stress ratings were not normally distributed and showed several outliers. However, in the total and sufficiently large sample, the standard parametric testing was assumed to be robust.

The manipulation of the stress-levels was successful. For the arithmetic stressor, the mean poststress-level (VAS: $M = 46.5$ and $SD = 28.1$) was significantly higher than the prestress-level (VAS: $M = 32.2$ and $SD = 28.8$), $t(103) = -5.215$, $p < .001$, and Cohen's $d = 0.5$. The participants' responses revealed a mean of 12.5 ($SD = 4.5$) correct answers, with a range from 2 to 25. Only two participants gave less than five correct answers (i.e., one per minute) and exclusion of these participants did not change the reported results. Similarly, for the social stressor, the poststress VAS scores ($M = 37.8$ and $SD = 29.5$) were significantly higher than the prestress VAS scores ($M = 31.2$ and $SD = 26.7$), $t(103) = -4.026$, $p < .001$, and Cohen's $d = 0.40$. A review of the content of the stated situations by the first author revealed that two participants did not describe a distinct social situation and four participants did not provide sufficient detail (i.e., only one or two short sentences). However, the exclusion of these six participants did not change the results reported in the main findings. Furthermore, the prestress VAS levels did not differ between the two stress conditions, indicating that the nonstress conditions in between were successful in reestablishing baseline values, $t(103) = -0.505$ and $p = .614$. In line with that, the pictures that we used for the nonstress condition were rated low in the VAS for eliciting emotions; the ratings after the social stressor, $M = 29.0$ and $SD = 17.2$, and after the arithmetic stressor, $M = 28.7$ and $SD = 17.0$, did not differ significantly, $t(102) = -0.365$ and $p = .716$.

Finally, the participants' overall concentration on the tasks was rated with a mean of 68.8 ($SD = 25.4$), indicating acceptable concentration. Including concentration as a covariate did not change the reported results.

3.2. Construct Validity: Hypotheses (1a) and (1b). The two APS groups that were used for the analyses consisted of $n = 31$ participants in the lower tercile (i.e., APS_{low}) and $n = 35$ participants in the upper tercile (i.e., APS_{high}). Within the possible range of 12–60, APS_{low} showed a mean total score of 24.1 (SD = 2.9, range 18–28) and APS_{high} of 40.4 (SD = 4.7, range 35–56).

The repeated-measures ANOVAs for the arithmetic stressor showed a significant main effect of group, $F(1, 64) = 14.67$, $p < .001$, and $\eta^2_p = .186$, with APS_{low} revealing lower general stress estimates than APS_{high}. Similarly, for the social stressor, a main effect of group was found, $F(1, 64) = 25.33$, $p < .001$, and $\eta^2_p = .284$, confirming hypothesis (1a) (see Figure 3).

Contrary to hypothesis (1b), no significant time × group interaction was found, neither for the arithmetic, $F(1, 64) = 0.34$, $p = .564$, and $\eta^2_p = .005$, nor for the social stressor, $F(1, 64) = 1.23$, $p = .272$, and $\eta^2_p = .019$ (see Figure 3).

3.3. Arousal Predisposition as a Vulnerability Factor: Hypothesis (2). As reported in Table 1, there was a significant correlation between the CAPE symptoms and the APS score. Also, all three CAPE subscales were significantly associated with the APS.

3.4. Stress as a Potential Mediator: Hypotheses (3a) and (3b). There was a significant association of the CAPE symptoms with the sum of the prestressor stress-levels ($r = .35$ and $p < .001$). The regression model for hypothesis (3a) revealed a decrease in the β-weight when the stress-level was also considered. However, the change in R^2 and the β-weight for the model including stress-level showed a nonsignificant trend only, while the APS was still a significant predictor for the mean score in the CAPE (see Table 2).

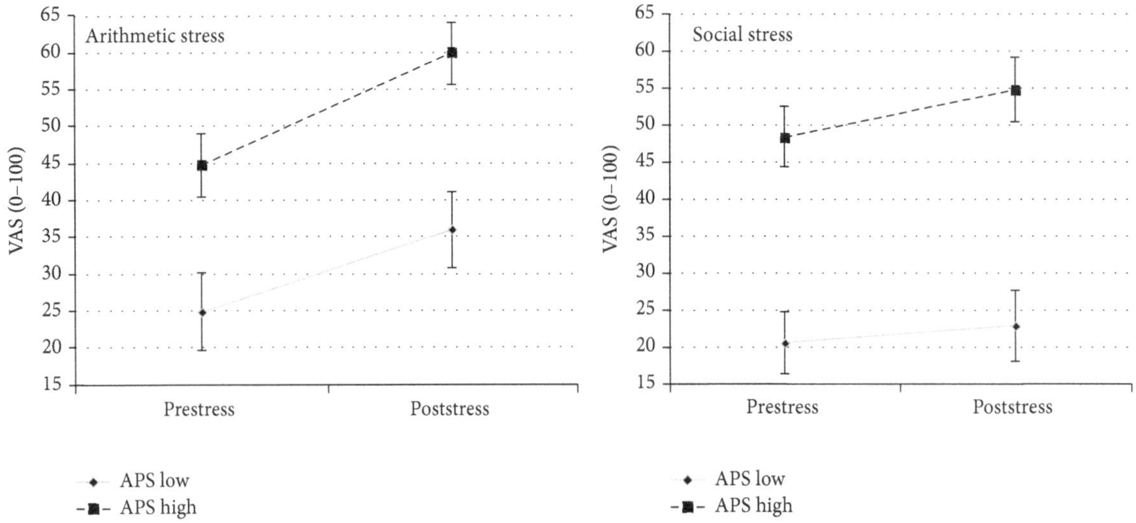

Figure 3: Repeated-measures ANOVA for stress-response in low versus high APS groups. APS: Arousal Predisposition Scale; VAS: visual analogue stress scales.

Table 1: Pearson's correlation coefficients, psychometric data, and scale properties.

Measure	1	2	3	4	M (SD)	α
(1) APS total score	—				32.4 (7.3)	.83
(2) CAPE total score	.51***	—			69.8 (10.4)	.87
(3) CAPE positive	.35***	.66***	—		27.6 (4.1)	.71
(4) CAPE negative	.28**	.87***	.34***	—	26.8 (5.9)	.86
(5) CAPE depressive	.60***	.71***	.23*	.47***	15.5 (3.7)	.84

Note. $N = 104$; α = Cronbach's α; CAPE: Community Assessment of Psychic Experiences; APS: Arousal Predisposition Scale.
$^{*}p < .05$. $^{**}p < .01$. $^{***}p < .001$, one-tailed.

Table 2: Multiple regression analyses predicting psychotic symptoms from arousal predisposition and general levels of stress.

Predictor	CAPE total score		
	ΔR^2	β	p
Step 1	.256		<.001
APS total score		.506	<.001
Step 2	.021		.093
APS total score		.438	<.001
VAS stress-level		.159	.093
Total R^2	.277		<.001

Note. $N = 104$; CAPE: Community Assessment of Psychic Experiences; APS: Arousal Predisposition Scale; VAS: Visual Analogue Scales (here: mean of the prelevels before both stressors).

The present data did not confirm hypothesis (1b). Thus, the mediation hypothesis (3b) was not pursued further.

3.5. Exploratory Analyses of Potential Confounders. A potential confounding of age was investigated by including age as a covariate in partial correlations of APS with stress-levels and CAPE as well as in the regression analysis of APS and stress-level predicting symptoms. However, this did not affect any of the results.

To investigate the generalizability of the effects further, we conducted several subgroup analyses (i.e., subsample without the outliers, male participants and female participants only, and participants without reported mental disorders). The following slightly different patterns of results emerged: (a) for the male participants hypothesis (1a) was not confirmed for the arithmetic stressor ($n = 17$ and $p = .328$) and hypothesis (2) was not confirmed for the CAPE subscales for negative and depressive symptoms, and (b) for the subsamples without mental disorders and without outliers, the regression models to test hypothesis (3) were significant for APS as a predictor for subclinical symptoms and also showed a significant predictive value for the general stress-level ($p \leq .040$). All other results remained unchanged.

4. Discussion

The present study investigated whether the construct of a predisposition to arousal is an indicator of vulnerability to psychosis. We expected that individuals with high arousal predisposition would report higher general stress-levels, show an increased response to stressors, and have higher levels of psychotic symptoms compared to individuals with low arousal predisposition. To clarify possible mechanisms, we analyzed whether the latter association is mediated by the general stress-level or the stress-response.

As expected we found that the group with increased arousal predisposition scores reported higher general levels of subjective stress, before as well as after the stressor. This is in line with studies showing increased autonomic arousal and increased subjective stress-estimates, even at rest, for individuals with clinical psychosis [22]. Previously, this was not found for a group with attenuated psychotic symptoms [22]. Importantly, these findings are not a result of the extreme group approach we used in the study as the correlations between general, pre-, and poststress-levels with arousal predisposition were also significant (all $r > .32$, $p < .001$). Also, in exploratory analyses, the results were robust to differences in the engagement in the task or the presence of a mental disorder. However, some associations were no longer significant in the group of the male participants only. Even though this may be attributed to a lack of power for this analysis, further investigations of gender differences in stress-responses are warranted. Concluding, the Arousal Predisposition Scale seems to be a promising indicator of vulnerability beyond clinical symptoms.

Contrary to what we expected from a trait that describes a person's responsiveness to the environment [10], we did not find arousal predisposition to be associated with the distinct responses to either of the stressors. Thus, arousal predisposition was only relevant to the subjective perception of "generally feeling stressed." At first glance, this appears surprising because previous studies found an association of arousal predisposition with stress-levels [13] and negative affect [12] after the exposure to stress. However, a closer look reveals that in the studies by Dinzeo et al. [12, 13] this was evident only for the participants with schizophrenia, not for their healthy controls. More importantly, in one study [13] the prestress values were not considered, making it difficult to ascertain whether the association refers to the general level of self-reported stress or to the distinct stress-response. Also in contrast to the expected validity of the construct, Docherty et al. [5] did not find arousal predisposition to interact significantly with life events to predict symptoms. They did, however, show an interaction of other reactivity measures such as emotional reactivity and trait anxiety with stressors to increase symptoms. Following from these findings, they propose that the items of the arousability predisposition scale emphasize the reactivity to sensory stimuli rather than to social stimuli [5]. This could be another explanation for the nonsignificant association of the predisposition to arousal with the online stressors in our study. Furthermore, there may have been ceiling effects due to the generally elevated stress-levels. It is also important to note that responses to our stressors were very heterogeneous. Our design may have left a wide range of ways to engage in the task. One could speculate that participants who are easily aroused may have been more tempted to avoid high engagement with the stressor than participants with low arousability. In sum, arousal predisposition seems to be related to the general level of subjective stress. The predictive value for the stress-response may be limited to distinct stressors only, may occur in more controlled or natural situations only, and may be stronger in clinical samples.

As hypothesized, we found the degree of arousal predisposition to be positively and moderately associated with the extent of psychotic symptoms. This finding is consistent with research in clinical psychosis that showed an association of arousal predisposition with positive and affective symptom severity of a similar extent [13]. It also confirms the importance of high arousal for symptom formation that has been proposed before [2, 23]. The fact that we found this association to be present in a population sample with only subclinical psychotic symptoms adds further support to the assumption that arousal predisposition may be a vulnerability indicator for psychosis.

In our mediation analyses, we were able to replicate the known association between general levels of stress and psychotic symptoms (e.g., [8, 24]). However, neither general levels of stress nor stress-sensitivity explained the association between arousal predisposition and symptoms. Excluding outliers and participants with mental disorders even corroborated this finding, with both arousal predisposition and general stress-levels predicting the occurrence of symptoms but not explaining the association. Future research should attempt to further elucidate the mechanisms that could explain why arousal predisposition may be predictive of psychotic symptoms. A possible mechanism could be that characteristic cognitive biases may lead to a premature interpretation of the increased arousability. In turn, this may enhance the formation of a threat belief as stated in cognitive models of persecution [4]. Moreover, by leading to an increase in emotional and physical responsiveness, arousal predisposition may interact with a decreased ability of emotion regulation and less efficient recovery after stress. In order to investigate the validity of this hypothesized causal chain, longitudinal observation of arousal predisposition, emotion regulation, and stress-sensitivity (emotionally and physically) is required, most efficiently within natural environments.

To our knowledge, the present study is the first to investigate arousal predisposition as a trait related to vulnerability for psychosis. Arousal predisposition is easily accessible via self-report, which has clear advantages compared to other possible predictors such as psychophysiological measurements. However, the study has some shortcomings that should be amended in future research. Firstly, the proposed association to subclinical symptoms needs to be confirmed in a more representative sample of the general population, as our sample mainly consisted of female, highly educated, and young participants, limiting its generalizability. Secondly, the predictive value of arousal predisposition for the stress-response should be approached in real-life assessments of stress. In the online stress induction we were not able to prevent external disturbances or avoidance behavior which may have influenced the task, leading to a variance of possibilities to engage in it. In addition, for future online studies, it might be helpful to further ensure continuous engagement by adapting the tasks (e.g., timing each arithmetic problem separately). Thirdly, one could argue that an acquiescence bias may have led to the positive associations, as few items were reversely coded. However, none of the participants' scores yielded a particular or systematic answering pattern. Future research should also include a follow-up on symptom change to disentangle causality. If it can be shown that arousal predisposition particularly predicts psychotic symptoms and response to stress in a longitudinal design, this would support its value as a vulnerability indicator. Moreover, the specificity of the association of increased arousal predisposition with psychosis in comparison to other disorders is interesting, because a strong association to depressive symptoms was shown in our study and in previous research [12].

5. Conclusions

In the present study, we found that individuals with higher levels of subclinical psychotic symptoms also showed a higher predisposition to arousal. Thus, the predisposition may be a relevant indicator of vulnerability to psychosis. We also found that arousal predisposition was associated with general levels of self-reported stress. However, it was not associated with specific responses to discrete stressors. A clinical implication of the presented findings is the need to detect and target elevated stress-levels early. In line with this, the increase of stress-resilience has been proposed as a possible goal in psychosis therapy (e.g., [6, 25]) and early at-risk interventions (e.g., [26]). Taken together with our finding that an increased predisposition to arousal is already indicative of subclinical psychotic symptoms, early intervention modules within stress-management programs seem promising and could potentially target hyperarousal specifically (see also [9]). Further studies are needed to confirm the value of arousal predisposition as an indicator of vulnerability to psychosis and its potential to enhance the development and implementation of stress-resilience trainings.

Conflict of Interests

The authors declare that there is no conflict of interests regarding the publication of this paper.

References

[1] T. J. Dinzeo and N. M. Docherty, "Normal personality characteristics in schizophrenia: a review of the literature involving the FFM," *The Journal of Nervous and Mental Disease*, vol. 195, no. 5, pp. 421–429, 2007.

[2] K. H. Nuechterlein and M. E. Dawson, "A heuristic vulnerability/stress model of schizophrenic episodes," *Schizophrenia bulletin*, vol. 10, no. 2, pp. 300–312, 1984.

[3] J. Zubin and B. Spring, "Vulnerability. A new view of schizophrenia," *Journal of Abnormal Psychology*, vol. 86, no. 2, pp. 103–126, 1977.

[4] D. Freeman, P. A. Garety, E. Kuipers, D. Fowler, and P. E. Bebbington, "A cognitive model of persecutory delusions," *The British Journal of Clinical Psychology*, vol. 41, no. 4, pp. 331–347, 2002.

[5] N. M. Docherty, A. St-Hilaire, J. M. Aakre, and J. P. Seghers, "Life events and high-trait reactivity together predict psychotic symptom increases in Schizophrenia," *Schizophrenia Bulletin*, vol. 35, no. 3, pp. 638–645, 2009.

[6] I. Myin-Germeys, F. Peeters, R. Havermans et al., "Emotional reactivity to daily life stress in psychosis and affective disorder: an experience sampling study," *Acta Psychiatrica Scandinavica*, vol. 107, no. 2, pp. 124–131, 2003.

[7] J. E. Palmier-Claus, G. Dunn, and S. W. Lewis, "Emotional and symptomatic reactivity to stress in individuals at ultra-high risk of developing psychosis," *Psychological Medicine*, vol. 42, no. 5, pp. 1003–1012, 2012.

[8] H. D. Trotman, C. W. Holtzman, E. F. Walker et al., "Stress exposure and sensitivity in the clinical high-risk syndrome: initial findings from the North American Prodrome Longitudinal Study (NAPLS)," *Schizophrenia Research*, vol. 160, no. 1-3, pp. 104–109, 2014.

[9] T. M. Lincoln, U. Köther, M. Hartmann, J. Kempkensteffen, and S. Moritz, "Responses to stress in patients with psychotic disorders compared to persons with varying levels of vulnerability to psychosis, persons with depression and healthy controls," *Journal of Behavior Therapy and Experimental Psychiatry*, vol. 47, pp. 92–101, 2015.

[10] S. Coren and K. B. Mah, "Prediction of physiological arousability: a validation of the arousal predisposition scale," *Behaviour Research and Therapy*, vol. 31, no. 2, pp. 215–219, 1993.

[11] A. Mehrabian, "Theory and evidence bearing on a scale of trait arousability," *Current Psychology*, vol. 14, no. 1, pp. 3–28, 1995.

[12] T. J. Dinzeo, A. S. Cohen, T. M. Nienow, and N. M. Docherty, "Arousability in schizophrenia: relationship to emotional and physiological reactivity and symptom severity," *Acta Psychiatrica Scandinavica*, vol. 117, no. 6, pp. 432–439, 2008.

[13] T. J. Dinzeo, A. S. Cohen, T. M. Nienow, and N. M. Docherty, "Stress and arousability in schizophrenia," *Schizophrenia Research*, vol. 71, no. 1, pp. 127–135, 2004.

[14] R. J. Linscott and J. van Os, "An updated and conservative systematic review and meta-analysis of epidemiological evidence on psychotic experiences in children and adults: on the pathway from proneness to persistence to dimensional expression across mental disorders," *Psychological Medicine*, vol. 43, no. 6, pp. 1133–1149, 2013.

[15] N. C. Stefanis, M. Hanssen, N. K. Smirnis et al., "Evidence that three dimensions of psychosis have a distribution in the general population," *Psychological Medicine*, vol. 32, no. 2, pp. 347–358, 2002.

[16] M. Konings, M. Bak, M. Hanssen, J. Van Os, and L. Krabbendam, "Validity and reliability of the CAPE: a self-report instrument for the measurement of psychotic experiences in the general population," *Acta Psychiatrica Scandinavica*, vol. 114, no. 1, pp. 55–61, 2006.

[17] S. Coren, "Prediction of insomnia from arousability predisposition scores: scale development and cross-validation," *Behaviour Research and Therapy*, vol. 26, no. 5, pp. 415–420, 1988.

[18] A. J. Saliba, R. D. Henderson, F. P. Deane, and D. Mahar, "The arousability predisposition scale: validity and determinants of between-subject variability," *The Journal of General Psychology*, vol. 125, no. 3, pp. 263–269, 1998.

[19] M. N. Castro, D. E. Vigo, H. Weidema et al., "Heart rate variability response to mental arithmetic stress in patients with schizophrenia. Autonomic response to stress in schizophrenia," *Schizophrenia Research*, vol. 99, no. 1–3, pp. 294–303, 2008.

[20] J. Gaab, N. Blättler, T. Menzi, B. Pabst, S. Stoyer, and U. Ehlert, "Randomized controlled evaluation of the effects of cognitive-behavioral stress management on cortisol responses to acute stress in healthy subjects," *Psychoneuroendocrinology*, vol. 28, no. 6, pp. 767–779, 2003.

[21] F. Faul, E. Erdfelder, A. Buchner, and A.-G. Lang, "Statistical power analyses using G*Power 3.1: tests for correlation and regression analyses," *Behavior Research Methods*, vol. 41, no. 4, pp. 1149–1160, 2009.

[22] A. Clamor, M. M. Hartmann, U. Köther, C. Otte, S. Moritz, and T. M. Lincoln, "Altered autonomic arousal in psychosis: an analysis of vulnerability and specificity," *Schizophrenia Research*, vol. 154, no. 1–3, pp. 73–78, 2014.

[23] R. Dudley, G. Dodgson, G. Sarll, R. Halhead, H. Bolas, and S. McCarthy-Jones, "The effect of arousal on auditory threat detection and the relationship to auditory hallucinations," *Journal of Behavior Therapy and Experimental Psychiatry*, vol. 45, no. 3, pp. 311–318, 2014.

[24] T. M. Lincoln, N. Peter, M. Schäfer, and S. Moritz, "Impact of stress on paranoia: an experimental investigation of moderators and mediators," *Psychological Medicine*, vol. 39, no. 7, pp. 1129–1139, 2009.

[25] D. Ben-Zeev, J. Larson, and M. Sarratt, "A possible role for Progressive Muscle Relaxation in the treatment of persecutory ideation," *Medical Hypotheses*, vol. 75, no. 6, pp. 568–571, 2010.

[26] J. E. DeVylder, S. Ben-David, S. A. Schobel, D. Kimhy, D. Malaspina, and C. M. Corcoran, "Temporal association of stress sensitivity and symptoms in individuals at clinical high risk for psychosis," *Psychological Medicine*, vol. 43, no. 2, pp. 259–268, 2013.

11

Long-Term Risperidone Treatment Induces Visceral Adiposity Associated with Hepatic Steatosis in Mice: A Magnetic Resonance Approach

Florent Auger,[1,2,3,4] Patrick Duriez,[1,2,4,5] Françoise Martin-Nizard,[1,5,6,7] Nicolas Durieux,[1,4] Régis Bordet,[1,2,4] and Olivier Pétrault[1,4,8,9]

[1] *Université Lille Nord de France, 59000 Lille, France*
[2] *Département de Pharmacologie Médicale, CHULille, EA 1046, 59000 Lille, France*
[3] *Inserm, U837, 59000 Lille, France*
[4] *IMPRT-IFR114, 59000 Lille, France*
[5] *Faculté de Pharmacie, 59006 Lille, France*
[6] *Inserm, U1011, 59000 Lille, France*
[7] *Institut Pasteur de Lille, 59019 Lille, France*
[8] *UArtois, 62300 Lens, France*
[9] *Laboratoire de Pharmacologie Médicale, EA 1046, Faculté de Médecine, Université Lille2, Pôle Pecherche, 1 Place de Verdun, 59045 Lille Cedex, France*

Correspondence should be addressed to Olivier Pétrault; olivier.petrault@univ-artois.fr

Academic Editor: Sonia Dollfus

Although atypical antipsychotic drugs (APDs) have led to significant advances in the treatment of psychotic disorders, they still induce metabolic disturbances. We aimed at characterizing the metabolic consequences of a risperidone treatment and at establishing a link with noninvasive MR markers, in order to develop a tool for predicting symptoms of the metabolic syndrome. Fat deposition and liver morphometry were assessed by T1-weighted imaging. Fatty acid composition and fat accumulations in tissues were determined using MR spectroscopy with and without water suppression, respectively. Risperidone treatment induced a weight gain accompanied with metabolic disturbances such as hyperglycemic status, an increase in visceral adipose tissue (VAT), and liver fat depositions. Correlations using Methylene-Water Ratio (MWR) and Polyunsaturated Index (PUI) demonstrated a concomitant increase in the weight gain, VAT and liver fat depositions, and a decrease in the quantity of polyunsaturated fatty acids. These results were consistent with a hepatic steatosis state. We evaluated the ability of MR techniques to detect subtle metabolic disorders induced by APDs. Thus, our model and methodology offer the possibility to investigate APDs side effects in order to improve the health conditions of schizophrenic patients.

1. Introduction

Antipsychotic drugs (APDs) are widely used in current psychiatric practice and are commonly classified as typical (conventional) or atypical (second generation). Atypical APDs have been introduced in clinical practice after 1990, including clozapine, olanzapine, quetiapine, and risperidone. Atypical APDs cause less extrapyramidal symptoms (tremors) than typical APDs. However, both of them produce a weight gain [1–3], which increases the risk to develop a metabolic syndrome [4] associating several disorders such as diabetes mellitus, hypertension, hyperglycemia, dyslipidemia, and abdominal fat deposition [4, 5].

The excess of visceral adipose tissue (VAT) mass is particularly correlated to the prevalence of metabolic syndrome and insulin resistance [6]. Indeed, abnormal VAT depositions lead to the storage of lipids in undesired organs such as pancreas, skeletal muscle, heart, and liver. This so-called "ectopic fat deposition" contributes to the development of metabolic syndrome [6–12]. VAT accumulation could thus represent a biomarker of metabolic disturbances, as used in clinic through the measurement of waist circumference in replacement of the body mass index [5]. Nevertheless, the susceptibility to develop a metabolic syndrome is not systematically linked to risk factors as fat distribution in other compartments (i.e., visceral *versus* subcutaneous fat), insulin-resistance, or sedentary lifestyle [7–11]. The relative independence of these factors points out the difficulty to find reliable biomarkers. "Ectopic fat deposition" remains the most relevant process for diagnosing early metabolic disturbances, thus justifying the use of new noninvasive techniques to characterize body fat repartition.

Several techniques are widely used for the *in vivo* assessment of body fat, such as anthropometry [13], hydrodensitometry, air displacement plethysmography, bioelectric impedance, and dual energy X-ray absorptiometry [14, 15]. Their common limitation arises from their inefficiency in distinguishing subcutaneous adipose tissue (SAT) from VAT and in establishing an accurate body fat repartition. Computerized Tomography (CT) and Magnetic Resonance (MR) scans have the capability to distinguish SAT from VAT [16–21]. CT and MR techniques enable quantification of ectopic fat [16, 22–26]. MR imaging (MRI) and Magnetic Resonance Spectroscopy (MRS) are noninvasive techniques which are suitable for fat quantification and fat nature identification [27]. T1-weighted images and Dixon sequence are usually recorded to quantify SAT and VAT [7, 19, 26, 28]. They allow the segmentation of adipose tissues by dedicated post-treatment software [17, 29]. MRS enables the *in vivo* hepatic triglyceride (TG) quantification in order to diagnose hepatic steatosis in clinical practice. Due to its good correlation with histological data from liver biopsies [30], MRS is now considered as a reference for the quantification of noninvasive hepatic fat [7, 28].

Previous work showed the relevance of a mouse model for assessing weight gain induced by risperidone treatment [31]. In the present study, and for a translational purpose, we aimed at: (i) characterizing the metabolic disturbances associated with the weight gain induced by a long-term risperidone treatment and (ii) establishing a link with noninvasive MR markers, in order to develop a tool for predicting symptoms of the metabolic syndrome.

2. Materials and Methods

2.1. Animals. The Ethic community approved all protocols for animal experiments. Twelve seven-week- old female mice of C57BL/6N strain were purchased from Charles River laboratories (L'Arbresle, France).

2.2. Drug Treatment. Twenty-four female mice were examined in this study. Two groups of twelve animals were randomized by weight. One group was treated weekly over 24 weeks with intraperitoneal (IP) injection of 12.5 mg kg^{-1} of long-acting risperidone (Risperdal Consta, Janssen, USA) (risperidone group). The other group received IP injections of the vehicle of long-acting risperidone (control group). Mice were housed in a cage and maintained under a 12 h light-12 h dark cycle with free access to food and water. MR examinations were performed on the twenty-four mice. Pelleted food was weighted weekly to assess total grams of food consumed per cage and per day, and then divided by six to estimate the average weekly food consumption per mouse. Following MR examinations, the twenty-four mice were sacrificed by an overdose of pentobarbital. Biological samples were collected for histological examination.

2.3. MRI. All MR examinations were done after the 24 weeks of risperidone treatment on a 7 T Bruker Biospec (Ettlingen, Germany) imaging system equipped with a 40 cm horizontal bore magnet. Anesthesia was induced by 2% isoflurane and maintained at 1%–1.5% along acquisition, depending on respiration frequency. A pneumatic pillow (SA Inc. Stony Brook, NY) was used to perform and monitor triggered respiratory gating. Each mouse was placed in a cylindrical coil (39 mm inner diameter). Multislice gradient echo sequence was triggered with respiration and performed to assess mouse position inside the magnet, with the following sequence parameters: TR/TE (Repetition Time/Echo Time) = 200/3 ms, FA (Flip Angle) = 30°.

Liver and adipose tissue images were acquired by T1-weighted imaging, using axial and coronal Rapid Acquisition with Relaxation Enhancement (RARE) sequence, which was gated with respiration. Multislice coronal (FOV = 3.6 × 3.6 cm, 14 contiguous slices of 1.5 mm thick) and axial (FOV = 3 × 3 cm, 18 contiguous slices of 2 mm thick) RARE images were collected with a TR of 400 ms, a TE of 9 ms, a 256 × 256 data matrix, and a number of repetitions (NEX) of 2. Reconstructions were done to evaluate the volumes of liver, Inguinal Adipose Tissue (IAT, characterizing the subcutaneous compartment), and VAT (defined as the sum of perirenal fat, gonadal fat, and mesenteric fat, Figure 1(a)). Reconstructions were manually drawn on ITKSnap software [32] for each set of T1-weighted images.

2.4. MRS. Single-voxel localized 1H MR spectra were acquired using the PRESS sequence (respiratory gated) with the following parameters: voxel volume 3 × 3 × 3 mm; TR = 10,000 ms; TE = 20 ms. To avoid obvious blood vessel and subcutaneous fat contributions, the voxel was carefully placed on previous anatomic axial and coronal T1-weighted images (Figure 1(b)). The magnetic field homogenization remains a critical step, and the local shimming was performed until the water line width achieves less than 50 Hz conditioning the spectral resolution. Spectral data were processed on Topspin 2.0 (Bruker, Germany).

2.5. Methyl Water Ratio (MWR). The MWR was assessed from localized proton spectroscopy performed without water suppression. *In vivo,* hepatic fatty acid proportion is determined as the percentage of the bulk methylene resonance to water [33]. So, MWR is defined as the ratio of the intensity of the lipid proton peak (methylene bulk) with the intensity of

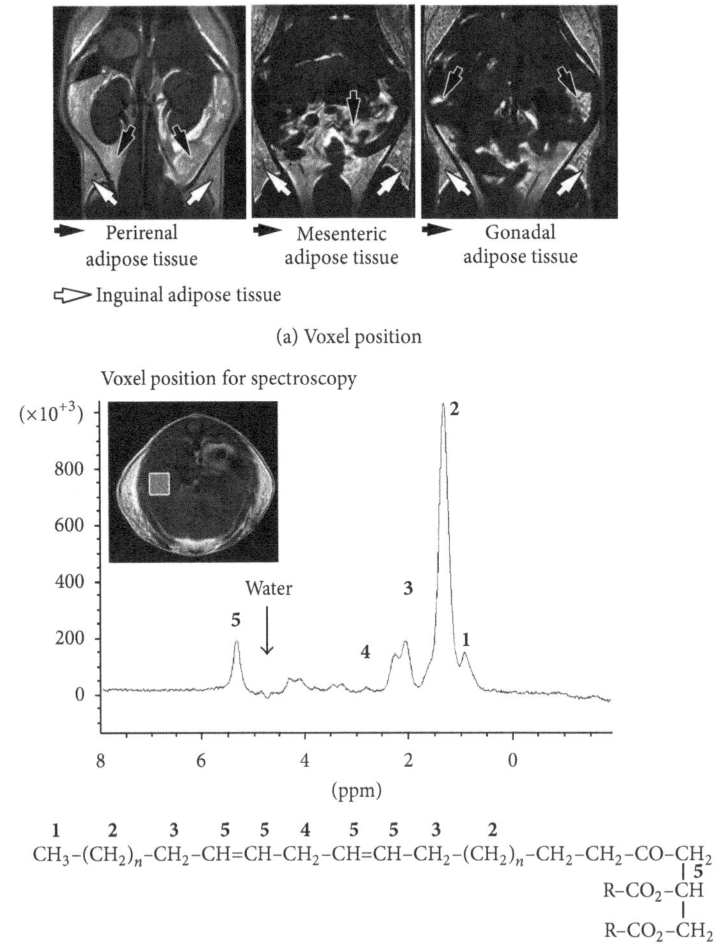

(a) Voxel position

(b) Hepatic MRS (water suppressed)

FIGURE 1: Hepatic lipids composition. (a) Three coronal T1-weighted MR images displaying inguinal, perirenal, mesenteric, and gonadal adipose tissues. These images were used to perform volumetric analyses. (b) Axial T1-weighted liver image with the voxel position used for MRS analyses and an example of a water suppressed MRS spectrum. Each peak corresponds to a particular chemical group described as follows: **1** = terminal methyl (CH_3) at 0.9 ppm; **2** = methylene groups of saturated fatty acids and the "saturated" components of mono- and poly fatty acids $(CH_2)_n$ at 1.3 ppm; **3** = allylic as the methylene adjacent to methene groups (CH_2) at 2.1 ppm; **4** = diallylic as the methylene inserted between sequential methene groups of fatty acid ($CH-CH_2-CH$) at 2.8 ppm; **5** = methene as the olefinic groups (CH=CH) at 5.3 ppm.

the water proton peak, allowing the estimation of the quantity of intracellular fat accumulation in the tissue.

2.6. Lipid MR Spectroscopy. The localized proton spectroscopy was acquired with manual water suppression using VAPOR (VAriable Power and Optimized Relaxation delays) sequence module and a signal accumulation amounted to 64. The different ratios were calculated from peak intensities of the lipid spectra. Previous works reported that the T1 relaxation values of liver methylene and methene groups were respectively between 0.39 to 1.20 s and 0.60 to 1.16 s [34, 35]. In order to fully relax all resonances (up to 5 × T1), we set the TR parameter of the PRESS sequence to 10 s and no further T1 correction was necessary. Depending on spectral resolution, the MR lipid spectrum profile is characterized by nine peaks but only five of them were usually considered for the lipid index calculation (see Figure 1(b)): **1** = terminal *methyl* (CH_3) at 0.9 ppm; **2** = *methylene* groups of saturated fatty acids and the "saturated" components of mono- and poly fatty acids $(CH_2)_n$ at 1.3 ppm; **3** = *allylic* as the methylene adjacent to methene groups (CH_2) at 2.1 ppm; **4** = *diallylic* as the methylene inserted between sequential methene groups of fatty acid ($CH-CH_2-CH$) at 2.8 ppm; **5** = *methene* as the olefinic groups (CH=CH) at 5.3 ppm.

Calculation of hepatic lipid indexes was based on the proportion of constitutive saturated mono- and poly unsaturated fatty acids according to Johnson and colleagues' study [36]. Using MR spectroscopy, four indexes can be calculated: the unsaturated index (UI), the unsaturated index surrogate (UIs), the saturated index (SI), and the polyunsaturated index (PUI). The formulas were as follows:

$$UI = \frac{I_{\text{methene}}}{I_{\text{methene}} + I_{\text{allylic}} + I_{\text{methylene}} + I_{\text{methyl}}}, \qquad (1)$$

where I_{methene}, I_{allylic}, $I_{\text{methylene}}$, and I_{methyl} are, respectively, the signal amplitude of the methene, allylic methylene, bulk methylene, and terminal methyl peaks.

UIs formula is based on the principle that methene functional group is always next to allylic methylene group in monounsaturated fatty acids and with both allylic and diallylic methylene groups in Poly Unsaturated Fatty Acids (PUFAs). Thus UIs formula is as follows:

$$\text{UIs} = \frac{I_{\text{allylic}} + I_{\text{diallylic}}}{I_{\text{allylic}} + I_{\text{diallylic}} + I_{\text{methylene}} + I_{\text{methyl}}}, \quad (2)$$

where $I_{\text{diallylic}}$ is the signal amplitude of the diallylic methylene peak. SI is calculated as the complemented index of UI_s and can be easily assessed as follows:

$$\text{SI} = 1 - \frac{I_{\text{allylic}} + I_{\text{diallylic}}}{I_{\text{allylic}} + I_{\text{diallylic}} + I_{\text{methylene}} + I_{\text{methyl}}}. \quad (3)$$

Lastly, the diallylic peak is detected only in PUFAs (18 : 2, 18 : 3, 20 : 4, 20 : 5, and 22 : 6) in liver. Thus the measure of PUI is

$$\text{PUI} = \frac{I_{\text{diallylic}}}{I_{\text{allylic}} + I_{\text{diallylic}} + I_{\text{methylene}} + I_{\text{methyl}}}. \quad (4)$$

As the methene signal could not be correctly detected when water suppression pulses are applied, we decided to omit UI according to the method described by Johnson and colleagues [36] and the unsaturated index was therefore calculated with UIs. A spectrum with a low signal noise ratio (<2) for the diallylic peak at 2.8 ppm was excluded from the study.

2.7. Spontaneous Locomotor Activity. Spontaneous motor activity was measured using an actimeter (Panlab, Barcelona, Spain). This apparatus allowed horizontal motor activity (traveled distance, in centimeters), rearing behavior (number of rears), and mean velocity (in centimeters per second). These parameters gave clues about ability of mice to explore a new environment. Motor activity was recorded for ten minutes.

2.8. Glucose Tolerance Test. After fasting in fresh cages for 6 hours, approximately 25 μL of tail tip blood was collected to assess fasting glucose levels. Thereafter, mice received 2 g/kg of 15% dextrose by ip injection. Sample tail tip blood glucose levels were measured using a glucometer (Accu-Check performa, Roche Diagnostics GmbH, Mannheim, Germany) at 10, 20, 30, 60, 90, and 120 min.

2.9. Histology. IAT and livers were collected and weighted. Livers were then fixed in 4% paraformaldehyde for Oil Red O (ORO) staining. Analysis of lipid deposition was made by ORO staining on 7 μm-thick frozen-liver sections, using Harris haematoxylin for nucleus coloration. The surface of liver lipid droplets was quantified using image J software (1.43, Wayne Rasband, NIH, USA). Lipid droplet volumes were calculated from the surface previously measured by the software. Results were presented as a volume variation relative to the control group.

2.10. Assays

2.10.1. Plasma. Dosage of cholesterol and TG was performed immediately after MR. Plasma levels of total cholesterol (TC), TGs, and high density lipoprotein cholesterol (HDLc) were determined using commercially available kits (BioMérieux, France). Non-HDL cholesterol (Non-HDLc) was calculated by subtraction of HDLc from TC.

2.10.2. Livers TG. Frozen liver tissue (50 mg) was homogenized in SET buffer (1 mL; sucrose 250 mM, EDTA 2 mM, and Tris 10 mM), followed by two freeze-thaw cycles and three times passages through a 27-gauge syringe needle, and a final freeze-thaw cycle. Protein content was determined using the BCA method (Interchim, France), and TG and cholesterol were measured as described above.

2.11. Statistical Analyses. All statistical analyses were performed using StatWiev software (SAS institute Inc., Version 5.0). Data are reported as mean ± standard deviation (SD).The criterion for statistical significance was $P < 0.05$.

Statistical analyses were performed as follows.

(1) When distributions were normal in each group, a Student's t-test was used. If one or more group was not normally distributed, the nonparametric Mann-Whitney was used.

(2) To assess differences on autopsy, MR volumetry, and MRS experimental datasets, we performed ANCOVA tests using mice weight as a covariate in order to adjust statistical analyses and suppress the influence of the weight gain.

(3) For correlations among data, a Spearman test was used.

(4) A two-way ANOVA was performed to test weight gain and food intake.

3. Results

3.1. Risperidone Induced a Long-Term Weight Gain in Mice. After 24 weeks, a greater weight gain was observed in mice treated by risperidone compared to the control mice. At the beginning of the experiment, the mean weight of the risperidone group was 16.75 ± 0.87 g and 16.00 ± 1.04 g for the control group to achieve, respectively, 31.33±2.42 g *versus* 24.58 ± 1.21 g ($P < 0.01$, $n = 24$) at the end of the experiment (Figure 2(a)). In addition, this weight gain was associated with a change in food intake in treated animals from the 13th week (Control: 3.90 ± 0.17 g/day/mouse *versus* Risperidone: 4.43 ± 0.47 g/day/mouse; $P < 0.05$; $n = 24$ Figure 2(b)) as well as with a modification in spontaneous locomotor activity (Table 1). Indeed, the treatment induced a reduction of the distance covered in the arena (Control: 6, 300 ± 687 cm *versus* Risperidone: 5, 041 ± 688 cm $P < 0.001$; $n = 24$; Table 1), in association with a diminution of the mean velocity of animals (Control: 12.11 ± 1.55 cm·s^{-1} *versus* Risperidone: 9.54 ± 1.27 cm·s^{-1}; $P < 0.01$, $n = 24$; Table 1). Moreover, the exploration behaviour was also modified by the treatment as revealed by the reduction of the rearing number (Control: 29.17 ± 10.07 *versus* Risperidone: 65.83 ± 11.68; $P < 0.01$, $n = 24$; Table 1). These results suggest that the risperidone-induced weight gain could at least in part be linked to an increase of appetite combined with a reduced spontaneous locomotor activity.

3.2. Could the Risperidone-Induced Weight Gain Be Associated with Metabolic Disturbances? We sought several metabolic disorders such as glycemic status, blood lipid analysis, and specific biological samples as the liver and fat depositions in order to identify peripheral consequences of the weight gain induced risperidone. The glucose tolerance test revealed that risperidone led to a hyperglycemic status as shown by the glucose tolerance test (Figure 3(a)) and by the area under the curve values (AUC: 27453 ± 2389 (mg/dL·120 min) *versus* 42276 ± 12999 (mg/dL·120 min); $P < 0.01$, $n = 20$; Table 2). Blood analysis showed that risperidone increased the non-HDLc level compared to control mice (26.90 ± 6.73 mg/dL *versus* 18.82 ± 7.61 mg/dL; $P < 0.01$, $n = 24$). But no significant difference was found concerning fasting TG (78.07±30.07 mg/dL *versus* 66.21±11.18 mg/dL, $P = 0.05637$, $n = 24$) and HDLc concentrations (44.20 ± 6.77 mg/dL *versus* 42.59 ± 5.121 mg/dL, $P = 0.8625$, $n = 24$; Figure 3(b)).

To test whether the risperidone treatment modified the fat deposition, we quantified subcutaneous inguinal and visceral fat from anatomic MR images as defined previously (Figure 1). Table 2 summarizes the volumetric analyses. The IAT and VAT volumes were, respectively, 2-fold and 3-fold higher in risperidone-treated mice than in the control group (IAT: 544.19 ± 127.20 mm^3 *versus* 232.40 ± 34.20 mm^3 and VAT: 1065.06 ± 383.76 mm^3 *versus* 317.89 ± 116.79 mm^3; $P < 0.001$, $n = 24$; Table 2). In addition, the best correlation between the adipose tissue accumulation and the glucose tolerance test was interestingly found for the VAT (correlation factor = 0.867, $P < 0.001$, $n = 20$; Table 3), suggesting that VAT could represent a good biomarker of the hyperglycemic status in our experimental model.

At the liver level, the autopsies revealed that risperidone treatment increased the liver weight (1.50 ± 0.17 g *versus* 1.10 ± 0.14 g; $P < 0.001$, $n = 24$; Table 2). This hepatomegaly was confirmed by the volumetric data from MRI, as demonstrated by the significant increase in liver volume after risperidone treatment (702.77 ± 32.01 mm^3 *versus* 635.74 ± 49.54 mm^3; $P < 0.01$, $n = 24$; Table 2). The ORO staining quantification showed a significantly higher lipid accumulation in the liver of mice treated by risperidone than in the control mice (100.00 ± 46.58% *versus* 210.96 ± 68.19%; $P < 0.001$, $n = 21$; Figure 3(c), left panel). Results from hepatic lipid analyses were expressed as the ratio of TG to the protein concentration. The risperidone treatment increased the TG/protein ratio, pointing out an intrahepatic accumulation of TG (0.327 ± 0.096 *versus* 0.225 ± 0.097; $P < 0.05$, $n = 24$; Figure 3(c), right panel). This histological pattern clearly shows an early hepatic steatosis.

3.3. Quantification of the Hepatic Fat by MR Spectroscopy. Spectroscopy can easily distinguish the quantities of water and fat in body tissues. This technique is based on the calculation of the methylene/water ratio (MWR; Figure 4(a)). The MWR values calculated from hepatic spectra were significantly higher in the risperidone-treated group than in the control group (3.57 ± 1.26% *versus* 1.10 ± 0.20%; $P < 0.001$, $n = 24$; Figure 4(a), histogram). This result was in good accordance with the histological pattern, pointing out the high sensitivity of the MRS technique for the detection of fat accumulation in the liver. We drew a correlation between the MWR/TG protein ratio (correlation factor = 0.798, $P < 0.001$, $n = 24$; Table 3) and ORO staining proportion (correlation factor = 0.747, $P < 0.01$, $n = 20$; Table 3), also found proportional to the fat accumulation in the liver.

Table 3 summarizes the link between MRS, MRI, and the postmortem data. We found a strong correlation between MWR/VAT volume (correlation factor = 0.798, $P < 0.001$, $n = 24$; Table 3) and MWR/mice weight (correlation factor = 0.859, $P < 0.001$, $n = 24$; Table 3). These correlations demonstrated a concomitant increase of weight gain, fat accumulation in the liver, and VAT deposition.

3.4. Qualitative Aspects of the Lipid MR Spectrum. Given the limit of 50 Hz for spectral resolution, 4 acquisitions had not been performed, 2 in each group. Therefore, 20 animals were considered in lipid indexes calculations described previously in the methods section and in Figure 1(b). In addition to the liver fat accumulation, the spectral analysis provides information on the realignment of the lipid chains. Compared to the control group, the risperidone treatment had an effect on UIs (Risperidone: 0.156 ± 0.016 *versus* Control: 0.182 ± 0.021; $P < 0.01$, $n = 20$), on SI (Risperidone: 0.844±0.016 *versus* Control: 0.818 ± 0.021; $P < 0.05$, $n = 20$), and on PUI (Risperidone: 0.017 ± 0.008 *versus* Control: 0.047 ± 0.023; $P < 0.001$, $n = 20$) as illustrated in Figure 4(b). The decrease in PUI and the concomitant increase in SI suggest a pathological state of the fatty acid availability in a suffering liver. The aggravation of hepatic steatosis was proportional to the decrease in PUI values. In our model, we found a closed correlation between PUI and mice weight (correlation factor = −0.868, $P < 0.001$, $n = 20$; Table 3).

4. Discussion

Two aspects are addressed in this study: first, our experimental model, which gradually developed a metabolic disturbance pattern associated with a long-term risperidone treatment, and second, our methodology, based on magnetic resonance, which evidenced that these noninvasive techniques were suitable for the detection of body fat alterations and the resulting hepatic steatosis.

In our experimental mouse model, the risperidone treatment induced a weight gain after 24 weeks. We concomitantly described here components of the metabolic syndrome [5] in mice treated by risperidone. Treated mice developed (i) a hyperglycemic status, (ii) an increase in non-HDL cholesterol plasma level, (iii) an abnormal deposition of fat in the inguinal and visceral areas, and (iv) a hepatomegaly related with early hepatic steatosis. The other advantages

TABLE 1: Spontaneous locomotor activity.

Data sets	Control group n	Control group Mean ± SD	Risperidone group n	Risperidone group Mean ± SD	Significance
Distance (cm)	12	6300 ± 687	12	5041 ± 688	S ($P < 0.001$)
Mean velocity (cm·s^{-1})	12	12.11 ± 1.55	12	9.54 ± 1.27	S ($P < 0.001$)
Numbers of rearing	12	65.83 ± 11.68	12	29.17 ± 10.07	S ($P < 0.001$)

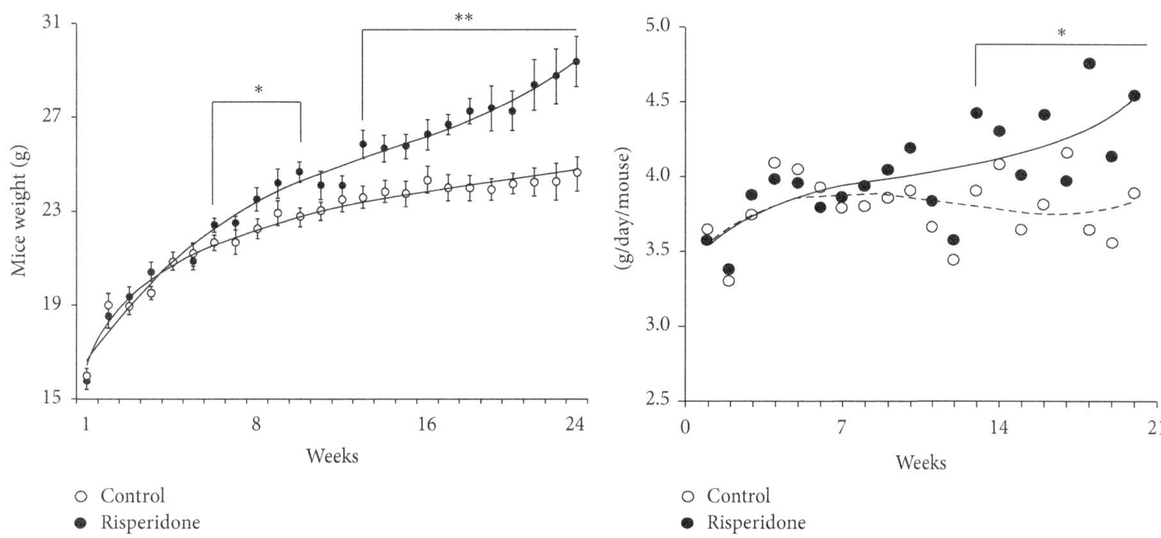

(a) Weight gain

(b) Food intake

FIGURE 2: Twenty-four week risperidone treatment increased mice weight and food intake. (a) Effect of risperidone on weight gain in female mice. Differences between both groups appeared significant after 7 weeks of treatment and remained significant at the end of the experiment (24 weeks: control (◦) 24.58 ± 1.21 g *versus* risperidone (•) 31.33 ± 2.42 g; $P < 0.01$, $n = 24$). (b) Effect of risperidone on food intake. Risperidone treatment increased food intake after 13 weeks (Control: 3.90 ± 0.17 g/day/mouse *versus* Risperidone: 4.43 ± 0.47 g/day/mouse $P < 0.05$; $n = 24$).

TABLE 2: Experimental parameters analysis.

Data Sets		Control group n	Control group Mean ± SD	Risperidone group n	Risperidone group Mean ± SD	Significance
AUC (mg/dL·120 min)		10	27,453 ± 2,389	10	42,276 ± 12,999	S ($P < 0.001$)
Tissue weight (g)	Liver	12	1.10 ± 0.14	12	1.50 ± 0.17	S ($P < 0.001$)
Tissue volume (mm^3)	Liver	12	635.74 ± 49.54	12	702.77 ± 32.01	S ($P < 0.01$)
	IAT	12	232.40 ± 34.20	12	544.19 ± 127.20	S ($P < 0.001$)
	VAT	12	317.89 ± 116.78	12	1,065.06 ± 383.76	S ($P < 0.001$)

TABLE 3: Correlations.

Correlations		n	R^2	Correlation factor	Significance
AUC/tissue volume	Liver	20	0.080	0.406	NS
	VAT	20	0.349	0.867	S ($P < 0.001$)
	IAT	20	0.269	0.772	S ($P < 0.001$)
MWR/hepatic lipid assay	TG/protein	24	0.440	0.798	S ($P < 0.001$)
	ORO staining	20	0.695	0.747	S ($P < 0.01$)
MWR/VAT		24	0.610	0.798	S ($P < 0.001$)
MWR/mice weight		24	0.651	0.859	S ($P < 0.001$)
MWR/AUC		20	0.611	0.798	S ($P < 0.001$)
PUI/mice weight		20	0.399	−0.868	S ($P < 0.001$)

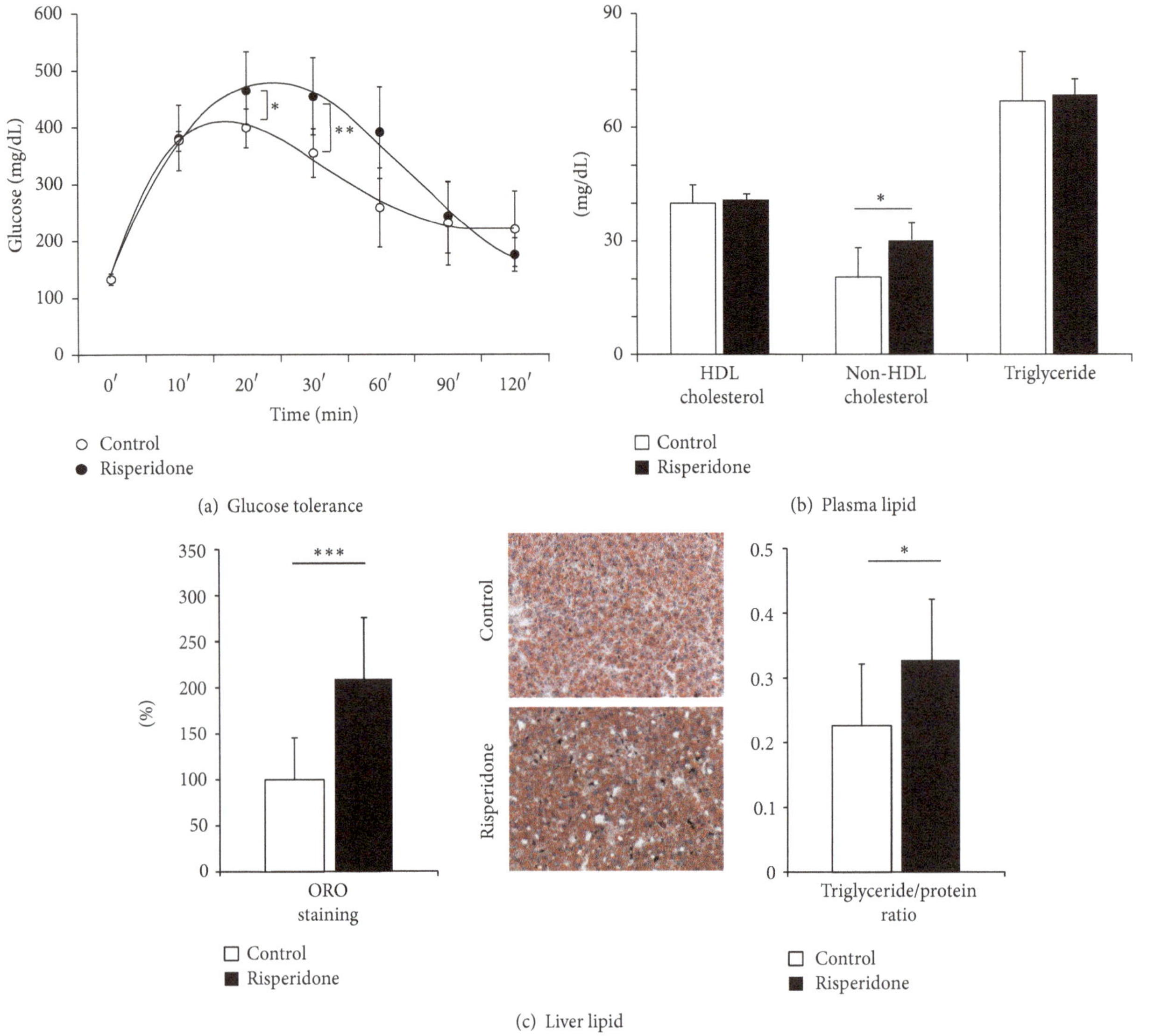

FIGURE 3: Metabolic disturbances induced by a 24-week treatment of risperidone on female mice. (a) Effect of risperidone on glucose tolerance in female mice. Risperidone treatment significantly decreased glucose tolerance. (b) Effect of risperidone on plasma lipid concentration. Risperidone treatment increased non-HDLc (26.90 ± 6.73 mg/dL *versus* 18.82 ± 7.61 mg/dL; $P < 0.01$, $n = 24$). (c) Effect of risperidone on liver fat accumulation. Risperidone treatment induced an increase in liver lipid accumulation as displayed by ORO staining (control (□) 100.00 ± 46.58% *versus* risperidone (■) 210.96 ± 68.19%; $P < 0.05$, $n = 21$; left histogram and central pictures) and TG/protein ratio (control (□) 0.225 ± 0.097 *versus* risperidone (■) 0.327 ± 0.096; $P < 0.05$, $n = 24$; right histogram).

of this model are based on the risperidone-induced change in behaviour of the animal in terms of food intake and spontaneous locomotor activity. Several pieces of evidence support the idea that ADPs-induced weight gain would result from an increase in appetite self-mediated by a histaminic pathway at the CNS level [37]. Furthermore, risperidone could reduce locomotor activity by blocking the dopaminergic system [38, 39]. All these aspects highlight the relevance of our experimental model for the study of metabolic dark-side effects of ADPs.

The second aspect of this study is the use of noninvasive MR techniques. The volumetric analysis was performed through the use of T1-weighted imaging and was allowed the quantification of fat deposition in subcutaneous and visceral areas. Our findings showed a closed correlation between VAT and hyperglycemic status, in good accordance with clinical evidences suggesting a link between the prevalence of metabolic syndrome and an abnormal visceral adiposity [6]. This is why the different components of fat had to be distinguished. Previous clinical works reported that the abnormal VAT development led to lipid storage in undesired sites such as pancreas, skeletal muscle, heart, and liver [6, 7, 12]. In this study, we assessed the liver fat quantity reflected by MWR using MR spectroscopy and established a link between the mice being overweight, the increase in VAT, and liver fat deposition. These findings demonstrated that the MR

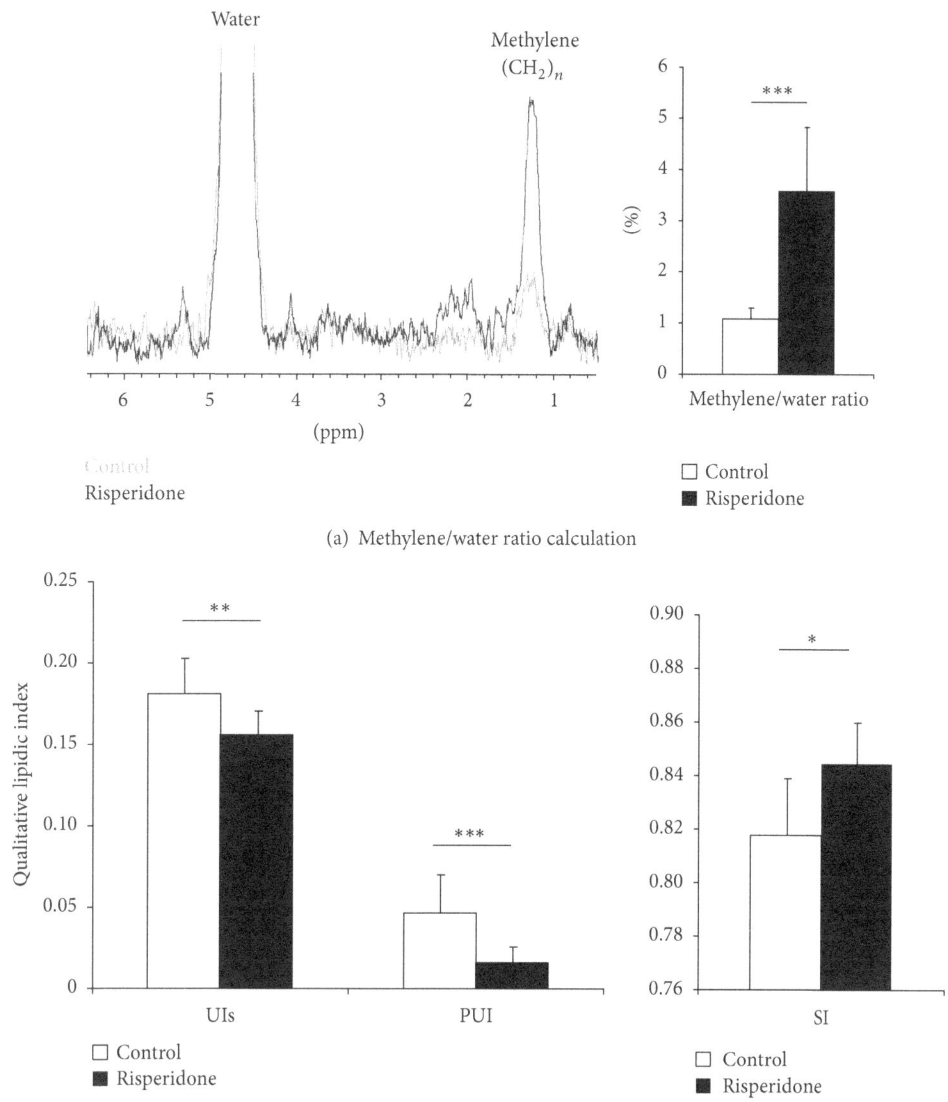

(a) Methylene/water ratio calculation

(b) Lipidic chain saturation indexes

FIGURE 4: Quantitative and qualitative *in vivo* lipid assessments. (a) Representative of water suppressed MR liver spectra (left; control: grey spectrum; risperidone: black spectrum). Spectra resulted from a voxel analysis positioned in liver as described in Figure 1(b). Water and methylene peaks were clearly visible and enabled the assessment of the methylene water ratio (MWR). MWR revealed that risperidone treatment increased the lipid accumulation in liver (right histogram: control (□) 1.10 ± 0.20% *versus* risperidone (■) 3.57 ± 1.26%; $P < 0.001$, $n = 24$). (b) Unsaturated Index surrogate (UIs), Poly Unsaturated Index (PUI), and Saturated Index (SI) reflecting the hepatic lipid composition. Compared to control mice, risperidone significantly induced an increase in UIs (control (□) 0.156 ± 0.016 *versus* risperidone (■) 0.182 ± 0.021; $P < 0.01$, $n = 20$), in SI (control (□) 0.844 ± 0.016 *versus* risperidone (■) 0.818 ± 0.021; $P < 0.05$, $n = 20$), and a decrease in PUI (control (□) 0.047 ± 0.023 *versus* risperidone (■) 0.017 ± 0.008; $P < 0.001$, $n = 20$).

methods constituted an accurate tool to study the possible fat reallocation from peripheral adipose tissue to the liver as suggested by clinical observations [40]. An interesting feature in our use of spectroscopy was the relatively low fat quantity in our model (MWR = 3.57 ± 1.26%) compared to other experimental models such as obese mice (ob/ob) or methionine choline deficient diet mice displaying a high fat level, respectively, MWR = 38% and MWR = 31% [41].

The low concentration of liver fat makes the hepatic steatosis difficult to diagnose by MR techniques. Clinical and preclinical studies showed modifications in nature and proportion of fatty acids in a suffering liver [42, 43]. The pathogenesis of steatohepatitis involves, at least in part, an oxidative process explaining the decrease in the PUFA level in steatotic liver. Indeed, assumptions indicate that polyunsaturated moieties within phospholipid membranes, the (n-3) species in particular, are most susceptible to free radical attacks leading to a reallocation of unsaturations [44, 45]. Using chromatographic techniques, two major markers have been identified as relevant for characterizing steatosis: the increase in saturated fatty acids and the depletion of polyunsaturated fatty acids [42, 46]. In our study, to validate the potential presence of this pathology, a water suppressed spectroscopy sequence was performed to estimate saturated and unsaturated fatty acid proportions. Compared to the control group, our spectrum analysis highlighted a significant decrease in PUI and an increase in SI in risperidone-treated mice. This result is in good agreement with previous works in which a similar variation of PUI was reported on obese patients with hepatic steatosis. This study concluded that hepatic steatosis potentiated the decrease in PUI [36]. Despite our less severe experimental model than an obesity model, our results clearly showed that the high sensitivity of the MR techniques enabled the diagnosis of early hepatic steatosis, as shown by the different correlations with PUI and MWR.

Nevertheless, these techniques have their own limitations, especially when the target organ for instance liver is subjected to respiratory motion. Although respiratory gating improves the quality of acquisitions, residual breathing artifacts may yield to uncertainty in amplitude and phase variations in localized MR spectra. These artifacts may induce bias on the spectral resolution which is dependent on the homogenization of the magnetic field (shim), and consequently modify the calculation of saturation/unsaturation indices. To minimize breathing artifacts, the ideal condition should define a TR value as close as possible to the steady state duration of breathing. Nevertheless, the use of low TR values leads to a T1-weighting at the expense of the signal/noise ratio. Compromisingly, we selected a high TR value to promote the signal/noise ratio. The magnetic field strength represents also a parameter which conditions a good signal/noise ratio, but depends only on the properties of the machine. The arrival of 3 T magnets for patients in clinical practice and 7 T magnets for clinical research may promote the use of these noninvasive techniques for diagnosis assistance through optimized signal/noise ratio and acquisition time.

Although our experimental model is far from obesity models, the subtle metabolic disturbances observed here demonstrated that MR approaches leave the opportunity to evaluate consequences of the risperidone treatment. We highlight three noninvasive markers to predict metabolic disturbances and hepatic steatosis severity when critical limits are reached and exceeded: mice weight up to 26 g, MWR up to 2.5%, and PUI down to 0.17. As a perspective to improve health conditions of schizophrenic patients, this experimental approach (model and methodology) could represent a relevant tool to (i) define the best effective dose of ADPs to maintain CNS effects and minimize metabolic dark-side effects; (ii) evaluate the benefit of a functional food such as dietaries supplemented with omega-3 [47] or curcuminoids [48]; (iii) develop new drugs through the validation of new therapeutic strategies using an active principle or a new pharmacological adjuvant targeting the CNS or not, in a view to reduce metabolic disturbances.

5. Conclusion

In this study, we proposed a pathophysiologic model of slight metabolic disturbances induced by a long-term risperidone treatment, which have been evaluated *in vivo* by MR methods. Three parameters have been selected: MWR, PUI, and mice weight as reliable factors to define the severity of the disturbances. Thus, our model and methodology offer the possibility to investigate APDs side effects more precisely, in order to improve health conditions of schizophrenic patients.

Conflict of Interests

The authors declare that there is no conflict of interests regarding the publication of this paper.

Acknowledgments

The authors would like to thank Anthony Lucas for his technical assistance in histology, Emmanuelle Vallez for her technical contribution to chemical assays, Camille Potey for her helpful assistance in animal autopsies, and Julia Salleron for her statistical analyses contribution (Department of Biostatistic, CHU Lille, EA 2694, Univ Lille Nord de France, F-59000 Lille, France). To end, The authors would like to thank Vincent Bérézowski for his helpful assistance in the English editing of the paper. The research leading to these results has received funding from the "Conseil regional du Nord-Pas-de-Calais," the "Fond Européen de DEveloppement Régional" (FEDER), and the ministry of "Recherche et de l'Enseignement Supérieur."

References

[1] M. de Hert, J. Detraux, R. van Winkel, W. Yu, and C. U. Correll, "Metabolic and cardiovascular adverse effects associated with antipsychotic drugs," *Nature Reviews Endocrinology*, vol. 8, no. 2, pp. 114–126, 2012.

[2] J. A. Lieberman, T. S. Stroup, J. P. McEvoy et al., "Effectiveness of antipsychotic drugs in patients with chronic schizophrenia," *The New England Journal of Medicine*, vol. 353, no. 12, pp. 1209–1223, 2005.

[3] W. W. Fleischhacker, R. D. McQuade, R. N. Marcus, D. Archibald, R. Swanink, and W. H. Carson, "A double-blind, randomized comparative study of aripiprazole and olanzapine in patients with schizophrenia," *Biological Psychiatry*, vol. 65, no. 6, pp. 510–517, 2009.

[4] C. U. Correll, J. M. Kane, and P. Manu, "Obesity and coronary risk in patients treated with second-generation antipsychotics," *European Archives of Psychiatry and Clinical Neuroscience*, vol. 261, no. 6, pp. 417–423, 2011.

[5] K. G. M. M. Alberti and P. Zimmet, "Metabolic syndrome—a new world-wide definition. A consensus statement from the International Diabetes Federation," *Diabetic Medicine*, vol. 23, no. 5, pp. 469–480, 2006.

[6] N. Rasouli, B. Molavi, S. C. Elbein, and P. A. Kern, "Ectopic fat accumulation and metabolic syndrome," *Diabetes, Obesity and Metabolism*, vol. 9, no. 1, pp. 1–10, 2007.

[7] B. J. Arsenault, E. P. Beaumont, J. P. Despres, and E. Larose, "Mapping body fat distribution: a key step towards the identification of the vulnerable patient?" *Annals of Medicine*, vol. 44, pp. 758–772, 2011.

[8] D. B. Carr, K. M. Utzschneider, R. L. Hull et al., "Intra-abdominal fat is a major determinant of the National Cholesterol Education Program Adult Treatment Panel III criteria for the metabolic syndrome," *Diabetes*, vol. 53, no. 8, pp. 2087–2094, 2004.

[9] C. S. Fox, J. M. Massaro, U. Hoffmann et al., "Abdominal visceral and subcutaneous adipose tissue compartments: association with metabolic risk factors in the Framingham Heart Study," *Circulation*, vol. 116, no. 1, pp. 39–48, 2007.

[10] S. R. Smith, J. C. Lovejoy, F. Greenway et al., "Contributions of total body fat, abdominal subcutaneous adipose tissue compartments, and visceral adipose tissue to the metabolic complications of obesity," *Metabolism*, vol. 50, no. 4, pp. 425–435, 2001.

[11] J. Tong, E. J. Boyko, K. M. Utzschneider et al., "Intra-abdominal fat accumulation predicts the development of the metabolic syndrome in non-diabetic Japanese-Americans," *Diabetologia*, vol. 50, no. 6, pp. 1156–1160, 2007.

[12] J.-P. Després and I. Lemieux, "Abdominal obesity and metabolic syndrome," *Nature*, vol. 444, no. 7121, pp. 881–887, 2006.

[13] A. S. Jackson and M. L. Pollock, "Steps towards the development of generalized equations for predicting body composition of adults," *Canadian Journal of Applied Sport Sciences*, vol. 7, no. 3, pp. 189–196, 1982.

[14] K. J. Ellis, "Human body composition: in vivo methods," *Physiological Reviews*, vol. 80, no. 2, pp. 649–680, 2000.

[15] S. Mattsson and B. J. Thomas, "Development of methods for body composition studies," *Physics in Medicine and Biology*, vol. 51, no. 13, pp. R203–R228, 2006.

[16] N. Abate, A. Garg, R. Coleman, S. M. Grundy, and R. M. Peshock, "Prediction of total subcutaneous abdominal, intraperitoneal, and retroperitoneal adipose tissue masses in men by a single axial magnetic resonance imaging slice," *American Journal of Clinical Nutrition*, vol. 65, no. 2, pp. 403–408, 1997.

[17] J. L. Lancaster, A. A. Ghiatas, A. Alyassin, R. F. Kilcoyne, E. Bonora, and R. A. DeFronzo, "Measurement of abdominal fat with T1-weighted MR images," *Journal of Magnetic Resonance Imaging*, vol. 1, no. 3, pp. 363–369, 1991.

[18] J. Kullberg, J. Brandberg, J.-E. Angelhed et al., "Whole-body adipose tissue analysis: comparison of MRI, CT and dual energy X-ray absorptiometry," *British Journal of Radiology*, vol. 82, no. 974, pp. 123–130, 2009.

[19] J. Berglund, L. Johansson, H. Ahlström, and J. Kullberg, "Three-point Dixon method enables whole-body water and fat imaging of obese subjects," *Magnetic Resonance in Medicine*, vol. 63, no. 6, pp. 1659–1668, 2010.

[20] H. Kvist, L. Sjostrom, and U. Tylen, "Adipose tissue volume determinations in women by computed tomography: technical considerations," *International Journal of Obesity*, vol. 10, no. 1, pp. 53–67, 1986.

[21] J. C. Seidell, C. J. G. Bakker, and K. van der Kooy, "Imaging techniques for measuring adipose-tissue distribution—a comparison between computed tomography and 1.5-T magnetic resonance," *American Journal of Clinical Nutrition*, vol. 51, no. 6, pp. 953–957, 1990.

[22] G. Brix, S. Heiland, M. E. Bellemann, T. Koch, and W. J. Lorenz, "MR imaging of fat-containing tissues: valuation of two quantitative imaging techniques in comparison with localized proton spectroscopy," *Magnetic Resonance Imaging*, vol. 11, no. 7, pp. 977–991, 1993.

[23] B. H. Goodpaster, V. A. Stenger, F. Boada et al., "Skeletal muscle lipid concentration quantified by magnetic resonance imaging," *American Journal of Clinical Nutrition*, vol. 79, no. 5, pp. 748–754, 2004.

[24] F. Schick, J. Machann, K. Brechtel et al., "MRI of muscular fat," *Magnetic Resonance in Medicine*, vol. 47, no. 4, pp. 720–727, 2002.

[25] E. L. Thomas, G. Hamilton, N. Patel et al., "Hepatic triglyceride content and its relation to body adiposity: a magnetic resonance imaging and proton magnetic resonance spectroscopy study," *Gut*, vol. 54, no. 1, pp. 122–127, 2005.

[26] H. H. Hu, K. S. Nayak, and M. I. Goran, "Assessment of abdominal adipose tissue and organ fat content by magnetic resonance imaging," *Obesity Reviews*, vol. 12, no. 501, pp. e504–e515, 2011.

[27] R. Ross, B. Goodpaster, D. Kelley, and F. Boada, "Magnetic resonance imaging in human body composition research. From quantitative to qualitative tissue measurement," *Annals of the New York Academy of Sciences*, vol. 904, pp. 12–17, 2000.

[28] S. B. Reeder, I. Cruite, G. Hamilton, and C. B. Sirlin, "Quantitative assessment of liver fat with magnetic resonance imaging and spectroscopy," *Journal of Magnetic Resonance Imaging*, vol. 34, no. 4, pp. 729–749, 2011.

[29] L. Wilhelm Poll, H.-J. Wittsack, J.-A. Koch et al., "A rapid and reliable semiautomated method for measurement of total abdominal fat volumes using magnetic resonance imaging," *Magnetic Resonance Imaging*, vol. 21, no. 6, pp. 631–636, 2003.

[30] A. P. Levene, H. Kudo, M. J. Armstrong et al., "Quantifying hepatic steatosis—more than meets the eye," *Histopathology*, vol. 60, no. 6, pp. 971–981, 2012.

[31] E. Lauressergues, F. Martin, A. Helleboid et al., "Overweight induced by chronic risperidone exposure is correlated with overexpression of the SREBP-1c and FAS genes in mouse liver," *Naunyn-Schmiedeberg's Archives of Pharmacology*, vol. 383, no. 4, pp. 423–436, 2011.

[32] P. A. Yushkevich, J. Piven, H. C. Hazlett et al., "User-guided 3D active contour segmentation of anatomical structures: significantly improved efficiency and reliability," *NeuroImage*, vol. 31, no. 3, pp. 1116–1128, 2006.

[33] L. S. Szczepaniak, P. Nurenberg, D. Leonard et al., "Magnetic resonance spectroscopy to measure hepatic triglyceride content: prevalence of hepatic steatosis in the general population," *American Journal of Physiology—Endocrinology and Metabolism*, vol. 288, no. 2, pp. E462–E468, 2005.

[34] R. Deslauriers, R. L. Somorjai, Y. Geoffrion, T. Kroft, I. C. Smith, and J. K. Saunders, "1H and 13C NMR studies of tissue from normal and diseased mice. Analysis of T1 and T2 relaxation profiles of triglycerides in liver," *NMR in Biomedicine*, vol. 1, no. 1, pp. 32–43, 1988.

[35] J. Ren, I. Dimitrov, A. D. Sherry, and C. R. Malloy, "Composition of adipose tissue and marrow fat in humans by 1H NMR at 7 Tesla," *Journal of Lipid Research*, vol. 49, no. 9, pp. 2055–2062, 2008.

[36] N. A. Johnson, D. W. Walton, T. Sachinwalla et al., "Noninvasive assessment of hepatic lipid composition: advancing understanding and management of fatty liver disorders," *Hepatology*, vol. 47, no. 5, pp. 1513–1523, 2008.

[37] S. F. Kim, A. S. Huang, A. M. Snowman, C. Teuscher, and S. H. Snyder, "Antipsychotic drug-induced weight gain mediated by histamine H1 receptor-linked activation of hypothalamic AMP-kinase," *Proceedings of the National Academy of Sciences of the United States of America*, vol. 104, no. 9, pp. 3456–3459, 2007.

[38] M. Rodríguez-Arias, I. Broseta, M. A. Aguilar, and J. Miñarro, "Lack of specific effects of selective D1 and D2 dopamine antagonists vs. risperidone on morphine-induced hyperactivity," *Pharmacology Biochemistry and Behavior*, vol. 66, no. 1, pp. 189–197, 2000.

[39] J. Arnt, "Differential effects of classical and newer antipsychotics on the hypermotility induced by two dose levels of D-amphetamine," *European Journal of Pharmacology*, vol. 283, no. 1-3, pp. 55–62, 1995.

[40] H. E. Bays, "Adiposopathy: is "sick fat" a cardiovascular disease?" *Journal of the American College of Cardiology*, vol. 57, no. 25, pp. 2461–2473, 2011.

[41] I. R. Corbin, E. E. Furth, S. Pickup, E. S. Siegelman, and E. J. Delikatny, "In vivo assessment of hepatic triglycerides in murine non-alcoholic fatty liver disease using magnetic resonance spectroscopy," *Biochimica et Biophysica Acta*, vol. 1791, no. 8, pp. 757–763, 2009.

[42] J. Araya, R. Rodrigo, L. A. Videla et al., "Increase in long-chain polyunsaturated fatty acid n-6/n-3 ratio in relation to hepatic steatosis in patients with non-alcoholic fatty liver disease," *Clinical Science*, vol. 106, no. 6, pp. 635–643, 2004.

[43] L. A. Videla, R. Rodrigo, J. Araya, and J. Poniachik, "Oxidative stress and depletion of hepatic long-chain polyunsaturated fatty acids may contribute to nonalcoholic fatty liver disease," *Free Radical Biology and Medicine*, vol. 37, no. 9, pp. 1499–1507, 2004.

[44] J. H. Song, K. Fujimoto, and T. Miyazawa, "Polyunsaturated (n-3) fatty acids susceptible to peroxidation are increased in plasma and tissue lipids of rats fed docosahexaenoic acid-containing oils," *Journal of Nutrition*, vol. 130, no. 12, pp. 3028–3033, 2000.

[45] J. H. Song and T. Miyazawa, "Enhanced level of n-3 fatty acid in membrane phospholipids induces lipid peroxidation in rats fed dietary docosahexaenoic acid oil," *Atherosclerosis*, vol. 155, no. 1, pp. 9–18, 2001.

[46] P. Puri, R. A. Baillie, M. M. Wiest et al., "A lipidomic analysis of nonalcoholic fatty liver disease," *Hepatology*, vol. 46, no. 4, pp. 1081–1090, 2007.

[47] C. P. F. Marinangeli and P. J. H. Jones, "Functional food ingredients as adjunctive therapies to pharmacotherapy for treating disorders of metabolic syndrome," *Annals of Medicine*, vol. 42, no. 5, pp. 317–333, 2010.

[48] A. Sahebkar, "Why it is necessary to translate curcumin into clinical practice for the prevention and treatment of metabolic syndrome?" *Biofactors*, vol. 39, no. 2, pp. 197–208, 2012.

12

Schizophrenia and Suicide Attempts: Findings from a Representative Community-Based Canadian Sample

Esme Fuller-Thomson and Bailey Hollister

Factor-Inwentash Faculty of Social Work, University of Toronto, Toronto, ON, Canada M5S 1V4

Correspondence should be addressed to Esme Fuller-Thomson; esme.fuller.thomson@utoronto.ca

Academic Editor: L. Citrome

This study examined factors associated with suicide attempts among those with schizophrenia (n = 101) versus those without (n = 21,643) in a representative sample of noninstitutionalized Canadians. The lifetime prevalence of suicide attempts among persons with schizophrenia was 39.2% versus 2.8% of nonafflicted individuals. After adjusting for sociodemographics, childhood adversities, substance abuse/dependence, depression/anxiety, and chronic pain, those with schizophrenia had 6 times the odds (OR = 6.47) of attempting suicide. Among persons with schizophrenia, suicide attempts were associated with female gender (OR = 4.59), substance abuse/dependence (OR = 6.31), depression (OR = 4.93), and childhood physical abuse (OR = 5.75). Community-dwelling persons with schizophrenia appear to be at high risk for suicide attempts.

1. Introduction

In conjunction with the complexities and difficulties of the symptoms of schizophrenia, individuals with schizophrenia are more likely to attempt suicide than those without schizophrenia [1]. The prevalence of lifetime suicide attempts in those with schizophrenia ranges from 20% to 40% [2–6]. A meta-analysis estimated that one in every 20 individuals with schizophrenia will commit suicide [7]. The average age at suicide is younger among those with schizophrenia than those without the disorder [8]. It is unclear whether men or women with schizophrenia are more likely to attempt suicide with some sources stating that men and women are equally likely [9] while others indicate that women with schizophrenia are more likely to attempt suicide as compared to men with schizophrenia [10]. As will be elaborated below, the direct relationship between schizophrenia and suicide attempts may be attenuated when adjusting for several factors including socioeconomic status, pain, substance use, depression, anxiety, and early adversities.

The evidence concerning the relationship between schizophrenia and socioeconomic status (SES) is mixed [11]. Some studies have demonstrated that growing up in a low income home is associated with increased rates of schizophrenia [12, 13]. In contrast, other studies report an association between growing up in a higher income home and increased rates of schizophrenia [11, 14]. Higher levels of education have been associated with a greater likelihood of suicide completion among those with schizophrenia [15]. The association between social class and suicide completion amongst those with schizophrenia is inconclusive with some studies indicating high social class as a risk factor, while others find homelessness as a risk factor [15].

It is well documented that individuals with schizophrenia experience pain differently compared to the general population [16, 17]. A systematic review found that when there is a clear medical cause for pain, individuals with schizophrenia report a lower prevalence and intensity of pain as compared to the general population [17]. Other studies, both experimental and population-based, support the idea that individuals with schizophrenia experience a decrease in pain sensitivity [16, 18].

A strong association between substance abuse disorders and schizophrenia has been documented [19, 20]. Almost half of Americans with schizophrenia have had some form of substance abuse disorder [21]. A systematic review indicated that for individuals with schizophrenia, alcohol and drug misuse increased the risk of suicide [15].

Symptoms of depression and anxiety are common among individuals with schizophrenia [15, 22, 23]. It is estimated that approximately 50% of individuals with schizophrenia also experience comorbid depression [24]. As in the general population, individuals with schizophrenia who experience depressive symptoms have an increased risk of suicide [5, 15]. A recent systematic review estimated that one in ten (9.8%) of those with schizophrenia had Generalized Anxiety Disorder (GAD) [23]. In the schizophrenia population, individuals with a concurrent social anxiety disorder are more likely to have attempted suicide and to have a greater lethality of suicide attempts than those with schizophrenia without an anxiety disorder [25]. In addition, suicide among those with schizophrenia seems to be less likely a reaction to life events as compared to those without schizophrenia [26].

Early physical, emotional, and sexual abuse, as well as neglect, have been associated with the development of adult onset psychosis and schizophrenia [27–29]. In a systematic review, childhood adversity was indicated as a risk factor for the development of schizophrenia as compared to nonpsychiatric populations [28]. Physical and emotional abuse in childhood are also significantly associated with the development of disassociation symptoms in patients with schizophrenia and psychotic disorders [29]. Patients with schizophrenia who have a history of child maltreatment can experience worse peer relationships, difficulties in school, and more hospital visits at younger ages than those with schizophrenia without a history of child maltreatment [30]. Possibly because of these issues, those with schizophrenia who were maltreated in childhood are more likely than individuals without a history of maltreatment to express intentions of suicide and report depressive symptoms [30]. Childhood trauma in individuals with schizophrenia is associated with an increase in suicide attempts [31, 32], which is similar to findings of studies of the general population [33].

There are several gaps in the current literature. Most studies attempt to understand the relationship between suicidal behaviors and schizophrenia using clinical samples [4, 31, 34, 35]. Studies using representative samples of community dwellers are important too because they can provide information about individuals with schizophrenia who are relatively high functioning, rather than focusing only on those who are institutionalized and tend to be at the more extreme end of the illness continuum. However, the few population-based studies that do exist often use data from outside of North America [36, 37]. One Canadian population-based study found that schizophrenia is associated with an increased risk of suicide, particularly within the first 90 days of diagnosis [38]. An increased risk of suicide in those with schizophrenia has also been demonstrated immediately after discharge from hospitals [39].

A few population-based studies have been conducted with those diagnosed with schizophrenia outside of North America. For example, a Danish cohort study found that low birth weight, low IQ, and low socioeconomic status are associated with the development of psychiatric illnesses as well as drug and alcohol abuse in men later in life [40]. This drug and alcohol abuse was related to poorer survival rates [40]. A population-based study in Denmark found that younger people (<35) were most at risk for suicide as compared to other age categories [41]. This was true for both genders [41]. A Swedish population-based study concerning violent behavior and suicide indicated that, for men, alcohol use, drug use, previous self-harm, and previous violent offenses all increased suicide risk [42]. For women, self-harm was found to be associated with an increased suicide risk [42].

Another gap in the literature is that most studies analyze suicide risk, suicidal ideation, or suicide in general [1, 15, 43] and, thus, there is less known about suicide attempts, which are strongly associated with both future attempts and completed suicides [1, 3, 34]. To our knowledge, no studies have examined the role of witnessing parental domestic violence and its relationship to schizophrenia and suicide attempts. As witnessing domestic violence has been associated with several negative outcomes in adults, research to better understand its role and relationship to schizophrenia and suicide attempts is needed [44]. Our hypotheses are as follows: (1) noninstitutionalized people with schizophrenia will have higher odds of suicide attempts than those without the disorder, and this association will be partially attenuated when adverse childhood experiences, sociodemographics, and mental health and substance abuse are accounted for in the analysis and (2) among community-dwellers with schizophrenia the odds of suicide attempts will be associated with each of the three types of childhood adversity (childhood physical abuse, childhood sexual abuse, and witnessing parental domestic violence), substance abuse, depression, and anxiety disorders.

2. Methods

Data from the 2012 Canadian Community Health Survey-Mental Health (CCHS-MH) were analyzed in the current study. The CCHS-MH is a cross-sectional survey that collects information about the factors, influences, and processes that contribute to mental health through a multidisciplinary approach focusing on health, social, and economic determinants [45]. While the survey covers the population of individuals at age of 15 and older living in the 10 provinces, residents of the three territories, those living on reserves or other aboriginal settlements, full-time members of the armed forces, and the institutionalized population were excluded. The latter groups represent less than 3% of the target population [45].

2.1. Sample. Respondents for the CCHS-MH were sampled using a three-stage design, which began with selecting individuals from geographical areas and then households within each geographical area. Out of all eligible respondents, one individual within each household was randomly selected according to varying selection probabilities [45]. Based on the selected units, 36,443 were in-scope for the survey and, of these, 29,088 households agreed to participate in the survey, resulting in an overall household-level response rate of 79.8%. From responding households, 29,088 persons were selected to participate and 25,113 provided a valid questionnaire, which yielded an overall person-level response rate of 86.3%. At the national level, these figures result in a combined response rate of 68.9%.

The analysis for the current study is based on two subsamples of the full CCHS-MH. More specifically, the first analysis was restricted to those with complete data on each of the measures in the analyses (n = 21,744). It only contains respondents at age of 20 and older because younger respondents were not asked questions about adverse childhood experiences. The second analysis was a subsample of the first analysis restricted to respondents who reported that they had been diagnosed with schizophrenia (n = 101).

2.2. Measures. Schizophrenia was assessed based upon a list of "conditions diagnosed by a health professional that are expected to last or have already lasted 6 months or more." Those with a positive response to the question "do you have schizophrenia?" were coded as such.

Suicide attempt was ascertained by a positive response to the question: Have you ever "attempted suicide or tried to take your own life?" The questions were found in a section of the CCHS-MH that focuses specifically on suicide and beginning with a statement that "the questions may be sensitive to some people, but we have to ask the same questions of everyone."

Sociodemographic variables include gender, self-identified race (nonaboriginal White versus visible minority and/or aboriginal), age (in decades), and *Socioeconomic Position* (SEP) measured by the highest level of achieved education (less than high school, high school graduate, some postsecondary school, postsecondary diploma, or university degree). Statistics Canada's measure of household income as a ratio related to the national low-income cut-off, divided into deciles, was also used to assess SEP. This variable takes into account the number of people in the household and the size of the community.

Adverse Childhood Experiences (ACEs) included the following.

(i) Witnessing Parental Domestic Violence (PDV). Individuals were determined as having been exposed to intimate partner violence if they reported they had seen or heard 11 or more times one of their "parents, step-parents, or guardians hit each other or another adult" aged 18 or over in their home.

(ii) Childhood Sexual Abuse (CSA). Childhood sexual abuse was measured by the question "How many times did an adult force you or attempt to force you into any unwanted sexual activity, by threatening you, holding you down, or hurting you in some way?" This variable was coded never versus ever.

(iii) Childhood Physical Abuse (CPA). Individuals were ascertained as having been physically abused if they reported that, before they reached the age of 16, an adult had at least once kicked, bit, punch, choked, burned, or physically attacked them.

Mental health factors include lifetime anxiety and depression. Individuals were coded as having an anxiety disorder if they met the WHO-CIDI lifetime criteria for Generalized Anxiety Disorder. Similarly, respondents were ascertained as a depressive disorder if they met the WHO-CIDI lifetime criteria for Major Depressive Episode. For more details please see [45].

Chronic pain was assessed in a section of the survey focusing on pain and discomfort that began with the following statement: the next set of questions asks about the level of pain or discomfort you usually experience. They are not about illnesses like colds that affect people for short periods of time. Respondents were determined to be regularly in pain if they responded no to the question "Are you usually free of pain or discomfort?"

Substance abuse was measured based on the WHO-CIDI using a combination of the derived variables created by Statistics Canada "Drug Abuse or Dependence (including Cannabis)" and "Alcohol Abuse or Dependence." Both were derived using the lifetime algorithm. For more information, please see the Canadian Community Health Survey (CCHS) mental health derived variable specifications [45].

2.3. Statistical Analyses. The lifetime prevalence of suicide attempts among those with schizophrenia was calculated in SPSS 22. Chi-square analysis was conducted to examine gender difference in the lifetime prevalence of suicide attempts among those with and without schizophrenia. Two series of logistic regression analyses were conducted. In the first series of analyses, the outcome was lifetime suicide attempt and the key exposure variable was schizophrenia status. The goals of the analyses were to document the odds of suicide attempts among those with schizophrenia in comparison to those without and to calculate the degree to which inclusion of the potentially confounding factors attenuated the relationship. Age, race, income, and education were controlled for in the first model and each subsequent model. The second and third model adjusted for three early adversities (witnessing parental domestic violence, being physically abused, and being sexually abused as a child) and chronic pain, respectively. The fourth model controlled for drug and alcohol abuse. The fifth model accounted for lifetime depression and anxiety disorders. The sixth and final model controlled for all the above-named factors simultaneously.

A second series of logistic regression analyses was completed using the subsample of those diagnosed with schizophrenia (n = 101). The first model controlled for childhood adversities only, the next adjusted for gender and substance abuse/dependence, and a third accounted for mental health factors. A final model controlled for all the above-named variables simultaneously. Data from all the analyses were weighted to adjust for the probability of selection and nonresponse. Sample sizes are reported in their unweighted form. Odds ratios and 95% confidence intervals are reported.

3. Results

In our population-based sample of noninstitutionalized Canadians, the lifetime prevalence of suicide attempts among those with schizophrenia was 39.2% compared to 2.8% of individuals without schizophrenia. One-third of males (33%) with schizophrenia had attempted suicide in contrast to 2.2%

of males without schizophrenia ($p < 0.001$). Almost half of women (47.3%) with schizophrenia had attempted suicide in comparison to 3.5% of women without schizophrenia ($p < 0.001$).

When the data were adjusted for age, race, income, and education, noninstitutionalized individuals with schizophrenia had 15 times the odds of attempting suicide (OR: 15.74, 95% CI = 9.84, 25.2) in comparison to those without schizophrenia (please see Table 1). We conducted a series of logistic regression analyses all of which included the above variables in addition to several different clusters of risk factors that we anticipated would attenuate the association between schizophrenia and suicide attempts. When three early adversities (witnessing parental domestic violence, being physically abused, and being sexually abused as a child) were added to the equation, the odds of suicide attempts among those with schizophrenia declined to 12.92 (OR: 12.92, 95% CI = 7.96, 21.753). When drug and alcohol abuse were included, people with schizophrenia still had 13 times the odds (OR: 13.06) of attempting suicide as compared to individuals without schizophrenia. When pain was added to the sociodemographic variables, people with schizophrenia had 14.5 times the odds of attempting suicide (OR: 14.5, CI = 8.91, 23.74). The greatest attenuation in the schizophrenia-suicide attempt association was due to the inclusion of lifetime depression and anxiety disorders. Inclusion of these mental health characteristics reduced the odds of suicide attempts among those with schizophrenia to 7.22 (95% CI = 4.22–12.36). After adjusting for all of the factors discussed above, individuals with schizophrenia had 6 times the odds (OR: 6.47) of attempting to suicide as compared to individuals who did not have schizophrenia. Among the variables controlled for, mental health factors explained the largest share of the relationship between schizophrenia and suicide attempts at 58%, followed by childhood adversities at 20% and substance use at 18%. All the factors together accounted for 63% of the association.

In order to identify the key factors associated with suicide attempts among those with schizophrenia, we conducted additional analyses restricted to the 101 respondents in the CCHS-MH data set who reported that they had been diagnosed with schizophrenia by a medical professional (please see Table 2). In a model adjusting for all variables simultaneously, we found that suicide attempts were associated with female gender (OR = 4.59), substance dependence (OR = 6.31), depression (OR = 4.93), and a history of physical abuse in childhood (OR = 5.75). When only early adversities were included, exposure to chronic parental domestic violence was associated with almost 7 times the odds of suicide attempts (OR = 6.95). After adjustments for gender, substance abuse, and depression and anxiety, this number decreased to nonsignificance (OR: 2.58, 95% CI = 0.65, 10.30). Among those with schizophrenia, early adversity accounted for 24% of the variability in suicide attempts (Nagelkerke $R^2 = 0.24$). When gender, drug and alcohol abuse, and lifetime anxiety and depressive disorders were added to the analysis, 38% of the variability in suicide attempts was accounted for (Nagelkerke $R^2 = 0.38$).

4. Discussion

The purpose of this study was to examine the relationship between suicide attempts and schizophrenia using representative community-based data. In individuals with schizophrenia, 39.2% had attempted suicide as compared to 2.8% of individuals without schizophrenia. Previous studies have estimated the prevalence of suicide attempts in individuals with schizophrenia to range from 20 to 40% [2–6]. Although the percentage of individuals with schizophrenia who attempted suicide fell between previously estimated rates, it was theorized that, with population-based data of noninstitutionalized individuals, these numbers would be lower than in studies using clinical samples. The data suggest, however, that rates of suicide attempts in those with schizophrenia living within the community may be similar to those found in clinical settings.

We found that the odds of suicide attempt were over 6 times higher among those with schizophrenia compared to those without, even when accounting for lifetime depression and anxiety disorders, substance use, childhood adversities, pain, and sociodemographics. Among the latter factors, depression and anxiety explained the largest share of the relationship between schizophrenia and suicide attempts, which is consistent with research showing that as much as half of individuals with schizophrenia suffer from depressive symptoms and that these symptoms are associated with an increase in suicide attempts [5, 15, 24]. Among those with schizophrenia, we found that depression was associated with 7 times the odds of a suicide attempt and that depression and anxiety together explained 17.5% of the variability in suicide attempts. These findings suggest that it is important for health care professionals working in the community to be aware of the need to assess for the presence of other mental health problems alongside the symptoms of schizophrenia. Developing best practices to support individuals who are experiencing schizophrenia comorbid with other mental health conditions could help decrease the prevalence of suicide attempts among those living in the community.

Interestingly, in the fully adjusted model, those with an anxiety disorder were 69% less likely to attempt suicide. Rapp et al. [46] found that individuals with schizophrenia who also had anxiety demonstrated higher verbal IQ, better problem solving, attention, and verbal fluency. Possessing these qualities might indicate that individuals with both schizophrenia and anxiety may be more likely to have the necessary skills to express themselves verbally and communicate with those around them should they be experiencing suicidal ideation, increasing the chances of a successful intervention. More research is required to understand the differences in characteristics between those with schizophrenia with an anxiety disorder and those with schizophrenia without an anxiety disorder.

In the general population, women are more likely to attempt suicide than men [47]. Some research has also identified this trend for women with schizophrenia [10], which is in keeping with what we found in our data. When only sociodemographics and substance abuse history were included in the analysis, women's odds of suicide attempts were elevated

TABLE 1: Odds ratios and 95% confidence interval of lifetime suicide attempts among those with schizophrenia versus those without in a representative community-based sample ($n = 21744$).

	Model 1 Demographics + SES	Model 2 Demographics + SES + ACEs	Model 3 Demographics + SES + substance abuse	Model 4 Demographics + SES + mental health	Model 5 Demographics + SES + pain	Model 6 Fully adjusted
Has schizophrenia						
Yes	15.74 (9.84, 25.18)	12.92 (7.68, 21.75)	13.06 (7.95, 21.47)	7.23 (4.22, 12.36)	14.54 (8.91, 23.74)	6.47 (3.73, 11.20)
No (Ref)	1.00	1.00	1.00	1.00	1.00	1.00
Adverse childhood experiences						
Witnessed parental domestic violence						
>10 times	—	2.40 (1.88, 3.06)	—	—	—	2.21 (1.71, 2.86)
≤10 times (Ref)	—	1.00	—	—	—	1.00
Physical abuse						
Abused	—	3.35 (2.72, 4.13)	—	—	—	2.28 (1.84, 2.83)
None (Ref)	—	1.00	—	—	—	1.00
Sexual abuse						
Abused	—	4.21 (3.41, 5.21)	—	—	—	2.85 (2.28, 3.56)
None (Ref)	—	1.00	—	—	—	1.00
Demographics						
Sex						
Female	1.57 (1.33, 1.85)	1.44 (1.21, 1.72)	2.33 (1.95, 2.77)	1.25 (1.05, 1.48)	1.50 (1.27, 1.77)	1.49 (1.23, 1.80)
Male (Ref)	1.00	1.00	1.00	1.00	1.00	1.00
Race						
White only	1.33 (1.09, 1.61)	1.31 (1.07, 1.61)	0.97 (0.79, 1.19)	0.99 (0.81, 1.22)	1.22 (1.01, 1.49)	0.94 (0.76, 1.17)
Visible minority or aboriginal (Ref)	1.00	1.00	1.00	1.00	1.00	1.00
Age						
Age by decade	0.82 (0.78, 0.86)	0.80 (0.76, 0.84)	0.88 (0.84, 0.93)	0.84 (0.79, 0.88)	0.77 (0.73, 0.81)	0.82 (0.77, 0.87)
Socioeconomic status						
Education						
No high school graduation (Ref)	1.00	1.00	1.00	1.00	1.00	1.00
High school graduate	0.64 (0.50, 0.83)	0.73 (0.56, 0.96)	0.64 (0.50, 0.83)	0.58 (0.45, 0.76)	0.69 (0.54, 0.90)	0.64 (0.48, 0.85)
Postsecondary graduate	0.79 (0.64, 0.99)	0.93 (0.74, 1.18)	0.87 (0.70, 1.09)	0.73 (0.58, 0.91)	0.87 (0.70, 1.09)	0.93 (0.73, 1.19)
Household income (decile)	0.84 (0.81, 0.87)	0.87 (0.85, 0.90)	0.83 (0.80, 0.86)	0.86 (0.84, 0.89)	0.86 (0.83, 0.89)	0.89 (0.86, 0.92)
Drug or alcohol abuse						
Yes	—	—	5.57 (4.68, 6.64)	—	—	2.77 (2.29, 3.34)
No (Ref)	—	—	1.00	—	—	1.00

TABLE 1: Continued.

	Model 1 Demographics + SES	Model 2 Demographics + SES + ACEs	Model 3 Demographics + SES + substance abuse	Model 4 Demographics + SES + mental health	Model 5 Demographics + SES + pain	Model 6 Fully adjusted
Mental health						
Lifetime generalized anxiety disorder						
Yes	—	—	—	3.23 (2.66, 3.93)	—	2.13 (1.73, 2.63)
No (Ref)	—	—	—	1.00	—	1.00
Lifetime depression						
Yes	—	—	—	5.43 (4.51, 6.55)	—	3.85 (3.17, 4.68)
No (Ref)	—	—	—	1.00	—	1.00
Chronic pain						
Pain						
Moderate or severe	—	—	—	—	4.13 (3.46, 4.93)	1.82 (1.49, 2.22)
Less than moderate (Ref)	—	—	—	—	1.00	1.00
Nagelkerke R square value	0.070	0.193	0.140	0.201	0.112	0.303
−2 Log likelihood	5431.6	4787.3	5068.4	4747.6	5213.9	4194.1

SES = socioeconomic status, ACEs = adverse childhood experiences.

TABLE 2: Odds ratios and 95% confidence interval of lifetime suicide attempt among those with schizophrenia from a representative community-based sample (n = 101).

	Model 1 ACEs only	Model 2 Demographics and substance abuse	Model 3 Demographics, substance abuse, and mental health	Model 4 Fully adjusted
Adverse childhood experiences				
Witnessed parental domestic violence				
>10 times	6.95 (2.30, 20.99)	—	—	2.58 (0.64, 10.30)
≤10 times (Ref)	1.00	—	—	1.00
Physical abuse				
Abused	2.66 (0.94, 7.51)	—	—	5.75 (1.53, 21.58)
None (Ref)	1.00	—	—	1.00
Sexual abuse				
Abused	1.00 (0.33, 3.04)	—	—	0.45 (0.13, 1.61)
None (Ref)	1.00	—	—	1.00
Demographics				
Sex				
Female	—	2.13 (0.91, 4.98)	3.10 (1.19, 8.04)	4.59 (1.21, 17.35)
Male (Ref)	—	1.00	1.00	1.00
Drug or alcohol abuse				
Yes	—	2.24 (0.96, 5.22)	5.02 (1.77, 14.26)	6.31 (1.83, 21.72)
No (Ref)	—	1.00	1.00	1.00
Mental health				
Anxiety				
Lifetime anxiety disorder	—	—	0.37 (0.13, 1.02)	0.31 (0.10, 0.94)
No anxiety disorder (Ref)	—	—	1.00	1.00
Depression				
Lifetime depressive disorder	—	—	6.97 (2.37, 20.52)	4.93 (1.26, 19.28)
No depression (Ref)	—	—	1.00	1.00
Nagelkerke R square value	0.241	0.074	0.250	0.381
−2 Log likelihood	115.5	129.629	114.7	101.9

ACE: adverse childhood experience.

but failed to reach statistical significance (OR = 2.13; 95% CI = 0.91, 4.98). However, these odds increased and became statistically significant when histories of depressive disorders and anxiety disorders were included (OR = 3.10; 95% CI = 1.19, 8.04). In the final model we were surprised by the magnitude of the association in our sample: women with schizophrenia had four times the odds of suicide attempts compared to men with schizophrenia when adjustments were made for adverse childhood experiences, sociodemographics, substance abuse, depression, and anxiety disorder (OR = 4.59; 95% CI = 1.21, 17.35). It appears that women with schizophrenia are particularly at risk, even independent of these comorbid conditions. One potential factor to explain this is that females with schizophrenia tend to present with symptoms later than males [10, 47], and individuals with later onset schizophrenia have been shown to have an increased risk of suicide [48, 49].

Among those with schizophrenia, 24% of the variability in suicide attempts was explained by a history of early adversity. When only early adversities were used to predict suicide attempts among those with schizophrenia, those who had been exposed to chronic parental domestic violence had approximately seven times the odds of attempting suicide. To our knowledge, this is the first study to examine the role of exposure to parental domestic violence in those with schizophrenia and its relationship to suicide attempts. Our findings are in keeping with data from the general population which has shown that individuals who are exposed to parental domestic violence have an increased risk of suicide attempts [50]. Childhood physical abuse was associated with 2.66 higher odds of suicide in those with schizophrenia; however, it only reached borderline significance (model 1: $p < 0.065$). After adjustments for demographics, substance abuse, and history of depression and anxiety disorders, the relationship between parental domestic violence and suicide attempts decreased to nonsignificance but childhood physical abuse reached statistical signficance. Our findings are in contrast to a recent clinical study of suicide attempts before and after first episode of schizophrenia which found no association between childhood traumas and suicide attempts [51]. There were numerous design differences between Togay et al.'s study [51] and this study which may have led to the different findings including source of sample (clinical sample of first episode clients versus representative population-based study), study location (Turkey versus Canada), period of suicide attempts (average of 5 years after first episode versus lifetime), and different measures of early adversities (combined measure of 5 types of abuse using a standardized scale versus separate inclusion of 3 specific types of childhood adversities). Physical, emotional, and sexual abuse, neglect, and witnessing parental domestic violence have been associated with an increased risk in suicide attempts in the general population [31, 32]. In our Canadian study, early childhood adversities explained a large portion of the variability in suicide attempts among those with schizophrenia. These findings reinforce the need to develop targeted programs for individuals with schizophrenia who have experienced early childhood abuse [31, 32].

In the fully adjusted model, substance abuse/dependence was associated with 6 times the odds of suicide attempts among those with schizophrenia. Both in the general population and in the schizophrenia literature drug abuse and addictions have been associated with increased risk of suicide attempts [19, 20, 52, 53]. Interestingly, substance abuse/dependence explained just 7% of the variation in suicide attempts. A potential explanation for the finding rests in exploring the self-medication hypothesis [54]. It is theorized that part of the reason individuals with schizophrenia have such high rates of substance abuse is that they try to alleviate the pain and suffering they feel as a result of the symptoms of schizophrenia by using substances [54, 55]. It is possible that, due to our use of population-based data of noninstitutionalized individuals, our sample may not be experiencing the same level of intensity of symptoms as one would see in a clinical sample and, thus, is less likely to be using substances to cope and, subsequently, turn to attempting suicide.

There are a several limitations present in this study. It is possible that recall bias may have occurred considering the retrospective nature of reporting suicide attempts as well as early adversities. There has been a lack of research aimed at establishing the validity and reliability of self-report measures related to suicide attempts [56]. In the general population, the evidence concerning the validity and reliability of retrospective reporting of child maltreatment is mixed, with some studies finding the self-reports an accurate way of assessing child maltreatment [57], while others are finding significant instability in retrospective reports of child maltreatment [58]. In individuals with schizophrenia, concerns about memory and cognition could be cited as a potential challenge to relying on self-report data [59]. Although slower recall and deficits in recalling emotion laden memories have been reported in individuals with schizophrenia, most of these studies have relied on clinical samples, thus potentially skewing the understanding of memory deficits in those with schizophrenia [60–62]. Other research has found good validity in self-report measures of childhood abuse among patients with mental disorders [63]. There are some potential risk factors for suicide attempts in individuals with schizophrenia that were not included in our analysis. These include insight into disease, poor adherence to treatment, schizophrenia symptom profile, housing conditions, marital status, and living alone. The absence of these important potential confounds could have biased our findings.

Questions have also been raised as to whether self-report of a medical diagnosis of schizophrenia is a reasonable method to assess the presence or absence of this condition. Self-reports of a medical diagnosis of schizophrenia are a prominent technique used in large, population-based data sets [64]. The prevalence of schizophrenia based on self-report of a medical diagnosis in the current sample was in keeping with the systematic review by Saha and colleagues [65] which estimated that the lifetime prevalence of schizophrenia was approximately 0.44%. However, alternative techniques for assessing schizophrenia status, such as screening tools and self-report measures, also carry the risk of missing cases of psychiatric illnesses [66]. There is particularly the potential for missing those with negative symptoms [66, 67]. In a previous study using an earlier wave of the CCHS, self-report of a clinical diagnosis of schizophrenia was found to be a reasonable way to assess the existence of schizophrenia [64]. There have been few studies examining this phenomenon, and it has been suggested that more research is to be conducted using diagnostic interviewing as a comparison to produce better, more reliable data [64]. Although the overall response rate of 68.9% was quite good for a large population-based survey, it is possible that those with schizophrenia, particularly those with more severe symptoms, may be less likely to participate in a survey such as this. If the most severe cases are most likely to have had suicide attempts, it is likely that such an underrepresentation of these individuals would result in our analyses underestimating the magnitude of the relationship between schizophrenia and suicide attempts. Additionally, it is possible that the question *"How many times did an adult force you or attempt to force you into any unwanted sexual activity, by threatening you, holding you down, or hurting you in some way?"* does not adequately capture all types of sexual abuse, specifically forms that would be subtler in nature. Consequently, our study might underestimate the history of sexual abuse.

Our nationally representative sample suggests noninstitutionalized individuals with schizophrenia are 6 times more likely than individuals without schizophrenia to attempt suicide. The presence of depressive symptoms, as well as early childhood adversities, played significant roles in explaining the high rates of suicide within the schizophrenia population. With this information, it is important to recognize that individuals who are experiencing psychosis are also vulnerable to other serious mental health issues, which are related to suicide attempts. This, alongside targeted programs for those with schizophrenia who have experienced early adversity, could help reduce the suicide attempts by individuals with schizophrenia living in the community.

Disclaimer

The views expressed in this paper do not necessarily represent the CRDCN's or that of its partners.

Conflict of Interests

The authors declare that there is no conflict of interests regarding the publication of this paper.

Acknowledgment

The authors would like to thank Rafael Riviere for assistance with paper preparation. Esme Fuller-Thomson would like to gratefully acknowledge support received from the Sandra Rotman Endowed Chair in Social Work at the University of Toronto. The analysis presented in this paper was conducted at the Toronto RDC, which is part of the Canadian Research Data Centre Network (CRDCN). The services and activities provided by the Toronto RDC are made possible by the financial or in-kind support of the SSHRC, the CIHR, the CFI, Statistics Canada, and University of Toronto. The opinions expressed do not represent the views of Statistics Canada.

References

[1] K. Hawton, L. Sutton, C. Haw, J. Sinclair, and J. J. Deeks, "Schizophrenia and suicide: a systematic review of risk factors," *The British Journal of Psychiatry*, vol. 187, no. 1, pp. 9–20, 2005.

[2] M. Pompili, X. F. Amador, P. Girardi et al., "Suicide risk in schizophrenia: learning from the past to change the future," *Annals of General Psychiatry*, vol. 6, article 10, 2007.

[3] S. G. Siris, "Suicide and schizophrenia," *Journal of Psychopharmacology*, vol. 15, no. 2, pp. 127–135, 2001.

[4] A. C. Altamura, R. Bassetti, S. Bignotti, R. Pioli, and E. Mundo, "Clinical variables related to suicide attempts in schizophrenic patients: a retrospective study," *Schizophrenia Research*, vol. 60, no. 1, pp. 47–55, 2003.

[5] J. T. Suokas, J. Perälä, K. Suominen, S. Saarni, J. Lönnqvist, and J. M. Suvisaari, "Epidemiology of suicide attempts among persons with psychotic disorder in the general population," *Schizophrenia Research*, vol. 124, no. 1-3, pp. 22–28, 2010.

[6] M. Yildiz, A. Yazici, and O. Böke, "Demographic and clinical characteristics in schizophrenia: a multi center cross-sectional case record study," *Turkish Journal of Psychiatry*, vol. 21, no. 3, pp. 213–224, 2010.

[7] B. A. Palmer, V. S. Pankratz, and J. M. Bostwick, "The lifetime risk of suicide in schizophrenia. A reexamination," *Archives of General Psychiatry*, vol. 62, no. 3, pp. 247–253, 2005.

[8] F. Limosin, J.-Y. Loze, A. Philippe, F. Casadebaig, and F. Rouillon, "Ten-year prospective follow-up study of the mortality by suicide in schizophrenic patients," *Schizophrenia Research*, vol. 94, no. 1-3, pp. 23–28, 2007.

[9] J. M. Harkavy-Friedman, E. A. Nelson, and D. F. Venarde, "Suicidal behavior in schizophrenia and schizoaffective disorder," *Clinical Neuroscience Research*, vol. 1, no. 5, pp. 345–350, 2001.

[10] C. M. Canuso and G. Pandina, "Gender and schizophrenia," *Psychopharmacology Bulletin*, vol. 40, no. 4, pp. 178–190, 2007.

[11] S. Goldberg, E. Fruchter, M. Davidson, A. Reichenberg, R. Yoffe, and M. Weiser, "The relationship between risk of hospitalization for schizophrenia, SES, and cognitive functioning," *Schizophrenia Bulletin*, vol. 37, no. 4, pp. 664–670, 2011.

[12] C. Corcoran, M. Perrin, S. Harlap et al., "Effect of socioeconomic status and parents' education at birth on risk of schizophrenia in offspring," *Social Psychiatry and Psychiatric Epidemiology*, vol. 44, no. 4, pp. 265–271, 2009.

[13] B. Saraceno, I. Levev, and R. Kohn, "The public mental health significance of research on socio-economic factors in schizophrenia and major depression," *World Psychiatry*, vol. 4, no. 3, pp. 181–185, 2005.

[14] F. Mulvany, E. O'Callaghan, N. Takei, M. Byrne, P. Fearon, and C. Larkin, "Effect of social class at birth on risk and presentation of schizophrenia: case-control study," *British Medical Journal*, vol. 323, no. 7326, pp. 1398–1401, 2001.

[15] K. Hor and M. Taylor, "Suicide and schizophrenia: a systematic review of rates and risk factors," *Journal of Psychopharmacology*, vol. 24, no. 4, pp. 81–90, 2010.

[16] M. K. Singh, L. L. Giles, and H. A. Nasrallah, "Pain insensitivity in schizophrenia: trait or state marker?" *Journal of Psychiatric Practice*, vol. 12, no. 2, pp. 90–102, 2006.

[17] G. Engels, A. L. Francke, B. van Meijel et al., "Clinical pain in schizophrenia: a systematic review," *The Journal of Pain*, vol. 15, no. 5, pp. 457–467, 2014.

[18] T. Jochum, A. Letzsch, W. Greiner, G. Wagner, H. Sauer, and K.-J. Bär, "Influence of antipsychotic medication on pain perception in schizophrenia," *Psychiatry Research*, vol. 142, no. 2-3, pp. 151–156, 2006.

[19] G. Carrà and S. Johnson, "Variations in rates of comorbid substance use in psychosis between mental health settings and geographical areas in the UK. A systematic review," *Social Psychiatry and Psychiatric Epidemiology*, vol. 44, no. 6, pp. 429–447, 2009.

[20] I. L. Fowler, V. J. Carr, N. T. Carter, and T. J. Lewin, "Patterns of current and lifetime substance use in schizophrenia," *Schizophrenia Bulletin*, vol. 24, no. 3, pp. 443–455, 1998.

[21] D. A. Reiger, M. E. Farmer, D. S. Rae et al., "Comorbidity of mental disorders with alcohol and other drug abuse," *The Journal of the American Medical Association*, vol. 264, no. 19, pp. 2511–2518, 1990.

[22] C. Mulholland and S. Cooper, "The symptom of depression in schizophrenia and its management," *Advances in Psychiatric Treatment*, vol. 6, no. 3, pp. 169–177, 2000.

[23] A. M. Achim, M. Maziade, É. Raymond, D. Olivier, C. Mérette, and M.-A. Roy, "How prevalent are anxiety disorders in schizophrenia? A meta-analysis and critical review on a significant association," *Schizophrenia Bulletin*, vol. 37, no. 4, pp. 811–821, 2011.

[24] P. F. Buckley, B. J. Miller, D. S. Lehrer, and D. J. Castle, "Psychiatric comorbidities and schizophrenia," *Schizophrenia Bulletin*, vol. 35, no. 2, pp. 383–402, 2009.

[25] S. Pallanti, L. Quercioli, and E. Hollander, "Social anxiety in outpatients with schizophrenia: a relevant cause of disability," *The American Journal of Psychiatry*, vol. 161, no. 1, pp. 53–58, 2004.

[26] H. Heilä, M. E. Heikkinen, E. T. Isometsä, M. M. Henriksson, M. J. Marttunen, and J. K. Lönnqvist, "Life events and completed suicide in schizophrenia: a comparison of suicide victims with and without schizophrenia," *Schizophrenia Bulletin*, vol. 25, no. 3, pp. 519–531, 1999.

[27] F. Varese, F. Smeets, M. Drukker et al., "Childhood adversities increase the risk of psychosis: a meta-analysis of patient-control, prospective-and cross sectional cohort studies," *Schizophrenia Bulletin*, vol. 38, no. 4, pp. 661–671, 2012.

[28] S. L. Matheson, A. M. Shepherd, R. M. Pinchbeck, K. R. Laurens, and V. J. Carr, "Childhood adversity in schizophrenia: a systematic meta-analysis," *Psychological Medicine*, vol. 43, no. 2, pp. 225–238, 2013.

[29] D. W. Holowka, S. King, D. Saheb, M. Pukall, and A. Brunet, "Childhood abuse and dissociative symptoms in adult schizophrenia," *Schizophrenia Research*, vol. 60, no. 1, pp. 87–90, 2003.

[30] L. S. Schenkel, W. D. Spaulding, D. DiLillo, and S. M. Silverstein, "Histories of childhood maltreatment in schizophrenia: relationships with premorbid functioning, symptomatology, and cognitive deficits," *Schizophrenia Research*, vol. 76, no. 2-3, pp. 273–286, 2005.

[31] A. Roy, "Reported childhood trauma and suicide attempts in schizophrenic patients," *Suicide & Life-Threatening Behavior*, vol. 35, no. 6, pp. 690–693, 2005.

[32] J. Read, K. Agar, N. Argyle, and V. Aderhold, "Sexual and physical abuse during childhood and adulthood as predictors of hallucinations, delusions and thought disorder," *Psychology and Psychotherapy: Theory, Research and Practice*, vol. 76, no. 1, pp. 1–22, 2003.

[33] R. Gilbert, C. S. Widom, K. Browne, D. Fergusson, E. Webb, and S. Janson, "Burden and consequences of child maltreatment in high-income countries," *The Lancet*, vol. 373, no. 9657, pp. 68–81, 2009.

[34] Y. Barak, Y. Baruch, A. Achiron, and D. Aizenberg, "Suicide attempts of schizophrenia patients: a case-controlled study in tertiary care," *Journal of Psychiatric Research*, vol. 42, no. 10, pp. 822–826, 2008.

[35] A. Gut-Fayand, A. Dervaux, J.-P. Olié, H. Lôo, M.-F. Poirier, and M.-O. Krebs, "Substance abuse and suicidality in schizophrenia: a common risk factor linked to impulsivity," *Psychiatry Research*, vol. 102, no. 1, pp. 65–72, 2001.

[36] J. Tiihonen, J. Lönnqvist, K. Wahlbeck et al., "11-year follow-up of mortality in patients with schizophrenia: a population-based cohort study (FIN11 study)," *The Lancet*, vol. 374, no. 9690, pp. 620–627, 2009.

[37] J. Suokas, K. Suominen, E. Isometsä, A. Ostamo, and J. Lönnqvist, "Long-term risk factors for suicide mortality after attempted suicide—findings of a 14-year follow-up study," *Acta Psychiatrica Scandinavica*, vol. 104, no. 2, pp. 117–121, 2001.

[38] J. R. Randall, R. Walld, G. Finlayson, J. Sareen, P. J. Martens, and J. M. Bolton, "Acute risk of suicide and suicide attempts associated with recent diagnosis of mental disorders: a population-based, propensity score-matched analysis," *Canadian Journal of Psychiatry*, vol. 59, no. 10, p. 531, 2014.

[39] P. Qin and M. Nordentoft, "Suicide risk in relation to psychiatric hospitalization: evidence based on longitudinal registers," *Archives of General Psychiatry*, vol. 62, no. 4, pp. 427–432, 2005.

[40] M. Osler, E. Rostrup, M. Nordentoft, E. L. Mortensen, H. Bruunsgaard, and B. Fagerlund, "Influence of early life characteristics on psychiatric admissions and impact of psychiatric disease on inflammatory biomarkers and survival: a Danish cohort study," *World Psychiatry*, vol. 14, no. 3, pp. 364–365, 2015.

[41] P. Qin, "The impact of psychiatric illness on suicide: differences by diagnosis of disorders and by sex and age of subjects," *Journal of Psychiatric Research*, vol. 45, no. 11, pp. 1445–1452, 2011.

[42] S. Fazel, A. Wolf, C. Palm, and P. Lichtenstein, "Violent crime, suicide, and premature mortality in patients with schizophrenia and related disorders: a 38-year total population study in Sweden," *The Lancet Psychiatry*, vol. 1, no. 1, pp. 44–54, 2014.

[43] Y. P. S. Balhara and R. Verma, "Schizophrenia and suicide," *East Asian Archives of Psychiatry*, vol. 22, no. 3, pp. 126–133, 2012.

[44] J. L. Edleson, "Children's witnessing of adult domestic violence," *Journal of Interpersonal Violence*, vol. 14, no. 8, pp. 839–870, 1999.

[45] Statistics Canada, *Canadian Community Health Survey—Mental Health (CCHS)*, 2013, http://www23.statcan.gc.ca/imdb/p2SV.pl?Function=getSurvey&SDDS=5015.

[46] E. K. Rapp, M. L. White-Ajmani, D. Antonius et al., "Schizophrenia comorbid with panic disorder: evidence for distinct cognitive profiles," *Psychiatry Research*, vol. 197, no. 3, pp. 206–211, 2012.

[47] R. Lewine, "At issue: sex and gender in schizophrenia," *Schizophrenia Bulletin*, vol. 30, no. 4, pp. 755–762, 2004.

[48] J. Reutfors, L. Brandt, E. G. Jönsson, A. Ekbom, P. Sparén, and U. Ösby, "Risk factors for suicide in schizophrenia: findings from a Swedish population-based case-control study," *Schizophrenia Research*, vol. 108, no. 1–3, pp. 231–237, 2009.

[49] C.-J. Kuo, S.-Y. Tsai, C.-H. Lo, Y.-P. Wang, and C.-C. Chen, "Risk factors for completed suicide in schizophrenia," *Journal of Clinical Psychiatry*, vol. 66, no. 5, pp. 579–585, 2005.

[50] T. I. Herrenkohl, C. Sousa, E. A. Tajima, R. C. Herrenkohl, and C. A. Moylan, "Intersection of child abuse and children's exposure to domestic violence," *Trauma, Violence, & Abuse*, vol. 9, no. 2, pp. 84–99, 2008.

[51] B. Togay, H. Noyan, R. Tasdelen, and A. Ucok, "Clinical variables associated with suicide attempts in schizophrenia before and after the first episode," *Psychiatry Research*, vol. 229, no. 1-2, pp. 252–256, 2015.

[52] M. Backmund, K. Meyer, C. Schütz, and J. Reimer, "Factors associated with suicide attempts among injection drug users," *Substance Use & Misuse*, vol. 46, no. 12, pp. 1553–1559, 2011.

[53] A. Roy, "Characteristics of drug addicts who attempt suicide," *Psychiatry Research*, vol. 121, no. 1, pp. 99–103, 2003.

[54] E. J. Khantzian, "The self-medication hypothesis revisited: the dually diagnosed patient," *Primary Psychiatry*, vol. 10, no. 9, pp. 47–54, 2003.

[55] K. T. Mueser and S. R. McGurk, "Schizophrenia," *The Lancet*, vol. 363, no. 9426, pp. 2063–2072, 2004.

[56] N. D. Brener, J. O. G. Billy, and W. R. Grady, "Assessment of factors affecting the validity of self-reported health-risk behavior among adolescents. Evidence from the scientific literature," *Journal of Adolescent Health*, vol. 33, no. 6, pp. 436–457, 2003.

[57] R. Pinto, L. Correia, and Â. Maia, "Assessing the reliability of retrospective reports of adverse childhood experiences among adolescents with documented childhood maltreatment," *Journal of Family Violence*, vol. 29, no. 4, pp. 431–438, 2014.

[58] D. M. Fergusson, L. J. Horwood, and L. J. Woodward, "The stability of child abuse reports: a longitudinal study of the reporting behaviour of young adults," *Psychological Medicine*, vol. 30, no. 3, pp. 529–544, 2000.

[59] E. Stefanopoulou, A. Manoharan, S. Landau, J. R. Geddes, G. Goodwin, and S. Frangou, "Cognitive functioning in patients with affective disorders and schizophrenia: a meta-analysis,"

International Review of Psychiatry, vol. 21, no. 4, pp. 336–356, 2009.

[60] S. Raffard, A. D'Argembeau, C. Lardi, S. Bayard, J.-P. Boulenger, and M. Van Der Linden, "Exploring self-defining memories in schizophrenia," *Memory*, vol. 17, no. 1, pp. 26–38, 2009.

[61] A. D'Argembeau, S. Raffard, and M. Van der Linden, "Remembering the past and imagining the future in schizophrenia," *Journal of Abnormal Psychology*, vol. 117, no. 1, pp. 247–251, 2008.

[62] A. Aleman, R. Hijman, E. H. F. de Haan, and R. S. Kahn, "Memory impairment in schizophrenia: a meta-analysis," *American Journal of Psychiatry*, vol. 156, no. 9, pp. 1358–1366, 1999.

[63] H. L. Fisher, T. K. Craig, P. Fearon et al., "Reliability and comparability of psychosis patients' retrospective reports of childhood abuse," *Schizophrenia Bulletin*, vol. 37, no. 3, pp. 546–553, 2011.

[64] A. L. Supina and S. B. Patten, "Self-reported diagnoses of schizophrenia and psychotic disorders may be valuable for monitoring and surveillance," *Canadian Journal of Psychiatry*, vol. 51, no. 4, pp. 256–259, 2006.

[65] S. Saha, D. Chant, J. Welham, and J. McGrath, "A systematic review of the prevalence of schizophrenia," *PLoS Medicine*, vol. 2, no. 5, pp. 413–433, 2005.

[66] O. Nielssen and S. Misrachi, "Prevalence of psychoses on reception to male prisons in New South Wales," *Australian and New Zealand Journal of Psychiatry*, vol. 39, no. 6, pp. 453–459, 2005.

[67] S. Rosenman, A. Korten, J. Medway, and M. Evans, "Characterising psychosis in the Australian National Survey of Mental Health and Wellbeing study on low prevalence (psychotic) disorders," *Australian and New Zealand Journal of Psychiatry*, vol. 34, no. 5, pp. 792–800, 2000.

13

Delusional Disorder over the Reproductive Life Span: The Potential Influence of Menopause on the Clinical Course

Alexandre González-Rodríguez,[1] Oriol Molina-Andreu,[2] Rafael Penadés,[3,4] Marina Garriga,[5] Alexandre Pons,[3,4] Rosa Catalán,[3,4] and Miguel Bernardo[3,4]

[1] *Barcelona Clinic Schizophrenia Unit (BCSU), Neurosciences Institute, Hospital Clinic of Barcelona, University of Barcelona, 170 Villarroel Street, 08036 Barcelona, Spain*
[2] *Department of Mental Health, Hospital Universitari Mútua de Terrassa, 5 Doctor Robert Street, 08221 Terrassa, Spain*
[3] *Barcelona Clinic Schizophrenia Unit (BCSU), Neurosciences Institute, Hospital Clinic of Barcelona, Department of Psychiatry and Clinical Psychobiology, University of Barcelona, 170 Villarroel Street, 08036 Barcelona, Spain*
[4] *Centro de Investigación Biomédica en Red en Salud Mental (CIBERSAM), Institut d'Investigacions Biomèdiques August Pi i Sunyer (IDIBAPS), 149 Rosselló Street, 08036 Barcelona, Spain*
[5] *Barcelona Clinic Schizophrenia Unit (BCSU), Bipolar Disorders Unit, Neurosciences Institute, Hospital Clinic of Barcelona, University of Barcelona, 170 Villarroel Street, 08036 Barcelona, Spain*

Correspondence should be addressed to Rosa Catalán; rcatalan@clinic.ub.es

Academic Editor: Robin Emsley

Background and Objectives. Recent evidence supports an association between estrogen levels and severity of psychopathology in schizophrenia women. Our main goal was to investigate whether delusional disorder (DD) women with premenopausal onset and those with postmenopausal onset differ in demographic and clinical features. *Methods.* Psychopathological symptoms were assessed in 80 DD women (DSM-IV-TR), at baseline and after six and 24 months. Scores in the PANSS, PSP for functionality, HRSD 17 items, C-SSRS for suicide, and the SUMD were considered outcome variables. For comparison purposes, t- and χ^2-tests were performed and nonparametric tests when necessary. Analysis of Covariance (ANCOVA) was conducted for multivariate comparisons. *Results.* 57 out of 80 DD women completed the study. When unadjusted, DD with premenopausal onset had a longer DUP, higher educational level, and a tendency toward higher rates of gynaecological disorders. Erotomanic type was most frequent in DD women premenopausal onset, and somatic and jealous types were most frequent in those with postmenopausal onset. After 24 months, DD women with premenopausal onset showed higher depressive symptoms and a tendency toward higher rates of psychotic relapses. *Conclusions.* Our results support that some aspects of psychopathology and insight may differ according to the onset of DD and the reproductive status.

1. Introduction

In recent years, an increasing scientific evidence highlighted an influence of estrogens on the psychopathology in women diagnosed with chronic psychosis [1, 2]. Most of the existing studies support an inverse correlation between estrogen levels and severity of psychopathology in these women [1, 3], and estradiol has been postulated to have specific antipsychotic-like effects on these populations.

For instance, Bergemann and colleagues investigated the effects of the menstrual cycle phase and estradiol levels on psychotic symptoms by using the Positive and Negative Syndrome Scale (PANSS) and the Brief Psychiatric Rating Scale (BPRS) [1]. The authors found a significant improvement in psychotic symptoms during the luteal phase of the menstrual cycle.

In this line of clinical and epidemiological findings, and based on animal models, two hypotheses have been proposed: "the estrogen protection hypothesis" and "the hypothesis of hypoestrogenism" [4, 5]. Specifically, the first hypothesis supports the notion that estrogens have a positive influence on mental well-being in women diagnosed with schizophrenia, and these women would be protected against the onset of the disorder between puberty and menopause [3, 5]. The second hypothesis proposed that schizophrenia women show a phenotype associated with a dysfunction of the estrogen and gonadal axis, irrespective of the use of antipsychotic medications.

When focusing on the estrogen protection hypothesis, a recent review proposed that women are more likely to develop psychotic disorders at a later age and show higher psychotic symptoms over the perimenopausal period [4]. As it was mentioned above, some clinical trials found new types of estrogen compounds to be an effective potential treatment for schizophrenia, in particular for those suffering from negative and cognitive symptoms [4, 5].

In particular, menopause has been defined as a medical condition with a permanent hypergonadotrophic hypogonadism and amenorrhea that determines a follicular depletion and a decline in estrogen serum levels [5]. This loss of estrogens would contribute to a high risk of onset of schizophrenia and deterioration of course in psychotic women. Furthermore, this depletion would also imply a high vulnerability for the exacerbation of psychotic symptoms in women previously diagnosed with schizophrenia [5].

Although increasing evidence regarding this issue in schizophrenia is provided, few studies have investigated differences in the psychopathology and clinical course of delusional disorder (DD) women with premenopausal onset and those with postmenopausal onset. Our team has recently published preliminary results focused on postmenopausal women, in a sample formed by 25 DD women, by describing some gynaecological and clinical endocrinological aspects in a descriptive design [2].

Thus, our main objective therefore was to investigate whether DD women with premenopausal onset and those with postmenopausal onset differ in sociodemographic characteristics, as it is a well-established fact that menopause interacts with other psychosocial risk factors and aging. Further, after comparisons in terms of sociodemographic characteristics, we aimed to search for differences in clinical features and psychopathology that means a comparison of the clinical course of the disorder between those women who had a background of menopause and other potential risk factors (e.g., educational level, employment status, and marital status) and those who had an onset prior to the menopause. We also aimed to compare longitudinally changes in psychopathology, rates of relapses, and rehospitalization rates between those who had an onset of DD prior to the menopause and those with a postmenopausal onset.

2. Methods

2.1. Patients and Study Design. We carried out a prospective observational study with a 24-month follow-up in a clinical group of 80 DD women, who attended for a first time our outpatient Schizophrenia Unit. We included all consecutive cases of DD women at the time they attended at psychiatric appointments. Our unit is of reference in a representative catchment area in Barcelona in the diagnosis, treatment, and research of schizophrenia and related disorders. Patients were evaluated at baseline and after six and 24 months.

Patients were included in the study if they met our inclusion criteria: (1) being aged >18 years, (2) being diagnosed as having a DD according to DSM-IV-TR criteria, and (3) being under antipsychotic treatment for more than six months. Female patients with a previous diagnosis of psychotic disorder, affective disorders or mental retardation, organic psychosis, or substance abuse were not invited to participate.

Age at onset of DD was determined by using the SCID-I interview that was assessed by at least two senior psychiatrists. The psychotic screening module for SCID-I has been widely used for coding psychotic symptoms that have been present at any point in the person's lifetime and can be used for clinical and research settings. Substance use disorders, general medical conditions, and mood disorders were excluded according to DSM-IV-TR criteria for DD. Further, onset of the disorder was obtained irrespective of the intensity of delusions.

The present study is a part of an ongoing study on schizophrenia and related disorders, which was approved by the Ethics Committee of the Hospital Clinic.

2.2. Measures and Psychopathological Assessment. Baseline sociodemographic and clinical variables were recorded, such as age, marital and employment status, educational level, age at onset of DD, age at first psychiatric appointment, DD type, and frequency of sexual delusional content. Relapse was defined as the occurrence or worsening of psychotic symptoms leading to hospitalization or to the need of higher rates for clinical appointments.

To investigate psychopathological symptoms, we used the following assessment tools at baseline and after six and 24 months: the Positive and Negative Syndrome Scale (PANSS) [6], which is a validated and translated scale for the assessment of positive, negative psychotic symptoms, the Personal and Social Performance Scale for functionality (PSP) [7], the 17-item Hamilton Rating Scale for Depression (HRSD-17) [8], the Columbia Suicide Severity Rating Scale (C-SSRS) [9] to identify lifetime and follow-up suicidal ideation and suicidal behaviour, and the first three items of the Scale to Assess Unawareness of Mental Disorder (SUMD) [10] Spanish version. Mean scores of the assessment scales at the six- and 24-month evaluation were considered outcome variables.

The sample was divided into two groups according the illness onset and the reproductive stage of the patients: group 1 was formed by DD women with premenopausal onset, and group 2 consisted of DD women with postmenopausal onset. The analysis was not intention to treat as we carried out a naturalistic and longitudinal study by comparing two subgroups of DD women in a pragmatic design. Patients were not excluded according to the adherence to protocol, so patients were grouped into two categories irrespective of the final results.

To classify DD women in premenopausal or postmenopausal groups, we account for the definitions from the International Menopause Society and the American

Association of Clinical Endocrinologists, who have developed medical guidelines for clinical practice for diagnosis and treatment of menopausal women [11, 12]. According to these definitions, menopause was considered the permanent cessation of menstruation, defined by one year without menses, resulting from loss of ovarian activity. Postmenopause was the time period after menopause, and premenopause was the time period before this year without menstruations. DD women with a perimenopausal onset of the disease were not included in the study as the main aim of the study was to compare women with an onset disease prior to the menopause and those women with a postmenopausal onset of DD.

2.3. Statistical Analysis. All data were analyzed by using SPSS for Windows (Version 19.9; SPSS Inc., Chicago, Illinois, USA). Differences in sociodemographic and clinical characteristics and assessment scales between patient groups (DD women with premenopausal onset and postmenopausal onset) were tested by using t- and χ^2-tests for continuous or categorical variables and nonparametric tests when necessary. To investigate multivariate differences, Analysis of Covariance (ANCOVA) was applied. Mean scores of the assessment scales at six and 24 months served as dependent variables; patient's menopausal onset status as between-subject factor and duration of untreated psychosis (DUP), antipsychotic dosage in chlorpromazine equivalent doses, educational level, and baseline assessment scores were considered covariates.

Significance level was set at 0.05 (two-tailed).

3. Results

3.1. Description of the Total Sample. Eighty DD women were recruited, from those 25 (31.25%) had a premenopausal onset, and 55 (68.75%) had a postmenopausal onset. Seventy-four participants from the initial sample completed the 6-month assessment and 57 were evaluated after 24 months, being 28.75% of patients lost at follow-up.

At baseline, in the whole sample, 42.5% of DD women have been never married and 60% had no cohabiters when searching for social network. Near 70% of the total sample showed delusions of persecution, which was the DD type most commonly found, followed by erotomania (11.3%) and jealousy (7.5%). Other types of delusions were less frequent. Further, 45% of the sample reported having a history of gynaecological illness at lifetime.

Baseline demographic and clinical features are shown in Table 1.

3.2. Baseline Comparisons of Sociodemographic, Clinical Features, and Psychopathology between Groups. DD women with premenopausal onset showed a longer DUP ($p = 0.028$) and had higher educational level ($p = 0.026$) compared to female DD with postmenopausal onset. No statistically significant differences were found between both groups in terms of other sociodemographic variables. Erotomanic type was more frequent in DD women with premenopausal onset, whereas jealous and somatic contents were more common in women with postmenopausal onset ($p = 0.003$). When analyzing the presence of sexual content in all types of delusions, women with premenopausal onset had higher rates of sexual delusional content compared to those with postmenopausal onset ($p = 0.006$).

At baseline, DD women with postmenopausal onset showed lower scores in the SUMD total ($p = 0.023$) than women with premenopausal onset. There were no significant differences in psychotic and depressive symptoms, neither in functionality and lifetime suicidal ideation and behaviour nor in intensity of lifetime suicidal ideation.

Mean differences in sociodemographic and clinical variables between groups are presented in Table 1.

3.3. Comparisons of Clinical and Psychopathological Symptoms at Follow-Up between Groups. After six months, no statistically significant differences were found between both groups in psychopathological symptoms, even when adjusted by confounding factors.

Furthermore, after 24 months, when uncorrected for potential confounders, no significant differences were found between both groups in psychotic symptoms, except for a tendency toward higher negative symptoms in those women with premenopausal onset ($p = 0.057$). On the other hand, DD women with premenopausal onset had also higher depressive symptoms compared to the other group ($p = 0.008$).

At the end of the follow-up period, despite being not statistically significant, DD women with premenopausal onset had higher rates of psychotic relapses (70% versus 54%) (e.g., at least one relapse) than women with postmenopausal onset.

After controlling for potential confounders, postmenopausal DD women showed a tendency toward higher scores in item 3 of the SUMD scale (e.g., awareness of social consequences) and had lower scores in depressive symptoms ($p = 0.021$) when compared to DD women with premenopausal onset. Differences in negative symptoms did not withstand significantly after adjustment.

Mean scores of psychotic and depressive symptoms and insight scores at the 24-month assessment can be found in Table 2. Figure 1 also shows the multivariate comparisons of the PANSS between women with premenopausal onset and those women with postmenopausal onset.

4. Discussion

To date, the vast majority of gender specific literature has been focused on the study of gender differences in the psychopathology and clinical course of DD patients. The most recent study regarding this issue could not confirm that male and female DD patients differ in age at onset, age at first psychiatric consultation, or suicidal ideation and behaviour, even after controlling for potential confounders [13]. However, to the best of our knowledge, no studies have investigated differences in the psychopathology of DD women attending to their reproductive status at the onset of the illness.

Thus, we conducted a prospective observational study with a 24-month follow-up period in DD women for investigating whether DD women with premenopausal onset and

TABLE 1: Baseline sociodemographic and clinical features and psychopathology symptoms by clinical groups ($N = 80$).

Variable	Total sample $N = 80$	DD women premenopausal onset $n = 25$	DD women postmenopausal onset $n = 55$	p value
Sociodemographic variables				
DUP, mean years (SD)	5.40 (9.5)	8.84 (13.9)	3.84 (6.01)	$t = 2.243$, df = 80, $p = 0.028^*$
Marital status, n (%)				$\chi^2 = 1.482$, df = 2, $p = 0.477$
Never married	34 (42.5)	13 (52)	21 (38.2)	
Married/partner	17 (21.3)	5 (20)	12 (21.8)	
Divorced/separated/widowed	29 (36.3)	7 (28)	22 (40)	
Social network (cohabiters), n (%)				$\chi^2 = 1.273$, df = 3, $p = 0.735$
0	48 (60)	15 (60)	33 (60)	
1	23 (28.8)	6 (24)	17 (30.9)	
2	6 (7.5)	3 (12)	3 (5.5)	
3 or >	3 (3.8)	1 (4)	2 (3.6)	
Educational level (years), n (%)				$\chi^2 = 9.225$, df = 3, $p = 0.026^*$
<8	10 (12.5)	1 (4)	10 (12.5)	
8-9	29 (36.3)	7 (28)	29 (36.3)	
10-11	22 (27.5)	6 (24)	22 (27.5)	
12 or >	19 (23.8)	11 (44)	19 (23.8)	
Employment status, n (%)				$\chi^2 = 6.303$, df = 3, $p = 0.098$
Unemployed	6 (7.5)	2 (8)	4 (7.3)	
Employed	24 (30)	8 (32)	16 (29.1)	
Economic benefit	20 (25)	10 (40)	10 (18.2)	
Pensioner	30 (37.5)	5 (20)	25 (45.5)	
Clinical features				
DD type, n (%)				$\chi^2 = 6.315$, df = 4, $p = 0.003^*$
Persecutory	55 (68.8)	14 (56)	41 (74.5)	
Erotomanic	9 (11.3)	8 (32)	1 (1.8)	
Jealous	6 (7.5)	1 (4)	5 (9.1)	
Somatic	3 (3.8)	1 (4)	2 (3.6)	
Grandiose	7 (8.8)	1 (4)	6 (10.9)	
Sexual delusional content, n (%)	19 (23.8)	11 (44)	8 (14.5)	FET = 0.009^*
Lifetime suicidal behaviour, n (%)	14 (17.5)	5 (20)	9 (16.4)	$\chi^2 = 0.157$, df = 1, $p = 0.755$
Gynaecological disorders, n (%)	36 (45)	15 (60)	21 (38.2)	FET = 0.058
Psychopathological symptoms, mean (SD)				
PANSS total	88.04 (14.44)	86.48 (21.91)	88.75 (15.16)	$t = -0.536$, df = 78, $p = 0.642$
PANSS positive subscale	24.77 (6.69)	24.68 (7.53)	24.82 (6.34)	$t = -0.085$, df = 78, $p = 0.932$
PANSS negative subscale	17.86 (5.18)	18.40 (6.92)	17.62 (4.21)	$t = 0.624$, df = 78, $p = 0.605$
PANSS general subscale	45.4 (8.87)	43.40 (10.54)	46.31 (7.94)	$t = -1.367$, df =78, $p = 0.175$
PSP	48.74 (13.37)	51.36 (16.2)	47.55 (11.87)	$t = 1.186$, df = 78, $p = 0.724$
HRSD-17	9.74 (5.92)	10.72 (6.52)	9.29 (5.63)	$t = 1.001$, df =78; $p = 0.320$
SUMD total	14.25 (1.45)	14.72 (1.02)	14.04 (1.65)	$t = 2.329$, df = 66.9, $p = 0.023^*$
C-SSRS, suicidal ideation intensity	3.39 (7.01)	3.12 (6.53)	3.51 (7.38)	$t = -1.208$, df = 71, $p = 0.172$

$^*p < 0.05$.

C-SSRS: Columbia Suicide Severity Rating Scale; DD: delusional disorder; df: degrees of freedom; DUP: duration of untreated psychosis; FET: Fisher's exact test; HRSD: Hamilton Rating Scale for Depression; p: p value; PANSS: Positive and Negative Syndrome Scale; PSP: Personal and Social Performance Scale; SD: standard deviation; SUMD: Scale for Unawareness of Mental Disorder; t: Student t-test; χ^2: Chi-square test.

TABLE 2: Psychopathological scores after 24 months adjusted for covariates and multivariate comparisons by groups.

Dependent variables, mean scores (SD)	Premenopausal DD women	Postmenopausal DD women	Two-way ANCOVA
PANSS total	90.51 (5.28)	77.90 (2.99)	$F(1,41) = 0.089$, $p = 0.767$
PANSS positive subscale	22.48 (1.57)	18.99 (0.88)	$F(1,41) = 2.614$, $p = 0.114$
PANSS negative subscale	21.43 (1.99)	19.35 (1.12)	$F(1,41) = 9.192$, $p = 0.567$
PANSS general subscale	46.73 (2.45)	39.09 (1.38)	$F(1,41) = 3.971$, $p = 0.757$
SUMD total	9.88 (1.15)	10.78 (0.43)	$F(1,41) = 4.590$, $p = 0.291$
SUMD item 1	3.44 (0.46)	3.93 (0.18)	$F(1,41) = 0.054$, $p = 0.782$
SUMD item 2	3.71 (0.50)	3.43 (0.18)	$F(1,41) = 0.396$, $p = 0.467$
SUMD item 3	2.73 (0.49)	3.38 (0.18)	$F(1,41) = 2.236$, $p = 0.082$
HRSD-17	8.83 (1.09)	3.91 (0.62)	$F(1,41) = 2.708$, $p = 0.021^{*}$

$^{*}p < 0.05$.
DD: delusional disorder; HRSD: Hamilton Rating Scale for Depression, PANSS: Positive and Negative Syndrome Scale; PSP: Personal and Social Performance Scale; SD: standard deviation; SUMD: Scale to Assess Unawareness of Mental Disorder.

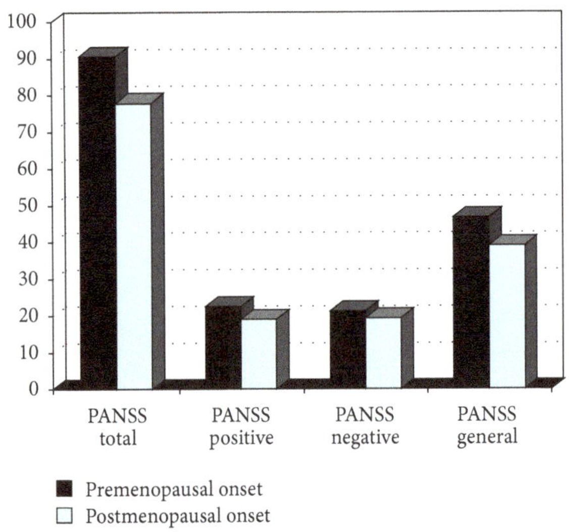

FIGURE 1: Assessment of psychotic symptoms after 24 months by groups.

those with postmenopausal onset differ in sociodemographic and clinical features and clinical course of the disorder. In this field, the only work focused on postmenopausal DD women was carried out by our team, as a first phase of an ongoing study [2]. This preliminary study evaluated gynecological variables in postmenopausal DD patients, and no correlations between age at menopause and clinical variables could be found.

In our study, surprisingly, DD women who presented a premenopausal onset of the disorder had a longer DUP and higher educational level compared to female DD patients with postmenopausal onset, suggesting that psychopathological and clinical course comparisons between groups should be controlled by these potential confounding variables. With regard to the content of delusions, erotomanic type was more frequent in women with premenopausal onset, and jealous and somatic themes were more frequent in those female DD patients with postmenopausal onset. The most representative study investigating gender differences in clinical symptoms in DD patients found no differences in DD type between men and women [14]. However, we hypothesized that these differences found in delusional content may be present when taken into account the reproductive status in women diagnosed with DD. In line with our findings, several authors have emphasized that psychotic phenomena, such as delusional content, may be related to sociodemographic and cultural variables and gender. For instance, delusional content can be related to social isolation in later life, an association not surprisingly found in women [15, 16]. In agreement with these findings, it has been reported that tactile and visual nonprominent hallucinatory phenomena may be related to late-onset psychosis, strongly associated with somatic delusional types, which were found to be more frequent in DD women with postmenopausal onset in our sample [17]. Further, some studies have highlighted that these well-established gender differences in the content of delusions can be interpreted by biological sex factors and cross-cultural factors, and not only by the age at onset of disease. In summary, different types of delusions between DD women with premenopausal onset and those with postmenopausal onset should be interpreted by the complex interactive contribution of biological, psychosocial, and cultural factors involved in the menopausal period, which is one of the most important social and biological changes in life span [16]. Further, the interface between aging and menopause should be considered, as aging can interact with the reproductive status, and menopause, defined as a loss of estrogen function, may have an influence on the process of aging [5]. For instance, estrogen withdrawal in the menopause has been associated with increased vulnerability of cerebrovascular disease, which several authors consider a risk factor for late-onset psychosis [17].

We found no baseline differences between both groups in terms of psychotic and depressive symptoms, functionality, and suicidality. To date, no studies have compared these clinical features in women with premenopausal and postmenopausal onset. de Portugal and colleagues [14] found that DD men showed a worse functioning and a more severe illness compared to women, but the potential effects of menopause on the clinical course in DD women were not specifically investigated.

Psychopathological symptoms, insight, rates for relapses, and admission rates at follow-up between both groups were also compared. After six months, these clinical variables did not seem to differ between DD women with premenopausal or postmenopausal onset. However, at the end of the study, when unadjusted for confounding factors, DD women with premenopausal onset showed a tendency toward higher negative symptoms compared to the other group. These findings are in agreement with previous studies that highlighted the potential vulnerability of women for an exacerbation of psychotic symptoms or a worsening of psychotic disorders in the menopause [4, 5, 18] and consistent with the fact that the loss of the protective effect of estrogens may be followed by a deterioration of course in women suffering from psychosis diagnosed in the reproductive period. In summary, this loss of protection after menopause may explain the presence of higher rates of relapses and higher depressive symptoms in women diagnosed with psychosis during the reproductive life span (e.g., DD women with premenopausal onset). On the other hand, lower depressive symptoms in DD women with postmenopausal onset compared to women with premenopausal onset can be explained by the fact that we did not include DD women in the perimenopausal period. In brief, the perimenopausal transition seems to be characterized by significantly higher intensity of depressive symptoms when compared to life span after menopause, and this fact may explain why DD women with postmenopausal onset did not achieve higher severity of depressive symptoms compared to postmenopausal women with an onset in the premenopausal period. In our study, no statistically significant differences in terms of positive psychotic symptoms were found between both groups. This finding is also in line with several studies that found patients who develop psychosis in later life to have similar intensity of positive symptoms compared with patients with an earlier onset of disease [19, 20].

Moreover, in our sample, DD women with premenopausal onset showed higher rates of relapses and higher depressive symptoms at the end of the study period compared to DD women with postmenopausal onset. This fact is also in line with the studies aforementioned [4, 5, 18]. Women with premenopausal onset showed a worse global insight at the time of the study inclusion that could have mediated the recovery or worsening of psychotic symptoms, specifically in negative symptoms. Gumley and coworkers [21] explored the relationship between DUP, insight, and psychotic recovery in a prospective sample of first-episode of psychosis. The authors found that recovery in negative symptoms was predicted by both DUP and insight, which is in line with our findings. However, these findings should be confirmed in larger samples comparing women diagnosed with schizophrenia with females individuals suffering from DD.

In a further step, we considered DUP, severity of baseline psychopathological symptoms, antipsychotic doses (i.e., chlorpromazine equivalent dosage), and educational level as potential confounders, so they were included as covariates in multivariate analyses. After controlling for these factors, postmenopausal DD women showed a tendency toward worse insight in terms of awareness of social consequences of the disorder compared to women with premenopausal onset, suggesting that a later onset of the disease would have an influence on insight. These results in our study are supported by a recent review [22] proposing trajectories of insight in schizophrenia across the life span. The authors concluded that insight may be worse at the first-episode of psychosis, shows a moderate improvement in midlife, and declines in the elderly. Further support for the influence of menopause in an indirect consideration (i.e., aging) comes from a recent study in late-life schizophrenia [23], which suggests that predictors of insight in schizophrenia differ across the life span, probably according to age-related changes in neurocognitive performance.

Strengths and Limitations. In our point of view, this study provides unique evidence in the field of delusional disorders, as to best of our knowledge; the vast majority of studies have been focused on the investigation of gender differences without taken into account the potential influence of menopause on the psychopathology or the clinical course.

However, in our study several limitations should be mentioned: (1) the first limitation would be the small sample size that could have limited the statistical power and the possibility of performing more complex statistical multivariate analysis and (2) the second limitation would be the lack of blood determinations of estrogen levels in these DD women; as this was not the aim of our study. Furthermore, perimenopause was not considered index episode in our study.

5. Conclusions

In summary, it is apparent that erotomanic, jealous, and somatic delusional contents may vary across the reproductive life in DD women.

DD women who presented a premenopausal onset attended later to our outpatient service and presented higher depressive symptoms compared to women with postmenopausal onset, suggesting a worse insight at the study entry and a worsening of symptoms after the menopause in women with premenopausal onset. Further, this group of DD women showed a tendency toward higher negative symptoms that may be mediated by the DUP and insight scores aforementioned. Larger studies should confirm these findings and propose a global model to better explain our results.

DD women with postmenopausal onset had a tendency toward a worse insight in social consequences after 24 months, suggesting that aging may have an influence on the course of insight in the direction of worse insight in the elderly.

Disclosures

Professor Bernardo has been a consultant for, received grant/research support and honoraria from, and been on the speakers/advisory board of ABBiotics, Adamed, AMGEN, Eli

Lilly, Ferrer, Forum Pharmaceuticals, Gedeon, Janssen-Cilag, Lundbeck, Otsuka, Pfizer, and Roche. Alexandre González-Rodríguez has received the First Juan José López-Ibor Grant for Young Researchers and honoraria or paid for travels from Pfizer, Janssen, Ferrer, and Lundbeck-Otsuka. Oriol Molina-Andreu has received honoraria or paid for travels from Pfizer, Janssen, Ferrer, and Lundbeck-Otsuka. Marina Garriga has received honoraria or paid for travels from Janssen-Cilag, Lilly, and Lundbeck-Otsuka. Alexandre Pons has provided consulting services to Janssen-Cilag, Johnson & Johnson, and he is speaker/advisory board member for Janssen-Cilag. Rosa Catalán has received honoraria or has been paid for travels from Lilly, Lundbeck, Janssen, Ferrer, Pfizer, and Bristol. Rafael Penadés has received honoraria or paid for travels from Otsuka-Lundbeck.

Conflict of Interests

The authors declare that there is no conflict of interests regarding the publication of this paper.

Acknowledgments

This study was supported by the Ministerio de Economía y Competitividad; Instituto de Salud Carlos III-Fondo Europeo de Desarrollo Regional; Unión Europea (Reference PI11/02006); Un manera de hacer Europa; Centro de Investigación Biomédica en Red de Salud Mental, CIBERSAM, by the Government of Catalonia, Secretaria d'Universitats i Recerca del Departament d'Economia i Coneixement (2014SGR441). This work was developed (in part) at the Centro Esther Koplowitz (Barcelona).

References

[1] N. Bergemann, P. Parzer, B. Runnebaum, F. Resch, and C. Mundt, "Estrogen, menstrual cycle phases, and psychopathology in women suffering from schizophrenia," *Psychological Medicine*, vol. 37, no. 10, pp. 1427–1436, 2007.

[2] A. González-Rodríguez, O. Molina-Andreu, R. Penadés Rubio, R. Catalán Campos, and M. Bernardo Arroyo, "Reproductive variables and gynaecological service use in delusional disorder outpatients," *Revista de Psiquiatría y Salud Mental*, vol. 8, no. 2, pp. 92–96, 2015.

[3] M. V. Seeman and M. Lang, "The role of estrogens in schizophrenia gender differences," *Schizophrenia Bulletin*, vol. 16, no. 2, pp. 185–194, 1990.

[4] A. Riecher-Rössler and J. Kulkarni, "Estrogens and gonadal function in schizophrenia and related psychoses," in *Biological Basis of Sex Differences in Psychopharmacology*, vol. 8 of *Current Topics in Behavioral Neurosciences*, pp. 155–171, Springer, Berlin, Germany, 2011.

[5] A. Riecher-Rössler, "Psychotic disorders and menopause: the untold story," in *The Menopausal Transition: Interface between Gynecology and Psychiatry*, C. N. Soares and M. Warren, Eds., vol. 175 of *Key Issues in Mental Health*, pp. 115–126, Karger, Basel, Switzerland, 2009.

[6] S. R. Kay, A. Fiszbein, M. Vital-Herne, and L. S. Fuentes, "The positive and negative syndrome scale—Spanish adaptation," *Journal of Nervous and Mental Disease*, vol. 178, no. 8, pp. 510–517, 1990.

[7] R. Apiquian, R. Elena Ulloa, M. Herrera-Estrella et al., "Validity of the Spanish version of the personal and social performance scale in schizophrenia," *Schizophrenia Research*, vol. 112, no. 1–3, pp. 181–186, 2009.

[8] J. A. Ramos-Brieva and A. Cordero-Villafafila, "A new validation of the Hamilton Rating Scale for depression," *Journal of Psychiatric Research*, vol. 22, no. 1, pp. 21–28, 1988.

[9] K. Posner, G. K. Brown, B. Stanley et al., "The Columbia-suicide severity rating scale: initial validity and internal consistency findings from three multisite studies with adolescents and adults," *American Journal of Psychiatry*, vol. 168, no. 12, pp. 1266–1277, 2011.

[10] A. Ruiz, E. Pousa, R. Duñó, J. M. Crosas, S. Cuppa, and C. García, "Spanish adaptation of the Scale to Asses Unawareness of Mental Disorder (SUMD)," *Actas Españolas de Psiquiatría*, vol. 36, no. 2, pp. 111–119, 2008.

[11] W. H. Utian, "The International Menopause Society menopause related terminology definitions," *Climacteric*, vol. 2, no. 4, pp. 284–286, 1999.

[12] N. F. Goodman, R. H. Cobin, S. B. Ginzburg, I. A. Katz, and D. E. Woode, "American Association of Clinical Endocrinologists. American Association of Clinical Endocrinologists Medical Guidelines for Clinical Practice for the diagnosis and treatment of menopause: executive summary of recommendations," *Endocrine Practice*, vol. 17, no. 6, pp. 949–954, 2011.

[13] A. González-Rodríguez, O. Molina-Andreu, V. Navarro, C. Gastó, R. Penadés, and R. Catalán, "Delusional disorder: no gender differences in age at onset, suicidal ideation, or suicidal behavior," *Revista Brasileira de Psiquiatria*, vol. 36, no. 2, pp. 119–124, 2014.

[14] E. de Portugal, N. González, V. Miriam, J. M. Haro, J. Usall, and J. A. Cervilla, "Gender differences in delusional disorder: evidence from an outpatient sample," *Psychiatry Research*, vol. 177, no. 1-2, pp. 235–239, 2010.

[15] V. A. Morgan, D. J. Castle, and A. V. Jablensky, "Do women express and experience psychosis differently from men? Epidemiological evidence from the Australian National Study of Low Prevalence (Psychotic) Disorders," *Australian and New Zealand Journal of Psychiatry*, vol. 42, no. 1, pp. 74–82, 2008.

[16] M. Sáenz-Herrero, *Psychopathology in Women: Incorporating Gender Perspective into Descriptive Psychopathology*, Springer, Cham, Switzerland, 2015.

[17] A. Hasset, "Schizophrenia and delusional disorders with onset in later life," *Revista Brasileira Psiquiatria*, vol. 24, supplement 1, pp. 81–86, 2002.

[18] O. P. Almeida, R. J. Howard, R. Levy, and A. S. David, "Psychotic states arising in late life (late paraphrenia) psychopathology and nosology," *British Journal of Psychiatry*, vol. 166, no. 2, pp. 205–214, 1995.

[19] G. D. Pearlson, L. Kreger, P. V. Rabins et al., "A chart review study of late-onset and early-onset schizophrenia," *American Journal of Psychiatry*, vol. 146, no. 12, pp. 1568–1574, 1989.

[20] M. V. Seeman, "Treating schizophrenia at the time of menopause," *Maturitas*, vol. 72, no. 2, pp. 117–120, 2012.

[21] A. I. Gumley, M. Schwannauer, A. Macbeth et al., "Insight, duration of untreated psychosis and attachment in first-episode psychosis: prospective study of psychiatric recovery over 12-month follow-up," *British Journal of Psychiatry*, vol. 205, no. 1, pp. 60–67, 2014.

[22] P. Gerretsen, E. Plitman, T. K. Rajji, and A. Graff-Guerrero, "The effects of aging on insight into illness in schizophrenia: a review," *International Journal of Geriatric Psychiatry*, vol. 29, no. 11, pp. 1145–1161, 2014.

[23] P. Gerretsen, B. H. Mulsant, A. Y. Liu et al., "Insight into illness in late-life schizophrenia: a function of illness severity and premorbid intellectual function," *Schizophrenia Research*, vol. 150, no. 1, pp. 217–222, 2013.

14

Irony and Proverb Comprehension in Schizophrenia: Do Female Patients "Dislike" Ironic Remarks?

Alexander M. Rapp, Karin Langohr, Dorothee E. Mutschler, and Barbara Wild

Department of Psychiatry, University of Tuebingen, Calwerstraße 14, 72076 Tuebingen, Germany

Correspondence should be addressed to Alexander M. Rapp; alexander.rapp@med.uni-tuebingen.de

Academic Editor: Robin Emsley

Difficulties in understanding irony and sarcasm are part of the social cognition deficits in patients with schizophrenia. A number of studies have reported higher error rates during comprehension in patients with schizophrenia. However, the relationships of these impairments to schizotypal personality traits and other language deficits, such as the comprehension of proverbs, are unclear. We investigated irony and proverb comprehension in an all-female sample of 20 schizophrenia patients and 27 matched controls. Subjects indicated if a statement was intended to be ironic, literal, or meaningless and furthermore rated the meanness and funniness of the stimuli and certainty of their decision. Patients made significantly more errors than controls did. Globally, there were no overall differences in the ratings. However, patients rated the subgroup of stimuli with answers given incorrectly as having significantly less meanness and in case of an error indicated a significantly higher certainty than controls. Across all of the study participants, performances in irony ($r = -0.51$) and proverb ($r = 0.56$) comprehension were significantly correlated with schizotypal personality traits, suggesting a continuum of nonliteral language understanding. Because irony is so frequent in everyday conversations, this makes irony an especially promising candidate for social cognition training in schizophrenia.

1. Background

Defective appraisal of the intention of others and difficulties with language are hallmark features of psychopathology in schizophrenia. Social cognition deficits have been previously identified and are currently being extensively researched. The results show that deficits in social cognition are relevant to real-world functioning and outcome [1]. Training of social cognitive skills has gained increasing interest in schizophrenia therapy. In this context, the comprehension of ironic remarks by patients with schizophrenia has become a research focus both as an outcome measure and as a training goal [1–5].

This is obvious, considering that the decision on whether a remark made by others is intended to be ironic or not is slightly artificial, but is instead required routinely in everyday interaction. Everyone is familiar with irony. It is remarkably frequently used, as shown by linguistic research [6, 7]. For example, Gibbs [8] showed that 1 out of 8 conversational turns in an everyday communication among college students was ironic. In the case of linguistic irony (which alone is discussed here), an ironic expression is usually incorrect and often the opposite of what the speaker intends to communicate [9]. Perhaps even more relevant to social cognition research is that irony serves important communicative functions [10, 11], such as expressing negative emotional content [12, 13], expressing anger [14, 15], creating an impression of being a humorous person [8, 16], disarming a difficult conversational situation [12, 17, 18], or—in the case of sarcasm—meaning the opposite and mocking someone. The fact that irony is more often used in difficult stages of communication [9, 16, 19] is also relevant in the context of schizophrenic impairment. Since ironic remarks are ambiguous per se, irony comprehension also poses challenges to ambiguity resolution [20, 21], which is a cognitive operation patients with schizophrenia are known to have difficulties with [22–24].

Previous research has shown that patients with schizophrenia, as a group, have difficulties in irony comprehension [3, 25–29], but not all patients show a deficit [30, 31]. However, given the increasing interest in irony for social cognition training and assessment, more profound knowledge of the difficulties faced by patients with schizophrenia in irony comprehension seems worthwhile [1]. Many studies on irony in schizophrenia are motivated by the intention to provide measurements of theory of mind (TOM) and perspective taking deficits [2, 5, 26] in schizophrenia because irony comprehension, essentially, requires building of a second-order TOM [32–34].

However, defective irony comprehension in schizophrenia is likewise influenced by numerous additional cognitive operations that individuals with schizophrenia are known to have difficulties with. For example, irony also relates to higher-level language comprehension [10, 34–37]. Traditionally [38–40], and as documented by a large body of research [41–45], schizophrenia is considered to lead to a deficit in comprehension of nonliteral language. Nonliteral language, such as proverbs, metaphors, and idioms, is interpreted "word by word" (literally) as either wrong or wrong in a particular context. The same applies to irony and sarcasm, because in many or even most cases, ironic statements taken literally state the exact opposite of what is intended (e.g., the remark "oh brilliant!" when something bad happens). Irony and sarcasm are therefore important subtypes of nonliteral language. Traditionally, it has been assumed that patients with schizophrenia show a cognitive bias towards literal interpretation of nonliteral expressions [46, 47]. In the case of irony, that would result in assuming the exact opposite of the intention. However, only limited research [2, 5, 25, 26] has been conducted on the relationship between irony comprehension and bias towards literal interpretation of other stimuli, such as metaphors, and even these studies have often used only small numbers of stimuli.

Another interesting point that has not received much attention in past research is how patients with schizophrenia appreciate ironic remarks. Most previous studies have addressed performance (i.e., whether patients fail to comprehend ironic remarks), while it is widely unknown if patients with schizophrenia "like" ironic remarks or they perhaps judge their intention as more mean than healthy controls would do. This relationship to the perceived "meanness" by patients with schizophrenia seems particularly interesting, because judging the intention of others as "mean" or "hostile" may relate to the origin of delusions in these patients [48, 49]. Indeed, it has been suggested (e.g., by [21, 50]) that misinterpretation of "ambiguous and hard-to-interpret communicative signals" such as "ironic comments" in combination with the above-mentioned factors may contribute to delusion formation in schizophrenia. Ironic comments are often intended to be funny [8, 11, 16]. Patients with schizophrenia showed aberrant ratings for the jocularity of stimuli in previous investigations [51–55]; however, to our knowledge, no research has addressed the funniness of ironic comments in schizophrenia.

There is consensus in the literature that the severity of irony comprehension deficit differs between individuals with schizophrenia. However, it is currently unclear whether this deficit depends on a continuum with schizophrenia and what the possible mediating factors could be. One possible mediating factor for deficits in sarcasm comprehension that has been discussed, but not consistently found, in the literature is schizotypal personality traits [35, 56–58]. A continuum is assumed for schizotypal personality traits between schizotypal traits in nonclinical subjects and symptoms manifested in patients with schizophrenia [21, 59, 60]. However, no studies have investigated irony comprehension in relation to schizotypal traits in both patients with schizophrenia and controls in a single study.

Our pilot study aimed to investigate both comprehension and appreciation of ironic remarks in a sample of patients with schizophrenia. On the one hand, we aimed to investigate comprehension and whether it was related to comprehension of proverbs, the most often applied measurement of concretism in schizophrenia. We applied an irony comprehension task recently developed by our group [35, 58]. In this task, which is a written task that is prosody-free, subjects decide by button press whether the statement of a protagonist in short text vignettes is intended, literal, ironic, or meaningless. In addition, the subjects rated their self-certainty for that decision in each stimulus and rated the "meanness" and "funniness" of the statements on a Likert scale.

We have several hypotheses concerning the results. Since lower performance in irony detection is documented in several previous investigations [25–29], our hypothesis was that patients may find the decision if a conversational remark is intended to be ironic more difficult and, therefore, would show lower certainty in their decisions, especially for ironic stimuli. We further assumed the supposed higher-level difficulty of the decision about their intention will result in schizophrenic patients judging the stimuli as more mean and less funny. Following the continuum hypothesis [60] and based on our previous functional magnetic resonance imaging findings [21, 35] we expected to find an association between schizotypal personality traits and performance across all subjects irrespective of the presence or absence of a schizophrenia diagnosis.

2. Materials and Methods

2.1. Subjects. 20 right-handed [61] individuals with DSM IV schizophrenia and 27 right-handed healthy control subjects gave written informed consent and participated in the study. All study subjects were female. Control subjects were recruited from the general population and were free from psychiatric illness. Groups were matched for age, educational level, and verbal intelligence (see Table 1).

Patients were recruited from the Department of Psychiatry, University of Tübingen, Germany. Patients were acute or subacute inpatients and predominantly of the paranoid subtype. All participants were native German speakers, had no other past or present medical illness, and had sufficient reading skills. A subgroup of the sample additionally participated in a functional magnetic resonance imaging study [21]. All patients were on stable medication, mainly with atypical antipsychotics (mean dosis [65] 534 (SD: 230) chlorpromazine equivalents).

TABLE 1: Clinical and sociodemographic characteristics of patient and control groups.

	Healthy controls $N = 27$	Schizophrenia $N = 20$	Significance
Age	38,9	34,1	n.s.
Education years[1]	15,1	14,2	n.s.
Digit span (digits)	6,2	6,1	n.s.
CPT errors	0,1	1,5	0.0026
Verbal intelligence[3]	31,3	30,6	n.s.
HAWIE picture sequencing test[2]	32,5	26,4	n.s.
SPQ cognitive perceptual[4]	10,1	22,3	0.00007
SPQ interpersonal[4]	5,7	14,8	0.00005
SPQ total score	15,6	36,7	0.00000
PANSS total score		70,3	
SANS total score		36,1	
SAPS total score		35,7	
Global assessment of functioning scale		37,9	

[1]In full-time education.
[2]Subtest 2 from [62].
[3]Multiple-choice vocabulary test [63].
[4]As defined by [64].

2.2. Procedure. First, all subjects received complete information about the study and ability to consent was ensured. Then, subjects underwent a practice session for the irony comprehension task with stimuli not used in the experiment and provided written informed consent. The study was approved by the local ethical committee (University of Tuebingen, Germany). Subjects then completed the irony comprehension task. The sequence of the other tests was counterbalanced between the subjects. If requested by the subject, a short break between the tests was possible.

2.3. Irony Comprehension Task. An irony comprehension and evaluation task was applied to all subjects. Stimuli and stimulus sequence are identical with a previous functional magnetic resonance imaging study [21, 35] from our group. However, comprehension assessment was modified. In addition, for each target sentence, subjects rated certainty of their decision, meanness of the statements, and jocularity of the statements.

The irony comprehension task consists of 56 short German text vignettes as stimuli, each consisting of an introductive context (2 sentences, 8–12 words) and two or more protagonists (e.g., "Petra hates fish. Her mother has cooked salmon for her."). The introductive context is then followed by a target part, in which one of the protagonists makes a statement (e.g., "Petra says: 'Oh brilliant, my favourite meal!'"). This statement has, in this context, either an ironic or a literal meaning or is meaningless.

The number of words and sentences, grammatical complexity, and word frequency are counterbalanced between literal, ironic, and meaningless context scenarios.

Corresponding literal and ironic target sentences are identical. For example, for the above ironic stimulus, the literal counterpart would be, "Katja loves spaghetti. Her mother has cooked a lot of spaghetti for her. Katja says: 'Oh brilliant, my favourite meal!'"

A comprehensive description of the stimuli and their development and evaluation process is given in [35, 58].

During the irony task, subjects were seated in front of a notebook computer (Dell Inspiron) next to one of the investigators (K.L.). In-house software was used to present the stimuli and measure the button press response. Stimuli were presented in a pseudorandomized order not foreseeable for the subject. The introductive context was both presented visually and read out by the investigator. To avoid any effect of prosody, target sentences were only presented visually. The task was to indicate by pressing one out of three buttons whether the target sentence was in this context most likely ironic, literally meaningful, or meaningless. After each stimulus and button press, subjects were asked by the investigator (K.L.) to rate the certainty of their decision on a 5-point Likert scale (from 0, very uncertain, to 4, very certain) as well as the meanness (from 0, not mean at all, to 4, very hurtful) and jocularity (from 0, not funny at all, to 4, very funny) of the protagonist's statement.

2.4. Proverb Comprehension Test. A multiple-choice German proverb test developed at the University of Münster [66, 67] was administered to all participants. It is a paper and pencil test without a time limit. This test has a higher than average number of test stimuli, as it consists of 32 salient German proverbs/idioms. A comprehensive description of the test and its development is given in Thoma et al. [66] and Uekermann et al. [67]. Some test proverbs/idiom stimuli are literally true, whereas others are not. The correct meaning cannot always be determined if a subject is unaware of the correct meaning. A major advantage of the test is that it enables an analysis of performance with respect to the subjects' familiarity. It consists of two procedures. First, the subject rates how familiar he or she is with the proverb given on a 5-point Likert scale (from 1, never, to 5, a lot of times). In a second procedure, the subject is presented with the proverbs again and asked to decide (multiple choice) which out of the 4 given answers best explains the meaning. Type I represents a definition that is based on the one given by the German dictionary of proverbs [68] and is subsequently referred to as the correct one. Type II (abstract/meaningless), Type III (concrete meaningful), and Type IV (concrete/meaningless) represent distractors.

Several scores were defined in our investigation. First a proverb familiarity score was calculated for each individual. It consists of the mean values of the familiarity ratings of all 32 proverbs. Secondly, mean values for numbers of proverbs rated as unfamiliar were compared between patients and controls. Here, we defined a proverb as "familiar" if its rating is above 1; that means it is ready counted as familiar if the subject indicates he has heard it once before. Each Type I answer given is counted as one point, whereas all other answers in multiple choice are counted zero. This results in a sum score for each participant. The higher the score is, the better the performance is. The highest reachable sum score is 32. All these scores were compared between the groups.

2.5. Other Assessment. After completion of the previous tests and the schizotypal personality questionnaire [69], German version by [64], a verbal intelligence test (Mehrfachwahl-Wortschatz test version B; [63]) and the subtest "picture sequencing" from the HAWIE-R intelligence test [62] were applied.

In addition, patients were interviewed by a psychiatrist (A.R.) to evaluate current psychopathology using the SAPS [70], SANS [71], and PANSS [72] and to evaluate functioning (GAF).

2.6. Statistical Analyses. SPSS 11.5 was used for all statistical analyses. Due to the exploratory character of the study and the small sample size, a significance level of 0.05 was chosen.

3. Results

3.1. Irony Comprehension

Performance. Regarding the percentage of correct answers, there was a significant difference between schizophrenia patients and healthy control subjects ($P < 0.001$, ANOVA): while the healthy control group had 95% correct answers on average, patients had only 85% correct answers. The error profile was also different between patients and controls (see Figure 1) ($P = 0.09$; Mann-Whitney U test).

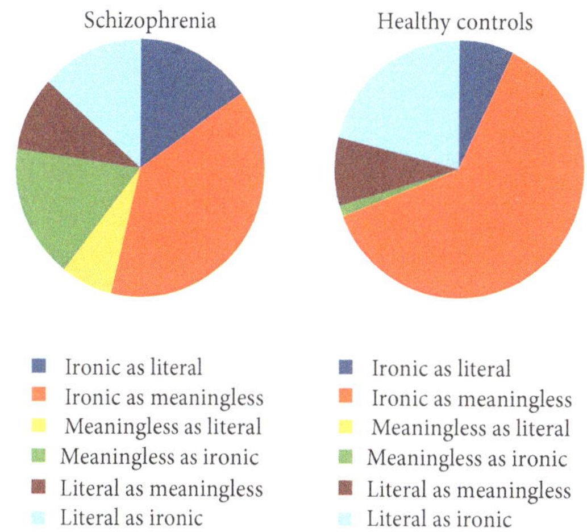

FIGURE 1: Pattern of errors in the irony comprehension test of patients (left) and control subjects (right).

3.2. Judgement/Appreciation of Ironic Remarks. For the whole task with all of the stimuli taken into account, the patient and control groups did not differ in their certainty, in their judgement of meanness, or in how funny they rated the stimuli (Table 2). The stimuli were then analysed in further detail. All of these results are shown in Table 2. First, the types of stimuli were analysed separately for ironic, literal, and nonsense stimuli. Neither the ratings for ironic nor those for literal sentences differed significantly. There was only a significant difference for the meaningless stimuli in funniness judgement in that patients with schizophrenia rated the meaningless sentences significantly more funny ($P = 0.002$).

In a next step, the ratings for answers given correctly and the answers given incorrectly were compared between the groups. Control subjects and patients with schizophrenia reported significantly lower certainty for the stimuli that they responded to with an error compared to those to which they replied correctly ($P = 0.004$ in patients with schizophrenia; $P < 0.0001$ in controls). However, the decline in perception was more enhanced in control subjects relative to patients (see Figure 2). Stimuli that they responded to with an error were rated as significantly less certain by controls than by patients.

In the case of meanness ratings, control subjects ($P > 0.0001$), but not patients with schizophrenia ($P = 0.26$), showed an increase in rated meanness for stimuli they responded to with an incorrect judgement as compared to ones they answered correctly.

There were no differences between correct and incorrect stimuli in either group for perceived funniness.

3.3. Association of Schizotypal Personality Traits with Performance. This analysis was calculated for all participants together, following the rationale that schizotypal traits represent a continuum [59]. There was a significant correlation between the performance in the irony comprehension test (% correct answers) and the total score of the SPQ (PEARSON $r = -0.51$; $P < 0.0001$) (Figure 3(a)). However, there was no correlation between the SPQ and the rating measures. There was also a significant correlation between proverb test performance and the SPQ total score (familiar stimuli $r = -0.46$; $P = 0.002$ (Figure 3(b)); all proverbs $r = -0.56$; $P = 0.00009$).

Table 2: Group differences in detection and appreciation of irony.

		Healthy controls	Schizophrenia	Significance
All stimuli	Certainty	3,81	3,73	0.26
	Meanness	0,58	0,52	0.58
	Funniness	0,57	0,51	0.54
Literal stimuli	Certainty	3,81	3,85	0.59
	Meanness	0,09	0,15	0.26
	Funniness	0,22	0,15	0.43
Ironic stimuli	Certainty	3,79	3,67	0.21
	Meanness	1,02	0,77	0.24
	Funniness	1,09	0,76	0.10
Meaningless stimuli	Certainty	3,88	3,60	**0.02**
	Meanness	0,70	0,69	0.95
	Funniness	0,19	0,70	0.002
Correct answers	Certainty	3,84	3,82	0.70
	Meanness	0,56	0,49	0.55
	Funniness	0,57	0,41	0.16
Incorrect answers	Certainty	2,34	3,34	**0.00002**
	Meanness	2,23	0,72	**0.000001**
	Funniness	0,52	0,60	0.64

4. Discussion

We investigated the comprehension and appraisal of higher-level language in female patients with schizophrenia and matched healthy control subjects. Subjects completed a German irony comprehension and appraisal test [58], which consists of text vignettes that end with a statement of one of its protagonists and this statement is (in this context) either ironic, literal, or meaningless. Congruent with our expectation, patients made significantly more errors in this test, as a group and relative to healthy controls.

4.1. Interpretation Ratings. Beyond investigating performance, a main goal of the study was to understand how patients with schizophrenia would evaluate and appreciate ironic remarks. As outlined in the introduction, we hypothesized that patients with schizophrenia would be less certain in their decision about intention and would indicate a higher degree of meanness for the stimuli, especially those intended to be ironic, and would rate them less funny. None of these hypotheses was clearly confirmed. Only meaningless stimuli were rated significantly higher in their funniness, a finding that is compatible with previous findings of differences in funniness ratings in patients with schizophrenia [55]. However, it must be noted that this was contrary to our hypothesis. Perhaps even more relevant was the finding that the overall difference was small and there was little variance. The data about certainty was less interesting, because although patients with schizophrenia made significantly more errors, they indicated equal certainty of their decisions. Since 85% of the correct answers could still be regarded as a positive performance, evaluation of irony could be impaired only to a small degree in schizophrenia. Therefore, it is possible that our sample size was insufficient to detect a significant effect. However, another possibility is that patients had difficulties with our metacognitive evaluation task since one of the instructions was to reflect about "self-certainty of their decision." Schizophrenia, however, may go along with a fundamental disturbance of self-certainty [73], and that may have altered ratings in our task. For example, delusions, doubtlessly one of the hallmark symptoms of schizophrenia, are unshiftable false beliefs and represent perturbance of certainty of an interpretation [74]. The pattern of response for certainty ratings for items judged wrong by the individual is compatible with such an effect while there is no significant difference in ratings between controls and patients with schizophrenia for items where performance was correct. There was a highly significant difference in items judged wrong; patients with schizophrenia were more certain in their (wrong) decisions, which is in line with previous findings and historical reports of a higher degree of unconcern in semantic judgment in schizophrenia. Moreover, they rated stimuli judged false as less mean. This may be interpreted as unconcern towards irony. However, our original hypothesis that female patients with schizophrenia may "dislike" ironic remarks is not supported.

4.2. Proverb Comprehension. An additional aspect to our investigation was the evaluation of performance in the multiple-choice proverbs test. As expected, we found an impairment in schizophrenia. Our finding of an impairment of proverb comprehension in schizophrenia mirrors numerous classical findings [40, 41, 45]. For example, similar to this study, a seminal investigation by Elmore and Gorham [75] found severe impairments in female patients with schizophrenia when they had to match proverbs with the appropriate alternative meaning in a multiple-choice test, a finding that is confirmed by a substantial number of

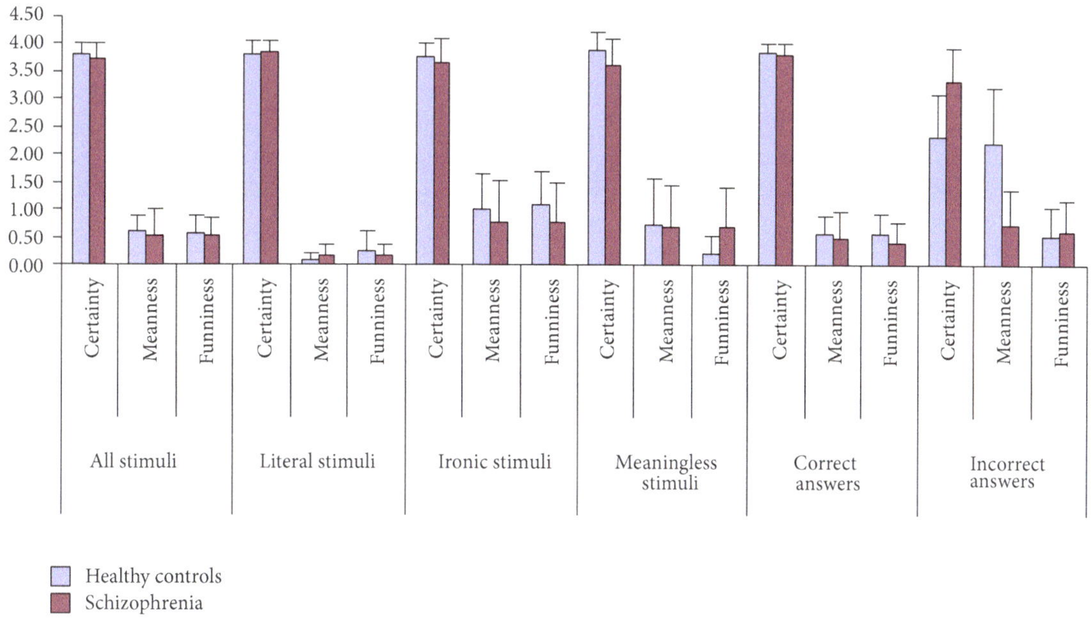

FIGURE 2: Detection and appreciation of irony. Group differences.

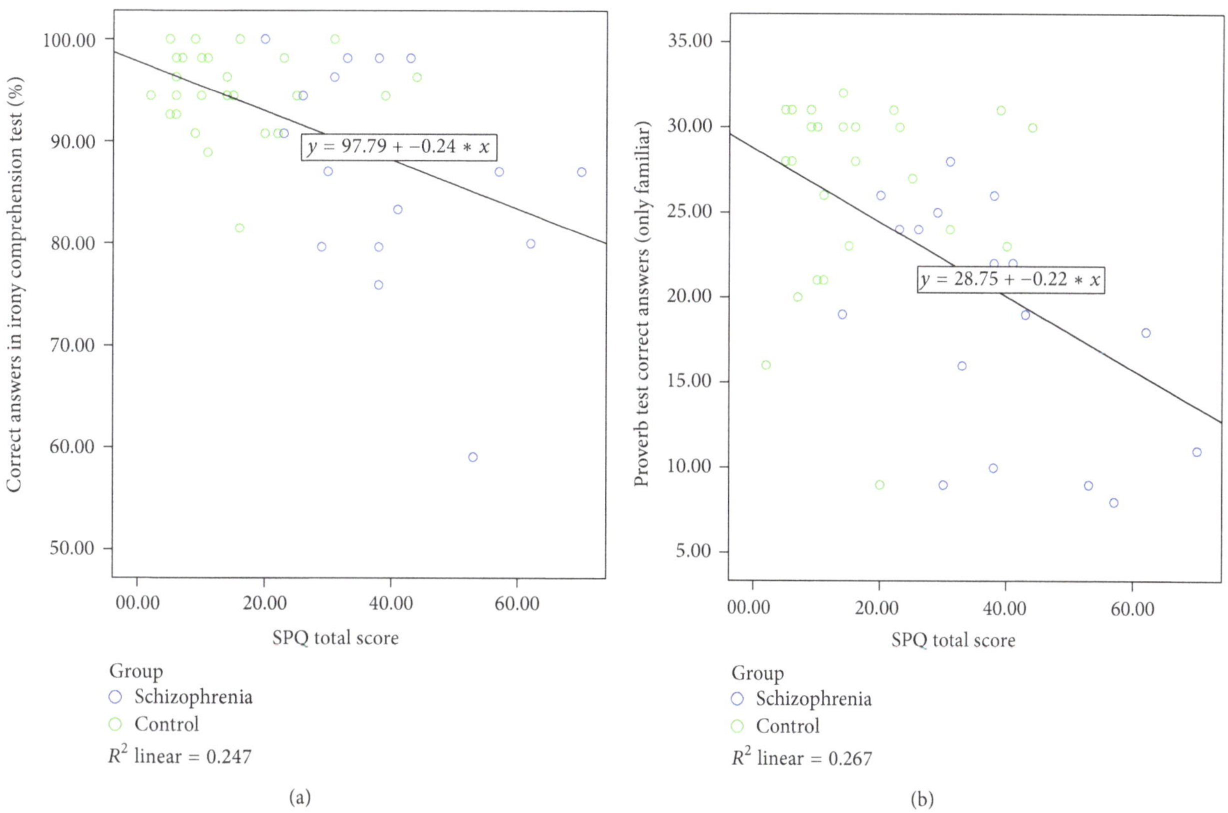

FIGURE 3: Correlation between performance in the (a) irony comprehension test and (b) proverb comprehension test and schizotypal personality traits.

studies [45]. However, research from both healthy and clinical populations indicates familiarity is a factor that critically interrelates with proverb test performance [37]. Familiar proverbs (that mean proverbs that the individual "knows") are much easier to interpret [45, 67]. Of note, this factor was not recommended in many previous investigations in schizophrenia; however our results indicate it is relevant: the impairment in schizophrenia was more pronounced when we analyzed only the stimuli that the subject said she was familiar with. This result was in line with the findings from the test developers of the German proverb test used here [66], which showed that patients with schizophrenia in a mixed gender sample are impaired in the test. However, in contrast to the investigation by Thoma et al. [66], in our sample, the difference in familiarity was not significant. Nevertheless, our results further underline the importance of familiarity for proverb comprehension described by this study.

4.3. A Possible Role of Schizotypal Personality Traits. Irrespective of the diagnosis when means were correlated across all study participants (patients and controls), the performance was correlated with schizotypal personality traits: the higher the total score of the schizotypal personality questionnaire (SPQ), the lower the performance in either the irony or proverb test. This result is in line with increasing evidence suggesting that schizotypal personality traits represent a continuum from healthiness to schizophrenia [59, 76] and, in a broader sense, our results further strengthen the increasing evidence of a continuum between healthiness and psychosis/schizophrenia. It has repeatedly been suggested that such a continuum might be present for language symptoms; however, our study is the first to demonstrate that, for nonliteral expressions, it is present for proverbs and ironic remarks. On the basis of our results, we conclude that schizotypal personality traits could possibly mediate nonliteral language impairment in schizophrenia. A possible cerebral correlate is a finding that brain activation in the medial prefrontal lobe/dorsal ACC during comprehension was associated with comprehension of ironic but not literal statements in our task in a recent fMRI study from our group [21]. It is important to note, however, that the patient sample from this study has overlap with our investigation.

Another limitation is that patients and control subjects significantly differ in their expression of schizotypal personality traits, although Figure 3 shows there is notable overlap between the groups. This limits the generalizability of our findings and makes future studies with a broader range of schizotypal symptoms in their nonclinical samples eligible, especially since the significant correlation between SPQ and proverb and irony comprehension performance reported here is in contrast to other studies with only nonclinical populations that failed to find such an association. For example, Langdon and Coltheart [56] found no association between irony and metaphor comprehension and psychometric schizotypy. In another nonclinical study [57], irony comprehension was assessed using the awareness of social inference test (TASIT); [77]; they also found no difference between high and low schizotypy. Using the same irony task as ours in a different sample of 15 healthy female subjects, Mutschler [58] found no performance difference between high and low expression of schizotypy. For other types of nonliteral stimuli, Humphrey et al. [78] failed to find a difference between high and low SPQ individuals on metaphor comprehension in a larger sample from New Zealand. However, compared to our study, all these investigations included a smaller range than our sample.

5. Limitations

We are aware of several limitations in our study. Several of them are related to the characteristics of our irony comprehension task [21, 35]. First, some relate to the characteristics of the stimulus material. Our stimulus material consisted of stimuli that were matched and counterbalanced for complexity, grammar, and word frequency. They were written material and therefore free from prosody and other social information like gesture and facial expressions. This may represent both a strength and a limitation of the study. Almost all factors mentioned above have been described to influence the decision whether intention is ironic or literal in previous studies and, importantly, each of them has been found impaired in schizophrenia previously. Our study makes clear that difficulties exist in schizophrenia even when prosody is eliminated and social context information reduced. However, our pilot study cannot answer whether adding such information improves irony comprehension in schizophrenia, so that studies systematically varying these factors become eligible. Current literature cannot answer these questions either. Studies differ in their amount of contextual and social cues: some are, like ours, prosody-free [79]; others used video clips, including gesture and prosody [27–29, 80]; and others even specifically addressed the effect of tone of voice [81]. However, these studies vary in schizophrenia disease severity and other factors as well. In our ironic text vignettes, protagonists made ironic comments towards another protagonist or about the environment. However, the reaction of patients with schizophrenia may be different when ironic statements are made towards the individual directly. In contrast to a real-world environment, where irony is not explicitly marked, subjects were informed that irony may occur during the stimuli and this priming may make the task less difficult. Affective connotation is a further limitation. Like those in most previous investigations, ironic and literal stimuli are not entirely matched for affective connotation in that ironic stimuli are more often negative than literal counterparts. It has been suggested that irony with positive connotations may be more difficult to comprehend, so that future investigations should investigate irony with positive connotation in patients with schizophrenia.

Sample size is another limitation of this study. Although it was within the range of comparable investigations [2, 5, 79, 81], the sample size is small given the heterogeneity of the disorder and gives our investigation the character of a pilot study.

In this study, we found a significant association of schizotypal personality traits with performance. However, SPQ values were significantly higher in patients with schizophrenia, and in our pilot study, we did not control for other personality variables. For example, other personality traits not measured here may be associated with irony comprehension as well [11, 82].

Another limiting factor in our study is gender. To enhance homogeneity of the sample, we investigated only female subjects. This point is relevant since gender differences have been reported for irony appreciation in healthy subjects [11, 83], in schizophrenia [84], and for schizotypal personality traits [85].

6. Conclusions/Implications

We see several implications from our study. Similar to a previous study [31], our study made it clear that the irony comprehension deficit in schizophrenia is not restricted to the "classical" symptom named concretism that claims a tendency towards the literal interpretations in schizophrenia. Instead, the error pattern also includes difficulties in disentangling the opposite direction, as a significant proportion of errors made by patients with schizophrenia are in misjudging the intention of meaningless and literal statements as ironic. Future schizophrenia research in the fields of pragmatic language comprehension and research on (mis)interpretation of the intention of others are warranted. In our pilot study, we cannot, due to the small sample size, disentangle which psychopathology dimensions are interrelated with this deficit. Positive symptoms, especially persecutory delusions, seem especially interesting in this context, as the relevance of capturing the intention (in this case linguistic) of others is impaired in these conditions, and the relationship between discriminating literal and ironic intention seems, therefore, a straightforward paradigm [21, 28, 32]. However, other schizophrenic symptomatologies, including cognitive deficits [30], altered theory of mind and perspective taking [2, 29], disorganized symptoms, negative symptoms [31, 79, 86], and formal thought disorder [31, 87], may be interrelated with irony comprehension as well.

Despite these limitations, we were able to demonstrate that female patients with schizophrenia are impaired in irony comprehension and show reduced insight and aberrant response, especially to those stimuli judged wrong. This, together with the observation that irony is so remarkably frequent in everyday conversations and is even more frequent in difficult communicative situations, which per se have a higher ambiguity, makes irony an especially promising candidate for social cognition training in patients.

Conflict of Interests

The authors declare that there is no conflict of interests regarding the publication of this paper.

References

[1] M. F. Green, C. E. Bearden, T. D. Cannon et al., "Social cognition in schizophrenia, part 1: performance across phase of illness," *Schizophrenia Bulletin*, vol. 38, no. 4, pp. 854–864, 2012.

[2] V. M. Drury, E. J. Robinson, and M. Birchwood, "'Theory of mind" skills during an acute episode of psychosis and following recovery," *Psychological Medicine*, vol. 28, no. 5, pp. 1101–1112, 1998.

[3] M. F. Green, G. Hellemann, W. P. Horan, J. Lee, and J. K. Wynn, "From perception to functional outcome in schizophrenia: modeling the role of ability and motivation," *Archives of General Psychiatry*, vol. 69, no. 12, pp. 1216–1224, 2012.

[4] M. M. Kurtz and C. L. Richardson, "Social cognitive training for schizophrenia: a meta-analytic investigation of controlled research," *Schizophrenia Bulletin*, vol. 38, no. 5, pp. 1092–1104, 2012.

[5] R. Herold, T. Tenyi, K. Lenard, and M. Trixler, "Theory of mind deficit in people with schizophrenia during remission," *Psychological Medicine*, vol. 32, no. 6, pp. 1125–1129, 2002.

[6] J. M. Whalen, P. M. Pexman, and A. J. Gill, "'Should be fun—not!": incidence and marking of nonliteral language in e-mail," *Journal of Language and Social Psychology*, vol. 28, no. 3, pp. 263–280, 2009.

[7] J. M. Whalen, P. M. Pexman, A. J. Gill, and S. Nowson, "Verbal irony use in personal blogs," *Behaviour & Information Technology*, vol. 32, no. 6, pp. 560–569, 2013.

[8] R. W. J. Gibbs, "Irony in talk among friends," *Metaphor and Symbol*, vol. 15, no. 1, pp. 5–27, 2000.

[9] R. W. J. Gibbs and H. L. Colston, *Interpreting Figurative Meaning*, Cambridge University Press, Cambridge, UK, 2012.

[10] H. L. Colston and A. N. Katz, Eds., *Figurative Language Comprehension: Social and Cultural Influences*, Lawrence Erlbaum Associates, Mahwah, NJ, USA, 2005.

[11] P. M. Pexman, "Social factors in the interpretation of verbal irony: the roles of speaker and listener characteristics," in *Figurative Language Comprehension: Social and Cultural Influences*, H. L. Colston and A. N. Katz, Eds., vol. 209–232, Lawrence Erlbaum Associates, Mahwah, NJ, USA, 2005.

[12] M. A. Creusere, "Theories of adults'understanding and use of irony and sarcasm: applications to and evidence from research with children," *Developmental Review*, vol. 19, no. 2, pp. 213–262, 1999.

[13] S. Kumon-Nakamura, S. Glucksberg, and M. Brown, "How about another piece of pie: the allusional pretense theory of discourse irony," *Journal of Experimental Psychology: General*, vol. 124, no. 1, pp. 3–21, 1995.

[14] A. N. Katz, D. G. Blasko, and V. A. Kazmerski, "Saying what you don't mean: social influences on sarcastic language processing," *Current Directions in Psychological Science*, vol. 13, no. 5, pp. 186–189, 2004.

[15] M. Harris and P. M. Pexman, "Children's perceptions of the social functions of verbal irony," *Discourse Processes*, vol. 36, no. 3, pp. 147–165, 2003.

[16] R. Kreuz, D. Long, and M. Church, "On being ironic: pragmatic and mnemonic implications," *Metaphor and Symbolic Activity*, vol. 6, no. 1, pp. 149–162, 1991.

[17] R. Giora, "On irony and negation," *Discourse Processes*, vol. 19, no. 2, pp. 239–264, 1995.

[18] S. Dews, J. Kaplan, and E. Winner, "Why not say it directly? The social functions of irony," *Discourse Processes*, vol. 19, no. 3, pp. 347–367, 1995.

[19] R. Giora, "Irony and its discontent," in *The Psychology & Sociology of Literature*, E. Ibsch, G. Steen, and D. Schram, Eds., John Benjamins, Amsterdam, The Netherlands, 2001.

[20] P. M. Pexman, "It's fascinating research: the cognition of verbal irony," *Current Directions in Psychological Science*, vol. 17, no. 4, pp. 286–290, 2008.

[21] A. M. Rapp, K. Langohr, D. E. Mutschler, S. Klingberg, B. Wild, and M. Erb, "Isn't it ironic? Neural correlates of irony comprehension in schizophrenia," *PLoS ONE*, vol. 8, no. 9, article e74224, 2013.

[22] D. Titone, D. L. Levy, and P. S. Holzman, "Contextual insensitivity in schizophrenic language processing: evidence from lexical ambiguity," *Journal of Abnormal Psychology*, vol. 109, no. 4, pp. 761–767, 2000.

[23] D. Salisbury, "N400 to lexical ambiguity and semantic incongruity in schizophrenia," *International Journal of Psychophysiology*, vol. 75, no. 2, pp. 127–132, 2010.

[24] D. Ketteler, A. Theodoridou, S. Ketteler, and M. Jäger, "High order linguistic features such as ambiguity processing as relevant diagnostic markers for schizophrenia," *Schizophrenia Research and Treatment*, vol. 2012, Article ID 825050, 7 pages, 2012.

[25] R. Langdon, M. Coltheart, P. B. Ward, and S. V. Catts, "Disturbed communication in schizophrenia: the role of poor pragmatics and poor mind-reading," *Psychological Medicine*, vol. 32, no. 7, pp. 1273–1284, 2002.

[26] S. Mo, Y. Su, R. C. Chan, and J. Liu, "Comprehension of metaphor and irony in schizophrenia during remission: the role of theory of mind and IQ," *Psychiatry Research*, vol. 157, no. 1–3, pp. 21–29, 2008.

[27] M. H. Kosmidis, E. Aretouli, V. P. Bozikas, M. Giannakou, and P. Ioannidis, "Studying social cognition in patients with schizophrenia and patients with frontotemporal dementia: theory of mind and the perception of sarcasm," *Behavioural Neurology*, vol. 19, no. 1-2, pp. 65–69, 2008.

[28] R. S. Kern, M. F. Green, A. P. Fiske et al., "Theory of mind deficits for processing counterfactual information in persons with chronic schizophrenia," *Psychological Medicine*, vol. 39, no. 4, pp. 645–654, 2009.

[29] A. Sparks, S. McDonald, B. Lino, M. O'Donnell, and M. J. Green, "Social cognition, empathy and functional outcome in schizophrenia," *Schizophrenia Research*, vol. 122, no. 1–3, pp. 172–178, 2010.

[30] M. Champagne-Lavau, A. Charest, K. Anselmo, J.-P. Rodriguez, and G. Blouin, "Theory of mind and context processing in schizophrenia: the role of cognitive flexibility," *Psychiatry Research*, vol. 200, no. 2-3, pp. 184–192, 2012.

[31] M. M. Hensler, *Sind konkretistische Denkstörungen eine homogene Entität? Untersuchungen zum Verständnis nicht-wortlicher Sprache bei schizophrenen Patienten [Dissertation]*, University of Tuebingen, Department of Psychiatry and Psychotherapy, 2009.

[32] R. Langdon, M. Davies, and M. Coltheart, "Understanding minds and understanding communicated meanings in schizophrenia," *Mind & Language*, vol. 17, no. 1-2, pp. 68–104, 2002.

[33] A. M. Rapp, "The brain behind nonliteral language: insights from brain imaging," in *The Handbook of the Neuropsychology of Language*, M. Faust, Ed., vol. 1, pp. 406–424, Wiley-Blackwell, West Sussex, UK, 2012.

[34] A. M. Rapp, D. E. Mutschler, and M. Erb, "Where in the brain is nonliteral language? A coordinate-based meta-analysis of functional magnetic resonance imaging studies," *NeuroImage*, vol. 63, no. 1, pp. 600–610, 2012.

[35] A. M. Rapp, D. E. Mutschler, B. Wild et al., "Neural correlates of irony comprehension: the role of schizotypal personality traits," *Brain and Language*, vol. 113, no. 1, pp. 1–12, 2010.

[36] R. Giora, *On Our Mind: Salience, Context, and Figurative Language*, Oxford University Press, 2003.

[37] A. M. Rapp and B. Wild, "Nonliteral language in alzheimer dementia: a review," *Journal of the International Neuropsychological Society*, vol. 17, no. 2, pp. 207–218, 2011.

[38] H. J. Wegrocki, "Generalizing ability in schizophrenia: an inquiry into the disorders of problem thinking in schizophrenia," *Archives of Psychology*, vol. 254, article 76, 1940.

[39] L. J. Chapman, "Confusion of figurative and literal usages of words by schizophrenics and brain damaged patients," *Journal of Abnormal and Social Psychology*, vol. 60, no. 3, pp. 412–416, 1960.

[40] D. R. Gorham, "Verbal abstraction in psychiatric illness: assay of impairment utilizing proverbs," *The Journal of Mental Science*, vol. 107, pp. 52–59, 1961.

[41] R. H. Goldstein and L. F. Salzman, "Proverb word counts as a measure of overinclusiveness in delusional schizophrenics," *Journal of Abnormal Psychology*, vol. 70, no. 4, pp. 244–245, 1965.

[42] M. de Bonis, C. Epelbaum, V. Deffez, and A. Feline, "The comprehension of metaphors in schizophrenia," *Psychopathology*, vol. 30, no. 3, pp. 149–154, 1997.

[43] P. Thoma and I. Daum, "Neurocognitive mechanisms of figurative language processing—evidence from clinical dysfunctions," *Neuroscience & Biobehavioral Reviews*, vol. 30, no. 8, pp. 1182–1205, 2006.

[44] A. M. Rapp, "The role of the right hemisphere for language in schizophrenia," in *Language Lateralization and Psychosis*, I. E. Sommer and R. S. Kahn, Eds., pp. 147–156, Cambridge University Press, Cambrigde, UK, 2009.

[45] A. M. Rapp and P. Schmierer, "Proverbs and nonliteral language in schizophrenia: a systematic methodological review of all studies published 1931–2010," *Schizophrenia Research*, vol. 117, no. 2-3, p. 422, 2010.

[46] C.-E. Brattemo, "Interpretations of proverbs in schizophrenic patients. Further studies," *Acta Psychologica*, vol. 20, no. 3, pp. 254–263, 1962.

[47] D. R. Gorham, "Additional norms and scoring suggestions for the Proverbs Test," *Psychological Reports*, vol. 13, no. 2, pp. 487–492, 1963.

[48] D. Freeman, "Suspicious minds: the psychology of persecutory delusions," *Clinical Psychology Review*, vol. 27, no. 4, pp. 425–457, 2007.

[49] A. Wittorf, K. E. Giel, M. Hautzinger et al., "Specificity of jumping to conclusions and attributional biases: a comparison between patients with schizophrenia, depression, and anorexia nervosa," *Cognitive Neuropsychiatry*, vol. 17, no. 3, pp. 262–286, 2012.

[50] G. Salvatore, P. H. Lysaker, R. Popolo, M. Procacci, A. Carcione, and G. Dimaggio, "Vulnerable self, poor understanding of others'minds, threat anticipation and cognitive biases as triggers for delusional experience in schizophrenia: a theoretical model," *Clinical Psychology & Psychotherapy*, vol. 19, no. 3, pp. 247–259, 2012.

[51] I. Falkenberg, K. Klügel, M. Bartels, and B. Wild, "Sense of humor in patients with schizophrenia," *Schizophrenia Research*, vol. 95, no. 1–3, pp. 259–261, 2007.

[52] V. P. Bozikas, M. H. Kosmidis, M. Giannakou et al., "Humor appreciation deficit in schizophrenia: the relevance of basic

neurocognitive functioning," *The Journal of Nervous and Mental Disease*, vol. 195, no. 4, pp. 325–331, 2007.

[53] B. Wild, *Humor in Psychiatrie und Psychotherapie: Neurobiologie, Methoden, Praxis*, Schattauer, Stuttgart, Germany, 2012.

[54] J. O. Polimeni, D. W. Campbell, D. Gill, B. L. Sawatzky, and J. P. Reiss, "Diminished humour perception in schizophrenia: relationship to social and cognitive functioning," *Journal of Psychiatric Research*, vol. 44, no. 7, pp. 434–440, 2010.

[55] M. Gelkopf, "The use of humor in serious mental illness: a review," *Evidence-Based Complementary and Alternative Medicine*, vol. 2011, Article ID 342837, 8 pages, 2011.

[56] R. Langdon and M. Coltheart, "Recognition of metaphor and irony in young adults: the impact of schizotypal personality traits," *Psychiatry Research*, vol. 125, no. 1, pp. 9–20, 2004.

[57] C. S. Jahshan and M. J. Sergi, "Theory of mind, neurocognition, and functional status in schizotypy," *Schizophrenia Research*, vol. 89, no. 1–3, pp. 278–286, 2007.

[58] D. Mutschler, *Funktionelle Neuroanatomie ironischer Sprache: zum Einfluss des Persönlichkeitsmerkmals Schizotypie auf die Sprachperzeption [Inaugural-dissertation]*, Universität Tübingen, 2010.

[59] M. Cochrane, I. Petch, and A. D. Pickering, "Aspects of cognitive functioning in schizotypy and schizophrenia: evidence for a continuum model," *Psychiatry Research*, vol. 196, no. 2-3, pp. 230–234, 2012.

[60] M. T. Nelson, M. L. Seal, C. Pantelis, and L. J. Phillips, "Evidence of a dimensional relationship between schizotypy and schizophrenia: a systematic review," *Neuroscience & Biobehavioral Reviews*, vol. 37, no. 3, pp. 317–327, 2013.

[61] M. Annett, "A classification of hand preference by association analysis," *British Journal of Psychology*, vol. 61, no. 3, pp. 303–321, 1970.

[62] U. Tewes, *Hawie-R: Hamburg-Wechsler Intelligenztest für Erwachsene, Revision 1991*, Hans Huber, Göttingen, Germany, 1994.

[63] S. Lehrl, G. Triebig, and B. Fischer, "Multiple choice vocabulary test MWT as a valid and short test to estimate premorbid intelligence," *Acta Neurologica Scandinavica*, vol. 91, no. 5, pp. 335–345, 1995.

[64] C. Klein, B. Andresen, and T. Jahn, "Erfassung der schizotypen Persönlichkeit nach DSM-III-R: Psychometrische Eigenschaften einer autorisierten deutschsprachigen Übersetzung des "Schizotypal Personality Questionnaire" (SPQ) von Raine," *Diagnostica*, vol. 43, no. 4, pp. 347–369, 1997.

[65] N. C. Andreasen, M. Pressler, P. Nopoulos, D. Miller, and B.-C. Ho, "Antipsychotic dose equivalents and dose-years: a standardized method for comparing exposure to different drugs," *Biological Psychiatry*, vol. 67, no. 3, pp. 255–262, 2010.

[66] P. Thoma, M. Hennecke, T. Mandok et al., "Proverb comprehension impairments in schizophrenia are related to executive dysfunction," *Psychiatry Research*, vol. 170, no. 2-3, pp. 132–139, 2009.

[67] J. Uekermann, P. Thoma, and I. Daum, "Proverb interpretation changes in aging," *Brain and Cognition*, vol. 67, no. 1, pp. 51–57, 2008.

[68] Duden, *Redewendungen und Sprichwörtliche Redensarten: Wörterbuch der Deutschen Idiomatik*, Duden, Mannheim, Germany, 2nd edition, 2002.

[69] A. Raine, "The SPQ: a scale for the assessment of schizotypal personality based on DSM-III-R criteria," *Schizophrenia Bulletin*, vol. 17, no. 4, pp. 555–564, 2001.

[70] N. C. Andreasen, *Scale for the Assessment of Positive Symtpoms (SAPS)*, University of Iowa, Iowa city, Iowa, USA, 1984.

[71] N. C. Andreasen, "Negative symptoms in schizophrenia. Definition and reliability," *Archives of General Psychiatry*, vol. 39, no. 7, pp. 789–794, 1982.

[72] S. R. Kay, A. Fiszbein, and L. A. Opler, "The positive and negative syndrome scale (PANSS) for schizophrenia," *Schizophrenia Bulletin*, vol. 13, no. 2, pp. 261–276, 1987.

[73] A. T. Beck, E. Baruch, J. M. Balter, R. A. Steer, and D. M. Warman, "A new instrument for measuring insight: the Beck Cognitive Insight Scale," *Schizophrenia Research*, vol. 68, no. 2-3, pp. 319–329, 2004.

[74] A. G. Guerrero and P. H. Lysaker, "Socially naïve self-appraisal moderates the relationship between cognitive insight and positive symptoms in schizophrenia," *Schizophrenia Research*, vol. 143, no. 1, pp. 97–101, 2013.

[75] C. M. Elmore and D. R. Gorham, "Measuring the impairment of the abstracting function with the Proverbs Test," *Journal of Clinical Psychology*, vol. 13, no. 3, pp. 263–266, 1957.

[76] M. Lenzenweger, *Schizotypy and Schizophrenia*, Guilford Press, New York, NY, USA, 2011.

[77] S. McDonald, S. Flanagan, J. Rollins, and J. Kinch, "TASIT: a new clinical tool for assessing social perception after traumatic brain injury," *The Journal of Head Trauma Rehabilitation*, vol. 18, no. 3, pp. 219–238, 2003.

[78] M. K. Humphrey, F. M. Bryson, and G. M. Grimshaw, "Metaphor processing in high and low schizotypal individuals," *Psychiatry Research*, vol. 178, no. 2, pp. 290–294, 2010.

[79] N. J. Mitchley, J. Barber, J. M. Gray, D. N. Brooks, and M. G. Livingston, "Comprehension of irony in schizophrenia," *Cognitive Neuropsychiatry*, vol. 3, no. 2, pp. 127–138, 1998.

[80] B. Casetta and V. Goghari, "Theory of Mind abilities in schizophrenia: a family study," *Schizophrenia Bulletin*, vol. 39, supplement 1, p. S258, 2013.

[81] D. Leitman, R. Ziwich, R. Pasternak, and D. Javitt, "Theory of Mind (ToM) and counterfactuality deficits in schizophrenia: misperception or misinterpretation?" *Psychological Medicine*, vol. 36, no. 8, pp. 1075–1083, 2006.

[82] D. G. Blasko and V. A. Kazmerski, "ERP correlates of individual differences in the comprehension of nonliteral language," *Metaphor and Symbol*, vol. 21, no. 4, pp. 267–284, 2006.

[83] S. L. Ivanko, P. M. Pexman, and K. M. Olineck, "How sarcastic are you? Individual differences and verbal irony," *Journal of Language and Social Psychology*, vol. 23, no. 3, pp. 244–271, 2004.

[84] H. Häfner, "Gender differences in schizophrenia," *Psychoneuroendocrinology*, vol. 28, supplement 2, pp. 17–54, 2003.

[85] J. Miettunen and E. Jääskeläinen, "Sex differences in Wisconsin Schizotypy Scales—a meta-analysis," *Schizophrenia Bulletin*, vol. 36, no. 2, pp. 347–358, 2010.

[86] I. Ziv, D. Leiser, and J. Levine, "Social cognition in schizophrenia: cognitive and affective factors," *Cognitive Neuropsychiatry*, vol. 16, no. 1, pp. 71–91, 2011.

[87] A. M. Rapp and A. E. Steinhäuser, "Functional MRI of sentence-level language comprehension in schizophrenia: a coordinate-based analysis," *Schizophrenia Research*, vol. 150, no. 1, pp. 107–113, 2013.

15

Parents' Experiences of Caring Responsibility for Their Adult Child with Schizophrenia

Ann Blomgren Mannerheim,[1] Ulla Hellström Muhli,[2] and Eleni Siouta[1,3,4]

[1]*Karolinska Institute, Division of Nursing, Department of Neurobiology, Care Science and Society, 171 77 Stockholm, Sweden*
[2]*Department of Sociology, Uppsala University, Box 624, 751 26 Uppsala, Sweden*
[3]*Department of Learning, Informatics, Management and Ethics (LIME), Karolinska Institute, 171 77 Stockholm, Sweden*
[4]*Sophiahemmet University, Box 5605, 114 86 Stockholm, Sweden*

Correspondence should be addressed to Ulla Hellström Muhli; ulla.hellstrom_muhli@soc.uu.se

Academic Editor: Markus Jäger

As a consequence of the latest psychiatry-related reform in Sweden and its implementation, relatives and family members have taken over from the formal healthcare system significant responsibility for the care of persons with a mental disability and illness. The aim of this study was to systematically describe and analyze the experiences of parents' informal care responsibility. The questions were, what are the experiences around parents' informal care activities and responsibilities and how do parents construct and manage their caring responsibility and with what consequences? Semistructured in-depth interviews were conducted (16 hours of recorded material) with eight parents who were all members of the Interest Association for Schizophrenia (*Intresseföreningen för Schizofreni* (IFS)) in Sweden. A mixed hermeneutic deductive and inductive method was used for the interpretation of the material. The parents endow their informal caring responsibility with meaning of *being a good*, *responsible*, and *accountable* parent with respect to their social context and social relationships as well as with respect to the psychiatric care representatives. In this tense situation, parents compromise between elements of struggle, cooperation, avoidance, and adaption in their interaction with the world outside, meaning the world beyond the care provision for their child, as well as with the world inside themselves.

1. Introduction

This study focuses on parents' experiences of informal care responsibility in relation to the responsibility for taking care of their adult child with a mental illness.

The term mental illness is often used as a collective term for less serious mental disorders such as anxiety. However, the term herein refers to severe mental illness that is expressed in a syndrome that can be verified on the basis of different criteria for psychiatric diagnosis [1].

Psychiatric care in Sweden has undergone several organizational changes after the mental health reform of 1995 [2]. Concretely, the changes were mainly decommissioning of large psychiatric institutions with a significant reduction in the number of inpatient care facilities in favor of the expansion of psychiatric outpatient care. This reform, from a policy perspective, meant that outpatient activities related to support and service, housing, employment, leisure, and the social needs of the mentally ill individuals were transferred from the county councils to the municipalities [3]. Thus, the reform was not a reform of specialized psychiatry but was instead an attempt to improve the lives of the mentally disabled and the sick in the community [4]. However, problems arose quickly since no sector entirely managed the needs that existed within the framework of the current outpatient care [3, 5–7]. A significant responsibility for care has also been transferred from the formal psychiatric care to related parties, that is, the families of the mentally ill individual. The definition of formal care here refers to "the healthcare organization," "healthcare professionals," "psychiatric institutions," "psychiatric care givers," and "formal care givers."

Under the policy framework described above, relatives constitute an important source of support for the care of individuals with mental illness. The family's informal care responsibility has been shown to have positive effects on the sick individual's rehabilitation, as well as on the patient's daily life, especially since relatives offer continuity in the care based on their knowledge of the sick individual [8–10].

However, at the individual level, the policy-formulation means that the parents of the adult child with schizophrenia (ACWS) have increased responsibilities for the care of their sick adult child, given that the child will now be treated either at the parental home or in some form of group housing [11]. The interdisciplinary field of caring studies has recently produced research showing that in many cases this responsibility represents an unacceptable burden on the family including social stigma, refusal of treatment, and stress [12–14]. The informal caregiving role puts a burden on the parents but also leads to economic problems, limitations in the parent's social life, and emotional problems [15–18]. Karanci [19] stresses increased incidences of family conflicts, divorces, and siblings who are maltreated. It has been shown that these care responsibilities affect the physical and mental health of the family member [15].

There have also been an increasing number of studies of the *welfare and mental health reform* in Sweden focused on the methods of planning and implementing the reform, the target group of the reform, and resulting deinstitutionalization [11, 20–24]. However, only a few studies in Sweden focus on parents' experiences and their perspectives on informal care responsibility for their ACWS. There is also a lack of knowledge about the formal psychiatric care support available for relatives taking care of the individuals with a mental illness [4, 10, 16, 25] and in particular support for relatives' own well-being [26, 27].

It is against this background that we framed our paper analyzing parents' experiences of their informal care responsibility related to their ACWS.

The questions posed are, what are the experiences around the parents' informal care activities and responsibilities and how do parents construct and manage their caring responsibility and with what consequences?

2. The Topic of Informal Care and Care Responsibility

Informal care is taken to mean care contributions made by relatives outside the framework of the public care services provided by state, the county council, or the municipality and in contrast to the formal care that refers to the services and care provided by the public system [12].

Unlike formal care, the specific nature of informal care depends on relatives being "available" practically around the clock [12]. Studies indicate that this constant accessibility is often the reason why relatives perceive informal care as an unacceptable burden [12, 14, 28].

International research has sought to distinguish between *objective* and *subjective* aspects of the burden of informal care. Objective aspects deal with giving up working, wholly or partly to be able to provide care, financial sacrifices, and sacrifices to the caregiver's own social relations and time [12, 15–18]. Subjective aspects refer to the caregivers' emotional and physical reactions to the situation [12].

The *concept of caring* captures the meaning of giving care to those who cannot perform a particular chore. Thereby it also captures the dimensions of a disadvantage in the caring relation. Accordingly, the specific logic of the care (the caring rationality) involves aspects of asymmetries, morality, and human values at the same time as the care must be planned, valued, and acted upon [29]. The objective of care is well-being and quality of life. Parental informal care responsibility to their ACWS can therefore be understood on the basis of this theoretical foundation, to increase the child's well-being and quality of life by being present in the existential as well as spatial and temporal meaning. According to Mayeroff [30], caring is about initiating a person's health and well-being processes by providing room for growth and development. In this study the authors intend to conceptualize this complex interplay of meaning-making, expectations, feelings, and attitudes, interpreted in interviews with parents to ACWS and related to their care responsibility.

Theoretically, the meaning-making can be traced to a social construction perspective when meaning-making of the parental caring responsibility is embedded in cultural meaning and the informal caring responsibility is perceived as parents' social reality and knowledge [31]. Furthermore, the parental caring responsibility is socially constructed at the experiential level, based on how individuals (here parents) come to understand and live with their parental and informal care responsibility. This approach can make a significant contribution to our understanding of the social and experiential dimensions of caring responsibility and it can help us broaden policy deliberations and decisions.

3. Methods

The aim of this study is to systematically describe and analyze the meaning of parents' care responsibility for their ACWS. This means that qualitative in-depth interviews were used to elicit parents' experiences and meaning-making, which were analyzed by a hermeneutic mixed deductive and inductive method [32]. This kind of hermeneutic interpretative perspective enables detailed analyses to be undertaken of the meaning of the parents' informal care responsibility as experienced (inductively) within the context of daily life and social interaction with others as well as with representatives of the psychiatric healthcare system. This analysis makes it possible to find interesting proposals for how various phenomena are related, here the parents' meaning-making incorporated in the social context or the everyday culture in which they live. This perspective also makes it possible to analyze parents' understanding of their own performance of self [33] and to analyze the data in regard to the theory of caring rationality [29] (deductively) and for confirming social construction as theoretical framework. This method extends understanding from what is called a hermeneutic circle. However, in this interpretative perspective it is also important to give an account of the researchers' prior understanding that may influence interviews and analysis. In addition, as researchers, our background qualifications in psychiatric care as well as in other care settings (work experience as a specialist nurse in psychiatric care, as a registered nurse in the cardiac care, and

Table 1: Characteristics of parents interviewed ($N = 8$).

Sex	Age	Child sex and age	Work time	Sickness degree	Retirement
Female	58	Son, 27	100%		
Female	58	Daughter, 25	100%		
Female	56	Son, 30	50%	50%	
Female	52	Daughter, 23	80%	20%	
Female	57	Son, 22		100%	
Male	63	Son, 31	80%		20%
Male	59	Son, 30		100%	
Male	59	Son, 27	100%		

as a manager of elderly care) contribute some ethnographic knowledge and preunderstandings of such a context. The understanding of the hermeneutic interpretative perspective toward the social construction perspective of the individual as a meaning-making subject also requires knowledge about the cultural context and knowledge that we possess to varying degrees.

3.1. Procedures and Data. The data corpus consists of eight interviews (a total of 16 hours of recorded interview material) with an equal number of parents of mentally disabled and ill persons who are members of an interest association for schizophrenia named (*Intresseföreningen för Schizofreni* (IFS)) *the Interest Association for Schizophrenia*, in Sweden. The association is a disability organization that organizes people with schizophrenia and related psychoses, their relatives, and other interested persons. The association works to increase understanding of schizophrenia and related psychotic disorders and the disabilities that the disease brings. The organization consists of about 50 local associations and districts with 3,500 members throughout Sweden [34]. A call for participants in the study went to one local association in the middle of Sweden.

To get participants for the study, the senior manager at the local association for schizophrenia was contacted by telephone and was provided with information about the study. The manager informed members about the study and she advertised for volunteer participants in the study. Eight members reported an interest in participating and represent the study participants. The purpose of the study was first presented orally and then in writing. An information letter describing the purpose of the study and its design was sent to those who expressed an interest in participating.

3.2. Participants. The participants—three men and five women between 52 and 63 years old—had all at least five years' experience of informal caring. Four of the eight parents were married at the time of the interviews (although one was in the process of getting divorced) and four lived as single parents. Only three of the eight participants worked full-time. The others were receiving sickness benefits to various degrees. The target group's ACWS consisted of six sons and two daughters aged 22–31 (Table 1).

3.3. Ethics and Data Collection. Ethical aspects were emphasized in accordance with the Helsinki Declaration of 1975, as revised in 2008 [35], and with the Swedish Government Proposition [36] and the Governmental Act [37]. The participants were informed that participation in the study was voluntary and that they could at any time cancel participation without giving any reasons. The participants were also assured of confidentiality during the interviews.

The interviews were conducted by the first author (Ann Blomgren Mannerheim). All the interviews took place at the time and place of the participant's choice: at the association's premises, their own workplace, or the participant's home. The interviews maintained a semistructured form, based on an interview guide. The interviews began by gathering general background information about age, working hours (full-time, part-time), and the child's age and gender, followed by main interview questions regarding (i) care responsibility, (ii) life situation, (iii) their own health, and (iv) manifesting confirmatory care from the psychiatric healthcare system. Each interview took about two hours and was conducted in an informal open dialogue, allowing interviewees to answer in many different ways and the interviewer to ask follow-up questions.

The parents interviewed during the research are seen primarily as informers, contributing knowledge of their experiences and of their meaning-making of the informal care responsibility. In our role as researchers, our interest focused on the information rather than the interaction, even though these aspects interlace, as the interview itself is an interactional activity. The interviews were tape-recorded and transcribed verbatim using a written and readable language. This resulted in a reduced level of detail in the transcriptions, but the purpose of this was to create more fluent text and description. The transcription excerpts in this paper have been translated from Swedish to English. Translating the parents' accounts is problematic as interpretation and cultural content within the accounts may be lost which is a limitation that should be considered.

3.4. Analysis of Data. Parents' experiences and meaning-making were central to the analysis [38]. The data was analyzed qualitatively by a hermeneutic deductive and inductive method for the interpretation. The analysis was done within the framework of the theory of social construction with emphasis on how meanings of phenomena do not necessarily inhere in the phenomena themselves (informal caring responsibility) but develop through interactions in a social context [31]. However, the analysis focused on how this was understood, what meaning it was given as described by the parents (inductively). This method interprets hermeneutics as the hypothetic-deductive and inductive mixed method used on meaning-carrying material created from the "insider's" view (parents') and how the parents come to understand and live with their informal caring responsibility based on their everyday knowledge [39]. The hypothesis that was set up had been created by an internal image of what one could expect to find in the material.

The hermeneutic approach is a constant movement between a part of a text and the contextual whole that it is part of. This method describes the hermeneutical spiral in the form of circles that touch the authors' understanding, the participants' meaning-making, and meaning of the text [38]. In this study, the movement between a part of the text and the contextual whole was to fit the part and the contextual whole into each other to form a meaningful unit. Using this approach, we (all three authors Ann Blomgren Mannerheim, Ulla Hellström Muhli, and Eleni Siouta) moved between understanding the persons, their actions, and ourselves and our horizon of understanding [32]. The data was read separately by each author. We started our analysis to find *statements and experiences* with focus on (i) the meaning of care responsibility and went on to find (ii) the social organization and strategies of the parents' world and further to find (iii) adaption to the caring responsibility. The final categorization was developed to summarize the results and the objectives as well as to create new descriptions and concepts that explain the main interpretation of the study. The analysis of the data is specified in following stages.

Stage 1. The transcripts were read thoroughly several times to obtain an overall representation and a comprehensive view of the material.

Stage 2. The data was then read with a first reflection on various themes related to the interview guide.

Stage 3. Then the data was read with a second reflection and the reflection was moved to the connection of the theoretical framework. This phase was the interpretative phase and meant to deepen our understanding.

Stage 4. In this stage, we took the first step towards the organization of the data with the help of a coding process. This coding process involved finding text that by its content was marked with a code. In this case, by color selections using different color pens, the coding continued with sorting of data as a thematic and code-driven grouping of the meaningful units in the data.

Stage 5. As mentioned above, the final categorization was developed to lead to a summary of the results and the objectives as well as to create new descriptions and concepts which explains the main interpretation of the study.

4. Findings

4.1. The Meaning of Informal Care Responsibility. In the following text, experiences and meaning-making of the parents' informal care responsibility are specified. The main findings were the parents' experience and that they present themselves as attentive and active parents, and they live with this responsibility by trying to create good social relations outside the home. They support and care for their ACWS in different ways and have good contact with the representatives of the formal psychiatric care. However, the most important meaning for parents seems to be to *experience themselves as good and responsible parents*, who care not only about their ACWS, but also about the whole family. This meaning-making is exemplified by the following extracts:

> *I have one task and that is to meet xx (her son) and sit and talk, and then... he has really talked about his situation every time and every week and it feels like I have his trust and then I think it's great that he wants to talk so much. I have a feeling that he also feels good about those talks, even if he talks to others as well; there is something special to talk to the mom who know him best.* (Informant)

> *The only thing that means something right now is to find some meaningful activity for her (her daughter), for she has not really had any over the last three, four years. It is vital for her actually, because otherwise I do not think she is able to cope with....* (Informant)

The parents take on their care responsibilities as a challenge and the paid work (employment) outside the informal care responsibility seems as stimulation or allows for "breathing," as one informant metaphorically put it. This challenge is expressed in the following extract:

> *I think I feel good, I feel myself quite happy, sleep well at night even though I have a big workload, now I have a full-time job, plus I take care of my dad who is 90 years plus I have xx (her son) to think about and I'm single, so it is much that lies on me.* (Informant)

Overall, the key issue here is that parents endow their informal caring responsibility with *meaning of being responsible and accountable* within the context of their personal and social relationships. Thus, the analysis shows that the importance of being a good parent with skills to care for his/her adult son or daughter means not only to be a capable parent to the child, but also to show the community and the formal mental health services that the parent takes his/her care responsibilities seriously. Table 2 summarizes the parents' meaning of their informal care responsibility in theme, categories, and subcategories.

4.2. The Social Organization of the Parent's World as Informal Carers in Form of Strategy Projects. The results from the analysis of strategies used for living with the informal care responsibility show four main categories: strategies such as (1) *parental projects*, (2) *work related projects*, (3) *recreational projects*, and (4) *repertoires of controlling the life situation*, on the one hand, and *feelings of being out of control*, on the other.

The parental project as a strategy was to be a good parent who felt responsible for their adult children. This was important even if it meant for some that they could not keep up with other works. Parents tried in various ways to support their children, for example, by teaching about finances, by encouraging independence, by offering companionship, and by finding employment.

The parent's own health as well as the child's health is also of importance in the parental project as strategy. The analysis

TABLE 2: The finding presented as theme, categories, and subcategories (theme: the meaning of being good, responsible, and accountable).

Categories	Subcategories
The social organization of the parent's world as informal carers in form of strategy projects	*Parental projects* *Work related projects* *Recreational projects* *Repertoires of controlling the life situation and feelings of being out of control*
Adaption to the caring responsibility	*Uncertainty facing all the unknowns* *Positive events that made life worth living* *Perception of health and activity* *Negative circumstances that made life difficult to live*

shows that the parents felt that they could relax more and feel better if their son or daughter was in a stable period of the disease process.

Other important health issues were to support the ACWS to follow the treatment plan with proposed activities and to get the child to feel commitment to the family. Another strategy was to support a daughter with companionship, and another strategy was to get the child to follow daily routines. Some of the parents' strategies were to fight for their child so that he/she could receive medical treatment. However, this took up all their time and energy and even contributed to thoughts of giving up life, as exemplified below:

> *The strength to fight...but it's not always that I have the strength to do that, sometimes I fall down and then I'll lie down for a couple of days and then I'll get up again ...now have they fucking done that again, now damn, I say to myself, and then I start over again, and then I fall down again, and sometimes I feel that I give up – now I'll take all my sleeping pills, now to hell with this, but I don't, but I feel like that sometimes.* (Informant)

In regard to the parental project strategy, results clearly show that parents are looking for various solutions to realize their goals and, on the whole, for existence that one is satisfied with based on the needs that may arise as a result of the child's illness. One important strategy was to uphold the relations within the family, between spouses, or with the child. Parents also report that they receive valuable knowledge about their own self and about their own abilities to realize their life through self-therapy or by consulting people and through psychiatric expertise about the disease affecting their child. The motivation for these strategies seems to be a greater readiness in their parenting, care responsibility, and understanding of their child's illness. In a constant search for knowledge and understanding of mental health and diseases, the parents test and process their own attitudes toward the illness as well as the general view in the society against persons with mental disabilities and illness. Alleviation of difficulties in their lives is also experienced by talking openly to others about their child being mentally ill.

The work related project objective was to use paid work as a source of internal development, stimulation, and appreciation. Thus it was an important strategy in their lives and not a burden in addition to the informal care responsibilities. Those parents who particularly emphasized the work as being challenging and stimulating also worked proportionally more, engaged in full-time service, and felt that they had a job that gave them the challenge, stimulation, and opportunities in life. This is expressed as follows:

> *No, the work is no problem, I've got a job after all; my boss jokes that now they have paid so much to me, so now I have to stay and work until I'm 67 years old, so from that aspect I am not concerned; that is really nice because it is really important.* (Informant)

In regard to the work and *recreational project* strategies, results show that *work and leisure time* are important assets and strategies in parenting and in the informal care responsibility. Parents stressed the importance of having a job that is stimulating. However, the job also allows space for breathing, which was expressed as follows:

> *Work became something to lean against; I simply fled to work, it was important for me to be able to go to work every day because then I switched off everything else.* (Informant)

As shown, work gives the opportunity to break with the everyday caring responsibility and creates contrasts between the role of parent and professional. Having a job cultivates a healthy distance with the informal caring responsibility helping to satisfy parents' own personal needs in the context of informal caring responsibility.

Another strategy was trying to *adapt their working conditions to the current life situation* by reducing the time at work in order to perform their caring responsibilities for their adult child. However, despite this change of life, work remains important and is explained as follows:

> *Then, when this clinical picture came of my son, I thought I could find some calmer work. I tried to adapt myself so I only needed to work three days a week. In that way, I had more time over for my son because he was still at home.* (Informant)

When it comes to *the recreational project*, the strategy is to pursue various hobbies or recreational activities. Such activities could be to walk in the mountains, bike, dance, or work with a holiday cottage or organizational activities. These parents have a variety of recreational activities that they describe as important, and such one is shown below:

> *We usually hike in the mountains a lot when we're up at the cottage, but this year we did not so much; mostly, there was berry picking and painting...well a little bit of hiking too.* (Informant)

The parents feel that having time to engage in diverse individual activities, from various forms of exercise to travel, is a valuable strategy to realize their own life in the caring responsibility. Social contact with openness about the disease with family, friends, and wider community is another strategy that also offers relief from shame and guilt.

Visiting the Interest Association for Schizophrenia is also viewed as a significant aspect of support for the parents' life circumstances. By joining the association, parents come into contact with other parents in the same situation, which is perceived as supportive of their existence. Parents also felt that they got knowledge and support through advice and lectures given by the association.

As shown, maintaining their social relationships and finding space and time for their own needs were emphasized by the parents as an important strategy to realize their life situation and circumstance and are expressed according to the following:

> *I've got my own home that I can go to, and I can meet my friends at my place. I even try to have some fun stuff so I can get some balance. I have done this consciously to feel good and I work with it consciously. I have history of difficult things happening in life; therefore, I feel proud that I have managed it – now I go and sing and make sure that I get out and away…dance and try to do the things that I'm good at and that's fun, to get some air under my wings. I've learned and I feel proud over this.* (Informant)

Overall, the analysis shows that parents' strategies for organizing their lives in regard to their informal care responsibility can be stated as strategies that make life worth living by providing room for own growth and development.

However, there are also negative *circumstances such as losses in life* related to the care responsibility of the ACWS, leading to the project and strategies to control life. These losses make life difficult to live or restrict the parents' actions. Such circumstances may be different kinds of losses in lives. One such unplanned life event was a break-up of a marriage, a life event that also had influenced parents not to remarry.

Other life circumstances related to the care responsibility are damaged relationships within the family or gnawing feelings about responsibility for the family and children. Feelings of powerlessness arose when the parents were unable to protect and support their children in different ways, as described below:

> *When xx (her daughter) got ill, my husband became very hateful toward me and also put the hatred on my children. I've never felt so hated; it was like his aggressions went over to my daughter and she kind of threw darts at me. I've never felt so bad, it felt horrible and unfair.* (Informant)

Negative life circumstances were also that one's own needs as an adult had to be put aside at the expense of the parental role and the responsibility to care for the adult daughter or son, as expressed below:

> *Life has become more and more limited with xx sickness. I can't even go abroad to work together with the new boyfriend; then, I live alone for months on end and that is not so fun.* (Informant)

Negative life circumstances are also the difficulties in finding time for activities and limited freedom to use their time for various options. These limitations are caused by making parenting the priority and addressing the adult child's needs with various support measures, rather than parents taking care of their own individual needs. In some cases, the limitations are only related to fatigue. The parents are simply too tired to engage in their own leisure activities. An example of such experience is expressed as follows:

> *His illness has also limited my daily freedom of action as well as weekends such as Saturday or Sunday, since half of the week xx and I eat dinner together. My social life is also limited because I get fewer free nights off to meet people.* (Informant)

As shown from the analysis, the main point here is that the care responsibility as informal carers is *having control over* their own life as well as over the child's life. Parents describe how they use strategies (parental project, works project, and recreational project) through different assessments that supported their goals and aspirations to be a good parent. They look for ways to parent and rely on relationships within and outside the family to find support for their parenting and care responsibility.

4.3. Adaption to the Caring Responsibility. The analysis shows that parents express feelings of great *uncertainty facing all the unknowns* that they encounter in their caring capacity as parent of an ACWS. This uncertainty leads to personal and social adaptions on different levels in order to be able to care. The parents describe how they lack the ability to be able to assess the decisions they make and feel uncertain about them. They do not know how they should act in relation to the children, family, friends, and formal psychiatric care providers. Their children behave abnormally and they do not know how to handle such a situation. The parents describe feelings of fear and fright when they were told that their daughter or son had been given a psychiatric diagnosis. The parents also describe feelings of great frustration when they did not get answers to their questions from the formal psychiatric care services or when they got fuzzy information regarding the proposed care or failed care. Lack of communication between the parents and the formal professional caregivers created many situations that contributed to the parents' insecurities. Such restricting aspects of experiences are exemplified as follows:

> *Nobody saw me, nobody told me anything; instead, it was only a shock to see all the people that were constantly sick, someone who just screamed right out and someone who just walked around like a zombie, and to know that there was my son. I thought that he would always be there and that he'd always be so crazy… "what a scream" the painting by Munch of the anxiety cry (scream). As a whole, I was like that painting.* (Informant)

However, the analysis shows also that the adaption to a life with caring responsibility can be supported by *positive events that made life worth living* and that developed the parents' own self-image.

The analysis shows how valuable it is to be met with positive attitudes from others, for the family to feel good, or to be able to see the child develop positively. The parents felt strengthened by the reaffirming social relationships and by increasing their own knowledge.

The parents in this study expressed in many different ways that they became positively involved in their caring responsibility when someone points out the merits of their children—for example, when the formal healthcare staff speaks positively about the son or daughter. This can be praise for the ability to cope with different things or expressing that the children are well liked within the staff group of service providers. All these aspects of social confirmation support the adaption to life with a caring responsibility.

It is also important for the parents' own well-being that the family, son, or daughter is doing well, that his/her condition is more stable, or that one can see a positive ongoing development. The parents say they are influenced by how different healthcare interventions work. When the situation is experienced as more stable, the parents feel safe in their adaption to the caring responsibility. Those who had experienced stabilization and perceived that their son or daughter was doing better expressed the impact that this had on themselves as follows:

> *I am so happy that he has been so good at taking his medicine and that he has insight into his illness.* (Informant)

The parents also talked about how their own self-image was influenced by their *perception of health and activity.* They stressed the importance of a good relationship with their child and the experience of working in a positive parental role.

Important for the adaption to the caring responsibility was repairing the relationship when the parents had accused each other of being at fault for the child's illness. Parents describe how stressful feelings of guilt had caused them to realize that mental illness can affect people just like any other disease and that one cannot find blame. Parents also expressed how the child's illness contributed to their own greater self-knowledge and strength and pride in being able to cope. Such positive self-image, personal growth, and dignity are described as follows:

> *I've gotten a whole new dimension in life, you could say, through a new way to see things about life and people. So after all, the disease has given me positive signals.* (Informant)

The formal healthcare provision was viewed often as supportive in the parents' informal care responsibility, when the healthcare workers provided the care, or when a meeting with a healthcare representative went well. This is expressed as follows:

> *I feel that the healthcare has been good for xx. He has gotten a lot of good support from hospitals, rehabilitation, the employment service, and the social insurance company. I give [them] 100 points. But support for family members, nothing exists.* (Informant)

Parents also give an account of *negative* aspects of the caring responsibility including *circumstances that made life difficult to live.* The analysis shows that the parents were strongly affected by the negative social attitudes directed toward the mentally ill in the community. Their own physical and mental health was, as the parents experienced it, affected by those attitudes. Parents described that some relationships with other people are difficult to manage. They even accused themselves of not being good enough as parents. Due to the accusations, the parents felt that they were the cause of their child's disease or that they were bad parents. Some parents were reluctant to talk about their child's illness with their relatives and friends. The son or daughter's diagnosis of schizophrenia was perceived as a negative stigma, and parents also felt relief when the child had not yet been diagnosed. Feelings of being questioned in their parental role by the health professionals were experienced as a lack of dignity, described as follows:

> *This diagnosis that he has gotten is extremely frightening. No one in society knows that there are subgroups of different types of psychoses. All these people don't chop someone with an axe or put a knife into people; not all of these people do that.* (Informant)

In regard to parents' adaption to the informal care responsibility, the analysis showed that the more strategies and goals the parents had in their care responsibility, the more they described their own health status as being better. Thinking that life was still worth living, feeling fine themselves, and being in good health were interpreted as indications of how the adult child was doing.

Parents described their physical and mental health as being good and then immediately supplemented this data with descriptions of both physical and psychological symptoms of ill health. Descriptions of illness that parents had experienced included, for example, obesity, insomnia, back pain, increased blood pressure, effects on the cardiovascular system, muscle inflammation, vocal cord inflammation, and breathing difficulties. The parents linked all of these symptoms to the fact that they were responsible as carers and that their son or daughter was mentally ill. These difficulties of the relationship were experienced as follows:

> *So, I've plugged up my ears shut so I won't hear so much, because otherwise my head starts to freeze. I get a headache and then I start to get nauseous, so physical stuff, so I'm in real bad shape...I've been extremely strong physically, but now it's hard to mow the lawn, I get injuries, so I have to think about what I'm doing. There are strains, inflammations. Really strange stuff. One can't believe it's true. The whole thing is because I can't get any deep sleep; I wake up every fifteen minutes. It has been like that for so long that the body has started to take a beating. First, came the lack of deep sleep,*

then came the problem with the muscles, and thereafter, came the problems to tolerate sounds. (Informant)

As shown, when the responsibility for care in daily life becomes too large, it is handled by switching off perceptions or by experiencing illness. In regard to experiencing mental illness, the parents described feelings of anxiety and uncertainty of what might happen with the adult child: if the son or the daughter would take their own life or set fire to their house. The parents described the anxiety that affects them and the insecurity they feel in terms of the help they received and did not receive as follows:

Now I can't handle it anymore, when I feel that stressed then I'm ready to/.../so I think that now I have to go in to the psychiatric emergency department. (Informant)

The experience of health problems was related to the parents' responsibility as carers and was often linked to the social situation as a whole. Some parents were divorced, and the relationship with the former husband/wife had not been the best, which also affected sibling relationships negatively. The guilt feelings were palpable when the parents blamed themselves for the bad relations within the family as well as for the external relations toward the nursing staff.

The fear of becoming sick themselves existed, but the most critical threats to the parents' health as was experienced were the feelings of powerlessness and anger about not being good enough, not being able to protect and help one's own child, and not being able to access healthcare or get sufficient healthcare.

The parents' own health was also adversely affected by the negative attitudes of the formal nursing staff toward the parents, as the parents experienced it. This, in turn, increased their own feelings of guilt when it came to their inadequacies in the caring responsibility, their parenting role, and contact with others, which is expressed by a parent as follows:

Well, everything is pretty week...very up and down, I don't feel a part of life, I have taken a step aside, I don't have the strength to be with people, I have stepped aside. (Informant)

Without professional healthcare support in the caring role, the social network has an even greater importance. The parents are critically of limited access to formal healthcare as well as limited choices of healthcare resources. They mentioned that a lack of trust in healthcare occurs when being unable to understand the behavior of nursing staff, the information provided, or the prescribed drug treatment. The lack of trust was expressed as follows:

That doctor that tells my son when he asks him about the medication, "well, if this doesn't help you, what should I do then?" (Nozinan, is that what that fucking rat poison is called)... "Well, then you'll have to pray to God," answers the doctor. I mean, how can someone answer in that way. (Informant)

As the analysis shows, the main point here is that the adaption to the caring responsibility and to being the parent of an ACWS is filled with uncertainty and is a process mixture of struggling, cooperation, and compromise. However, adaption is believed to contain an element of being involved in a social relationship with others. The parents felt strengthened by such involvement.

5. Discussion

The contributions of this paper will be discussed in relation to substantive, theoretical, methodological, and practical aspects.

Substantively, this analysis contributes to understanding the meaning that parents provide about their informal care responsibility. The expressed goal is to be a good, responsible, and accountable parent who cares not only about their ACWS, but also about the whole family. Furthermore, the study contributes to understanding how parents construct and manage their caring responsibility by adaption to it in a process that combines struggle, cooperation, and compromise, not only *outwardly* toward the social context in which they find themselves, but also *inwardly* toward the family and themselves.

So, what constitutes being a good parent and what are the consequences? *Inwardly*, the moral foundation of altruism and love as well as the rational consideration of their child is a crucial explanatory aspect when studying how parents understand being a good parent [12, 29]. This also explains why parents fight to get the child's different needs met and to get support for this care responsibility from the formal psychiatric healthcare system. Another perspective appears when one studies parents' personal motive of being a good parent. That means improving their readiness for parenting by searching for knowledge and understanding of mental illness and health. This readiness also involves parents' own growth and development. Parents need support and knowledge about mental illness. However, that support is not adequate if one looks at the formal psychiatric care support available for relatives who are taking care of individuals with a mental illness. The Interest Association for Schizophrenia (IFS) is of high importance in regard to supporting parents' readiness to care. We assert that support from the IFS is crucial not only for giving psychological and social support, but also to educate and serve as a knowledge center for parents and patients.

Outwardly, being a good parent living with the caring responsibility for everyday lives means to construct and perform the care by constructing an identity as a good responsible parent and by practicing accountability. In other words, the informal care responsibility is understood as being an accountable, good parent who also performs the accountability to the surrounding community, especially towards formal healthcare professionals. This kind of identity construction, of good and responsible parenthood in terms of altruism, love, and consideration, seems in terms of values to be faced as a moral self-identity in presentation of oneself [40, p. 9 and part II]. Gecas [41] supports these findings by emphasizing that identity has become a fertile ground for understanding personal experiences and the relationship between self and society. Values constitute an important location for identity construction, and "the self-conception starts with values and aspirations, and continues to be represented in value and aspiration terms." That is, values give meaning, purpose, and direction to our lives (ibid.).

However, this self-presentation is located in the social and cultural context and structural space between the informal and formal care service positions. The informal care position as parent, family member, and member of the Interest Association for Schizophrenia (IFS) deals with shared self-definition. This seems to be an important source of identity and of care rationality in the interaction with care professionals within the formal psychiatric care. Often, motivation to be a good parent also involves implicit expectations to fulfill the ascribed roles of a parent. However, is such self-identity and rationality presentation perceived and considered by the formal healthcare professionals? The question to be asked is, when it manifests, is extensive supportive and confirmatory care given to the parents? In this study, it seems that this interaction between parents and healthcare professionals is uneven, working very well in some cases and very poorly in others. However, there is still need of knowledge in this issue about whether these experiences differ from the fathers' versus the mothers' perspective.

A common feature of the meaning-making of the care responsibility as it is experienced is the centrality of both protective parenthood and accountable self-performance as a carer. The caring responsibility is understood as a link between the child, family, and the outside world. In this informal position, the parents' ability as an active parent with good social relations to family members and with the psychiatric care professionals is crucial.

The parents organize and use strategies to make sense of and endow their care responsibility by giving meaning within the context of their personal and social relationships and employment. The strategies used are parental projects, work related projects, and recreational projects. These projects are ways to control the life situation when feeling out of control. The key finding here is that the more projects the parents had, the more they seemed to experience well-being. This highlights the importance of considering parents' perspectives and subjective wishes and needs when formal psychiatric care professionals plan support for parents' informal care responsibilities.

Another important form of support from the formal care community is to acknowledge the relatives for the care they provide. It is also clear from findings presented here that life situations for parents are characterized by great uncertainty and, therefore, the parents find it valuable to encounter positive attitudes from others. However, there were many bitter complaints over how society responds to parents' caring responsibility, and the formal care representatives were indicated as approaching the parents with negative attitudes and with limited engagement. Previous studies support these findings [12, 14, 42–44]. According to Pejlert [43], the healthcare system's long patronizing history affects the health professionals' views on the relatives, which can create problems in the contacts between the relatives and the professionals. The relatives can be regarded as being unsuitable as carers for their sick children or healthcare professionals blame the family as a reason for the mental illness, based on theories developed by a group of influential American family therapists in the 1950s. Pejlert [43] writes that the view of the family as a cause of mental illness contributes to keeping the family outside the formal healthcare organization. As shown, the psychiatric care community's knowledge about care, illness, and disease is constructed and developed by claims-makers and interested parties. Therefore, a number of policy implications can be derived from the key findings concerning the social organization of the parents' world in their care responsibility for their ACWS.

Theoretically, the parents' meaning-making of their informal care responsibility and being a good parent not only is based on individual experiences of the parents' informal care responsibility, but is also embedded in the social and cultural meanings of the formal psychiatric care community. As shown, the parents' meaning-making of their care responsibility is also a communicative discursive negotiation with the psychiatric care community and the care professionals about accountability. This involves confirmation of the parents' self-definition and social interaction as responsible parents. This kind of confirmatory care or lack of the same can have long-term consequences for parents' health and well-being. One key finding from this study is that parents experience their caring responsibility with a great uncertainty which also gives them feelings of physical illness such as back pain, increased blood pressure, effects on the cardiovascular system, muscle inflammation, vocal cord inflammation, and breathing difficulties.

The parents' desire for information and knowledge is at stake in the discursive negotiations with the healthcare professionals. This study shows that parents have a great need to try to understand the illnesses and, above all, the knowledge that will enable them to provide appropriate support for their child. Instead of formal confirmatory care (e.g., information, social, emotional, and practical support), the parents expressed both frustration and anger over the construction of rigid rules and laws. They found themselves facing roadblocks. However, the information that was supportive could encourage the parents to regain or hold on to the social networks and thereby promote the informal care responsibility for the ACWS. Previous studies support these findings [10, 44–46].

The contribution of knowledge here is an insight into the complexity of parents' informal care responsibility as well as how its meaning is interactively produced. This is a key factor in the establishment of a functioning confirmation of care in order to support services to parents as informal carers. This knowledge contribution is also important to our understanding of the informal care position in mental health and illness in society. This theoretical perspective has guided us in suggesting political implementation of future informal care responsibility.

When it comes to new theoretical understanding based on this study, the parent's meaning-making involves a tension between care and concern for their own interests on the one hand and care and concern for the child's interests on the other. Being able to be a good parent and to handle the caring responsibility, the parent must compromise. In this tense situation, parents compromise between elements of struggle, cooperation, avoidance, and adaption in their interaction with the world outside as well as the world inside.

This approach can make a significant contribution to our understanding of the social and experiential dimensions of caring responsibility and it can help us broaden policy deliberations and decisions.

Methodologically, this paper reflects the special contribution that can be made by qualitative analysis to understand and uncover the micro and macro processes in psychiatric care and the relationship of formal care professionals with informal carers, here, parents. In other words, by giving voice to the parents' perspective, the experience of their care responsibility approach can lead to important clinical reforms and to changes in how society responds to related parties who are informal carers.

The perspective analysis shows that language use in the dialogues between the informants (the parents) and the interpretative analysts (the researchers) bridges the gap between the parents' meaning-making and the factual situation of being the informal carer. The question of validity implies that the interpretations in the study are checked against different criteria [47]. In this study, the main criterion is a valid interpretation that gives meaning to the phenomenon being studied, here the parents' informal care responsibility. In the chosen method, context, analysis, and interpretation have been made transparent so that the reader can follow and understand how these relate to each other.

When it comes to the limitations of this study, it can be concluded that the reported care responsibility experiences may not be reflective of carers in other settings because the sample used in this study was purposive. However, the main interpretation about parents' experiences as informal carers as being a good parent and their compromise between struggling, cooperation, avoidance, and adaption to the world outside as well as the world inside can be extended beyond its immediate context. This in turn increases the ability to apply it outside the study's context.

For practical considerations, however, these findings are of more than academic interest. They also point to significant psychiatric care policy from the perspective of confirmatory care, which are understood as care on a personal level. It is crucial for the healthcare professionals to be aware of the perspective that reflects the parent's perspective on informal care responsibility to be able to support care service to the parents. Similar findings were developed by Siouta et al. [48–51] and the Swedish Society of Nursing [52]. Creating an active role for the relatives requires knowledge based on the parents' preferences [53, 54]. This will give the healthcare providers a better understanding and willingness to cooperate with the relatives [48, 49, 54].

To that end, there is a need for an in-depth debate about formal psychiatric care's responsibility to support the relatives who are informal carers of psychiatric patients. It is most important to establish a policy for how the psychiatric care is to be divided between the formal and informal care givers.

There is a lack of research in the area investigated in this paper, and a number of issues regarding the informal care responsibility are still unexplored. One such area is in relation to what experiences the healthcare professionals have with parents who expect support from the mental healthcare system and examining how professionals support parents.

The Main Conclusions and Practical Considerations

(i) It is crucial for healthcare professionals to be aware of parents' perspectives as being responsible for informal care so as to be able to support a care service for parents.

(ii) There is a need for an in-depth debate about professional psychiatric care's responsibility to support the relatives who are informal carers of psychiatric patients.

(iii) It is most important to establish a policy for how psychiatric care is to be divided between the formal and informal care givers.

Conflict of Interests

The authors declare that there is no conflict of interests regarding the publication of this paper.

Authors' Contribution

Ann Blomgren Mannerheim and Ulla Hellström Muhli were responsible for the study design. Ann Blomgren Mannerheim collected and analyzed the data and drafted an early version of the paper. Ann Blomgren Mannerheim and Eleni Siouta made the revision of the background material. Eleni Siouta and Ulla Hellström Muhli both made critical revisions and Ulla Hellström Muhli drafted the last version of the paper.

Acknowledgments

The participants in the study are gratefully acknowledged. The authors also thank Professor Barry Saferstein for reading the English version of this paper and Professor Hannah Bradby for reading the revised version.

References

[1] S. Bremberg and C. Dalman, *Concepts, Methods and Prevalence of Mental Health, Mental Illness and Psychiatric Disorders in Children and Adolescents. A Review*, Swedish Research Council, Stockholm, Sweden, 2015.

[2] R. Lindqvist, S. Bengtsson, L. Fredén et al., "From reform intention to practice. How reforms in psychiatry and social care are transformed into concrete support in the Nordic countries," NHVs Rapportserie 2011:4R, Nordic School of Public Health NHV, The Nordic Council of Ministers, Göteborg, Sweden, 2011.

[3] R. Lindqvist, D. Rosenberg, and L. Fredén, "Den svenska psykiatrireformen i nordisk belysning," *Socialvetenskaplig Tidskrift*, vol. 88, no. 6, 2011.

[4] The National Board of Health and Welfare (Socialstyrelsen), *Välfärd och Valfrihet? Slutrapport från Utvärderingen av 1995 års Psykiatrireform*, The National Board of Health and Welfare (Socialstyrelsen), Stockholm, Sweden, 1999.

[5] Government Bill [Regeringens Proposition], *Ekonomisk Reglering Mellan Landsting och Kommuner med Anledning av Ökat Kommunalt Ansvar för Psykiskt Störda*, 96:72, Socialdepartementet, Stockholm, Sweden, 1995.

[6] L. Kjellin, O. Östman, Å. Rangford, and C.-G. Westrin, "Psykiskt långtidssjuka personers livssituation. En studie i Västmanland: bakgrund, syfte, metod och material," *Socialmedicinsk Tidskrift*, vol. 74, pp. 148–152, 1997.

[7] The World Health Report, *Mental Health: New Understanding, New Hope*, WHO Library Cataloguing-in-Publication Data, Geneva, Switzerland, 2001.

[8] A. Topor, *Managing the contradictions—recovery from severe mental disorders [Dr. Diss.]*, Department of Social Work, Stockholm University, Stockholm, Sweden, 2001.

[9] K. Persson, B. Axtelius, B. Söderfeldt, and M. Östman, "Association of perceived quality of life and oral health among psychiatric outpatients," *Psychiatric Services*, vol. 60, no. 11, pp. 1552–1554, 2009.

[10] J. A. Zauszniewski, A. K. Bekhet, and M. J. Suresky, "Relationships among perceived burden, depressive cognitions, resourcefulness, and quality of life in female relatives of seriously mentally ill adults," *Issues in Mental Health Nursing*, vol. 30, no. 3, pp. 142–150, 2009.

[11] H. Arvidsson, "Severely and persistently mentally ill—a changing group. Ten years after the 1995 Swedish mental health care reform," *Nordic Journal of Psychiatry*, vol. 63, no. 5, pp. 355–360, 2009.

[12] L. Johansson, "Caring for the next of kin. On informal care of elderly in Sweden," Doctoral Thesis from the Faculty of Medicine 330, Department of Social Medicine, University Hospital, Uppsala University, Reprocentralen, HSCm Uppsala, Uppsala, Sweden, 1991.

[13] H. P. Lefley, *Family Caregiving in Mental Illness*, Sage, Thousand Oaks, Calif, USA, 1996.

[14] A. Plank, V. Mazzoni, and L. Cavada, "Becoming a caregiver: new family carers' experience during the transition from hospital to home," *Journal of Clinical Nursing*, vol. 21, no. 13-14, pp. 2072–2082, 2012.

[15] N. J. K. Breitborde and V. H. Srihari, "Family work for first-episode psychosis: a service delivery protocol," in *Psychiatry—Theory, Applications and Treatments. Psychosis, Causes, Diagnosis and Treatment*, X. Anastassiou-Hadjicharalambous, Ed., Nova Science Publishers, New York, NY, USA, 2012.

[16] R. P. Cangelosi, "Caregiver burden or caregiver gain? Respite for family caregivers," *Journal of Psychosocial Nursing and Mental Health Services*, vol. 47, no. 9, pp. 19–22, 2009.

[17] F. Hjärthag, L. Helldin, U. Karilampi, and T. Norlander, "Illness-related components for the family burden of relatives to patients with psychotic illness," *Social Psychiatry and Psychiatric Epidemiology*, vol. 45, no. 2, pp. 275–283, 2010.

[18] H. L. Provencher and K.-T. Mueser, "Positive and negative symptom behaviors and caregiver burden in the relatives of persons with schizophrenia," *Schizophrenia Research*, vol. 26, no. 1, pp. 71–80, 1997.

[19] A. N. Karanci, "Caregivers of Turkish schizophrenic patients; causal attributions, burdens and attitudes to help from the health professionals," *Social Psychiatry and Psychiatric Epidemiology*, vol. 30, no. 6, pp. 261–268, 1995.

[20] H. Arvidsson, "Needs assessed by patients and staff in a Swedish sample of severely mentally ill subjects," *Nordic Journal of Psychiatry*, vol. 55, no. 5, pp. 311–317, 2001.

[21] H. Arvidsson, "Met and unmet needs of severely mentally ill persons—the psychiatric care reform in Sweden," *Social Psychiatry and Psychiatric Epidemiology*, vol. 38, no. 7, pp. 373–379, 2003.

[22] M. Carpenter, "'It's a small world': mental health policy under welfare capitalism since 1945," *Sociology of Health & Illness*, vol. 22, no. 5, pp. 602–620, 2000.

[23] U. Markström, *Den svenska psykiatrireformen: bland brukare, eldsjälar och byråkrater [Dr. Diss.]*, Umeå University, Umeå, Sweden, 2003.

[24] C.-G. Stefansson and L. Hansson, "Mental health care reform in Sweden, 1995," *Acta Psychiatrica Scandinavica*, vol. 104, supplement 410, pp. 82–88, 2002.

[25] The National Board of Health and Welfare & County Administrative Board (Socialstyrelsen & Länsstyrelserna), *Kommunernas Insatser för Personer med Psykiska Funktionshinder. Slutrapport Från en Nationell Tillsyn 2002–2004*, The National Board of Health and Welfare (Socialstyrelsen), Stockholm, Sweden, 2003.

[26] M. Östman, L. Hansson, and K. Andersson, "Family burden, participation in care and mental health—an 11-year comparison of the situation of relatives to compulsorily and voluntarily admitted patients," *International Journal of Social Psychiatry*, vol. 46, no. 3, pp. 191–200, 2000.

[27] M. Östman and L. Hansson, "The burden of relatives of psychiatric patients. Comparisons between parents, spouses, and grown-up children of voluntarily and compulsorily admitted psychiatric patients," *Nordic Journal of Psychiatry*, vol. 54, no. 1, pp. 31–36, 2000.

[28] A. Leinonen, "Informal family carers and lack of personal time: descriptions of being outside the sphere of formal help," *Nordic Social Work Research*, vol. 1, no. 2, pp. 91–108, 2011.

[29] K. Waerness, "The rationality of caring," *Economic and Industrial Democracy*, vol. 5, no. 2, pp. 185–211, 1984.

[30] M. Mayeroff, *On Caring*, William Morrow & Company, New York, NY, USA, 1999.

[31] P. L. Berger and T. Luckman, *The Social Construction of Reality. A Treatise in the Sociology of Knowledge*, Penguin Books, London, UK, 1966.

[32] D. Føllesdal, L. Wallöe, and J. Elster, *Argumentationsteori. Språk och Vetenskapsfilosofi*, Thales, Oslo, Norway, 1993.

[33] E. Goffman, *Asylums: Essays on the Social Situation of Mental Patients and Other Inmates*, Doubleday, Garden City, NY, USA, 1961.

[34] The Association for Schizophrenia, Schizofreniförbundet. Intresseförbundet för personer med schizofreni och liknande psykoser, 2015, http://www.schizofreniforbundet.se/.

[35] WMA, "World Medical association declaration of Helsinki, Ethical Principles for Medical Research Involving Human Subjects," 59th WMA General Assembly, Seoul, South Korea, 2008, http://www.wma.net/en/30publications/10policies/b3/17c.pdf.

[36] Reg. prop. (2002/03:50) [The government propel]. Etikprövning I forskning [The ethical probation]. Stockholm: Utbildningsdepartementet [The Department of Education].

[37] SFS, *Governmental Act (2003:460) on Ethical Review of Research Involving Humans*, Utbildningsdepartementet, Stockholm, Sweden, 2003.

[38] R. Buttny, *Social Accountability in Communication*, Sage Publications, London, UK, 1993.

[39] A. Schütz, *The Phenomenology of Social World*, Daidalos, Göteborg, Sweden, 1953/2002.

[40] S. Stryker, T. J. Owens, and R. W. White, Eds., *Self, Identity, and Social Movements*, University of Minnesota Press, Minneapolis, Minn, USA, 2000.

[41] V. Gecas, "Personal identity," in *Self, Identity, and Social Movements*, S. Stryker, T. J. Owens, and R. W. White, Eds., University of Minnesota Press, Minneapolis, Minn, USA, 2000.

[42] U. Hellström Muhli, "Accounts of pain experience in a Swedish elderly care context," *Communication & Medicine*, vol. 7, no. 1, pp. 55–64, 2010.

[43] A. Pejlert, "Leading a life with meaning and dignity in spite of suffering from long-term schizophrenia. Contributions of care," Medical Dissertations 653, Umeå University, Umeå, Sweden, 2000.

[44] B. Schulze and M. C. Angermeyer, "Subjective experiences of stigma. A focus group study of schizophrenic patients, their relatives and mental health professionals," *Social Science and Medicine*, vol. 56, no. 2, pp. 299–312, 2003.

[45] T. Orhagen, *Working with Families in Schizophrenic Disorders: The Practice of Psycho Educational Intervention*, vol. 363 of *Medical Dissertations*, Linköping University, Linköping, Sweden, 1992.

[46] L. Stein and A. Santos, *Psykiatriskt Arbete*, Studentlitteratur, Lund, Sweden, 2004.

[47] P.-J. Ödman, *Interpretation, Understanding, Knowing—Hermeneutics in Theory and Practice*, AWE/GEBERS, Borås, Sweden, 1994.

[48] E. Siouta, A. Broström, and B. Hedberg, "Content and distribution of discursive space in consultations between patients with atrial fibrillation and healthcare professionals," *European Journal of Cardiovascular Nursing*, vol. 12, no. 1, pp. 47–55, 2013.

[49] A.-M. Baronet, "Factors associated with caregiver burden in mental illness: a critical review of the research literature," *Clinical Psychology Review*, vol. 19, no. 7, pp. 819–841, 1999.

[50] A. Anell, A. H. Glenngård, and S. Merkur, "Sweden health system review," *Health Systems in Transition*, vol. 14, no. 5, pp. 1–159, 2012.

[51] L.-M. Sjöblom, A. Pejlert, and K. Asplund, "Nurses' view of the family in psychiatric care," *Journal of Clinical Nursing*, vol. 14, no. 5, pp. 562–569, 2005.

[52] Swedish Society of Nursing (Svensk Sjuksköterskeförening), *Närståendes Behov. Omvårdnad som Akademiskt Ämne*, Bromma Tryck, Stockholm, Sweden, 2004.

[53] I. Hellberg, V. Augustsson, and U. Hellström Muhli, "Elderly people's experiences of living in special housing accommodation," *International Journal of Qualitative Studies on Health and Well-Being*, vol. 6, no. 1, article 5894, 2011.

[54] E. Siouta, U. Hellström Muhli, B. Hedberg, A. Broström, B. Fossum, and K. Karlgren, "Patients' experiences of communication and involvement in decision-making about atrial fibrillation treatment in consultations with nurses and physicians," *Scandinavian Journal of Caring Sciences*, 2015.

16

Investigation of Anti-*Toxocara* and Anti-*Toxoplasma* Antibodies in Patients with Schizophrenia Disorder

Shahram Khademvatan,[1] Niloufar Khajeddin,[2] Sakineh Izadi,[3] and Elham Yousefi[4]

[1] *Health Research Institute, Infectious and Tropical Diseases Research Center, Department of Medical Parasitology, Ahvaz Jundishapur University of Medical Sciences, P.O. Box 613715794, Ahvaz, Iran*
[2] *Department of Psychiatry, Ahvaz Jundishapur University of Medical Sciences, Ahvaz, Iran*
[3] *Department of Psychology, Shahid Chamran University, Ahvaz, Iran*
[4] *Research Institute for Infectious Disease of Digestive System, Department of Medical Parasitology, Ahvaz Jundishapur University of Medical Sciences, Ahvaz, Iran*

Correspondence should be addressed to Shahram Khademvatan; khademvatan@yahoo.com and Elham Yousefi; elhamyousefi64@yahoo.com

Academic Editor: David C. Henderson

Objective. The aim of the present study was to examine the relationship between *Toxoplasma gondii* and *Toxocara* spp. infections in patients with schizophrenia disorder. *Method.* A total of 100 patients with schizophrenia disorder and 95 healthy individuals participated in the study. Participants were tested for the presence of anti-*T. gondii* and anti-*Toxocara* spp. antibodies by ELISA and Western blotting. Data were analyzed using Chi-square test and Fisher9s exact test. *Results.* There were no differences in *T. gondii* IgG seroprevalence between patients with schizophrenia and healthy individuals ($P = 0.1$), but there were differences in seroprevalence between males and females with schizophrenia ($P = 0.009$). In contrast, *Toxocara* spp. IgG seroprevalence was greater in patients with schizophrenia disorder than in healthy individuals ($P = 0.02$), but there were no differences in seroprevalence between men and women with schizophrenia ($P = 0.5$). Finally, there were no differences in seroprevalence of *T. gondii* or *Toxocara* spp. IgG among different subtypes of schizophrenia, various age groups, residential area, or clinical course of treatment ($P > 0.05$). *Conclusion.* The present study suggests that patients with schizophrenia disorder are at elevated risk of *Toxocara* spp. infection. Moreover, contamination with *T. gondii* is a risk factor for schizophrenia in women.

1. Introduction

Schizophrenia is a severe, disabling mental disorder with a devastating impact on patients, their family, and society [1]. Schizophrenia is a heterogeneous disorder characterized by a range of clinical features such as positive and negative symptoms [2], including a reduction in patients' health-related quality of life [3]. The prevalence of schizophrenia has been reported to be 1% of the adult population [4], developing in late adolescence or early adulthood, and most patients suffer from the disease throughout their lifetime [1].

Toxocariasis is a helminthozoonosis, caused by the Ascaridida nematodes, *Toxocara canis* and *Toxocara cati* [5]. Dogs and cats are the definitive hosts of *T. canis* and *T. cati*, respectively, although other mammals, such as humans and rodents, can be infected [6]. Humans are infected by ingestion of infectious eggs [6], often as a result of direct contact with pets or consumption of contaminated vegetables or undercooked meat [7]. *Toxocara* infection is also often transmitted by contact with the soil. Young children, people who live in rural areas, and people with soil-related occupation are at increased risk for toxocariasis [8–10]. The presence of *Toxocara* spp. larvae in the central nervous system may cause some neurological and psychiatric disorders including schizophrenia. Kaplan et al. [11] found more seroprevalence of *Toxocara* spp. infection in patients with schizophrenia than in healthy individuals (45.9% versus 2%). Further, in the study conducted by El-Sayed and Ismail [12], toxocariasis was detected in 23.3% of patients with schizophrenia disorder compared with that in 2.2% of healthy controls. In another study by Alvarado-Esquivel [13], 4.7% of psychiatric inpatients were positive for anti-*Toxocara* IgG antibodies compared with 1.1% of healthy controls. The difference was statistically significant.

Another parasite that is thought to be associated with schizophrenia is *Toxoplasma gondii*. Toxoplasmosis is one of the most common parasitic infections in human and other warm-blooded vertebrates including birds, livestock, and marine mammals [14, 15]. Humans usually become infected by consumption of undercooked meat, unwashed or poorly washed vegetables, or contaminated drinking water [16]. After a short phase of acute toxoplasmosis, the infection becomes latent and becomes encysted in the central nervous system and in muscle tissues, potentially for the life of the infected host [17, 18]. The parasite has the ability to alter the behavior of the host to increase transmission [19]. Some studies have found changes in infected individuals' personality characteristics [20–24].

There is much evidence to suggest that schizophrenia disorder is associated with toxoplasmosis [25–32]. Daryani et al. [33] and Hamidinejat et al. [34] from Iran also observed that higher titers of *T. gondii* IgG antibody was positively correlated with schizophrenia [33–35]. Some results however challenge the plausibility of this association [36, 37]. Because of these controversial findings and little knowledge about the prevalence of *Toxocara* spp. infection in patients with schizophrenia, the present study aimed to determine the seroprevalence of *Toxocara* spp. and *Toxoplasma* infections in patients with schizophrenia disorder and to compare it with healthy controls in Ahvaz, Southwest Iran.

2. Methods

Research was conducted over a period of 12 months from 2012 to 2013. A total of 100 patients diagnosed as having schizophrenia disorder and 95 matched healthy controls participated in the study. The patients had been admitted into Golestan hospital affiliated to Jundishapur University of Medical Sciences in Ahvaz, Iran. The diagnosis of schizophrenia disorder was performed by two psychiatrists following the DSM-IV-TR criteria. The control group consisted of blood donors who were tested at the laboratory in Jundishapur University of Medical Sciences. The controls were assessed by both a clinical psychologist and a psychiatrist and had no history of schizophrenia disorder. Neither of the 2 groups were immunodeficient nor were any other major psychiatric disorders or neurological diseases presentable.

To participate, subjects had to agree to comply with the requirements of study, and after describing the procedures and purposes of the study, written informed consents were obtained. The hospital's institutional review board approved all procedures.

A 5 mL blood sample was taken from each subject for serological analysis. Each subject was also asked to complete a questionnaire to obtain demographic data about ethnicity, gender, age, level of education obtained, marital status, and employment.

2.1. Serological Tests. Sera were separated by sample centrifugation at 3000 rpm for 5 min and then kept at −20°C until analysis. Anti-*Toxoplasma* antibodies (IgG and IgM) concentrations were measured by enzyme-linked immunosorbent assay (ELISA) (IgG and IgM: Trinity Biotech Captia, USA). In addition, all sera were examined by *Toxocara* IgG-ELISA test (IBL, International Gmbh, Hamburg, Germany) and *Toxocara* Western blot test (LDBIO Diagnostics, Lyon, France) for confirmation.

2.2. Statistical Analysis. Data were analyzed using Chi-square test, Fisher's exact test, and Student's t-test. Odds ratios (OR) with 95% confidence intervals (CI) were also determined. $P < 0.05$ was considered significant. Statistical analyses were carried out using SPSS v16 software.

3. Results

Demographic characteristics (sex, residence, marital status, level of education obtained, ethnicity, and age) of both patients and healthy controls are detailed in Table 1. Patient and control group seroprevalence for both *T. gondii* and *Toxocara* was evaluated. Anti-*Toxplasma* antibodies were detected in 34% of patients with schizophrenia disorder and 47.39% of healthy individuals ($P > 0.05$) (Table 2). Anti-*Toxoplasma* IgM antibodies were positive in 4 patients and 2 healthy individuals ($P > 0.05$).

Seroprevalence of anti-*Toxocara* IgG were higher in schizophrenia patients (14%) than in healthy controls (4.3%) ($P = 0.02$; Table 2). Western blot analysis confirmed *Toxocara* spp. infection, with low molecular weight bands (24–35 kDa) that are specific for *Toxocara* IgG present from all positive sera.

With respect to schizophrenia subtypes, anti-*T. gondii* antibodies were present in 35.82% (24 of 67) of patients with paranoid type of schizophrenia disorder, 42.85% (3 of 7) of patients with catatonic type, 33.3% (6 of 18) of patients with undifferentiated type, and 33.3% (1 of 3) of patients with residual type. None of the patients with disorganized type were seropositive. The difference in infection rate among the subtypes was not statistically significant ($P = 0.9$, Table 3). Anti-*Toxocara* antibodies were detected in 1.56% (10 of 64) of patients with paranoid type of schizophrenia disorder, 14.28% (1 of 7) of patients with catatonic type, 11.11% (2 of 18) of patients with undifferentiated type, and 20% (1 of 5) patients with disorganized type. None of the patients with residual type were seropositive. The difference in infection rate among the subtypes was not statistically significant ($P = 0.5$, Table 3). Serological analyses also confirmed that there were no significant increases in anti-*Toxocara* and anti-*Toxocara* antibody levels in patients with first-episode Schizophrenia disorder compared with those in patients with recurrent episodes ($P > 0.05$, Table 4).

The seroprevalence of anti-*T. gondii* IgG antibodies in male and female patients with schizophrenia disorder was 24.61% and 51.42%, respectively, ($P = 0.009$, Table 5). Anti-*Toxocara* antibodies were detected in 51.42% of females and 17.14% of males with schizophrenia disorder (nonsignificant).

Table 1: Demographic characteristics of the patient and control groups.

Feature	Frequency Patients' group	Control group	Total
T. gondii			
Positive	34 (34%)	45 (47.36%)	79 (40.51%)
Negative	66 (66%)	50 (52.63%)	116 (59.48%)
Toxocara			
Positive	14 (14%)	4 (4.39%)	18 (9.23%)
Negative	86 (86%)	91 (95.78%)	177 (90.76%)
Sex			
Female	35 (35%)	43 (45.74%)	78 (40.20%)
Male	65 (65%)	51 (54.25%)	116 (59.79%)
Residence			
Urban	76 (76%)	89 (93.98%)	165 (84.61%)
Rural	24 (24%)	6 (6.31%)	30 (15.38%)
Marital status			
Single	64 (64%)	77 (81.05%)	141 (72.30%)
Married	25 (25%)	18 (18.94%)	43 (22.05%)
Divorced/widowed	11 (11%)	0 (0)	11 (5.64%)
Level of education			
Grade school	74 (74%)	0 (0)	74 (37.94%)
12 years/high school	18 (18%)	9 (9.47%)	27 (13.84%)
University degree	8 (8%)	86 (90.52%)	94 (48.20%)
Ethnicity			
Fars	46 (48.42%)	15 (17.85%)	61 (34.07%)
Arab	15 (15.78%)	33 (39.28%)	48 (26.81%)
Lor	19 (20%)	34 (40.47%)	53 (29.60%)
Others	15 (15.78%)	2 (2.38%)	17 (9.49%)
Age (years)			
<20	0 (0)	4 (4.21%)	4 (2.05%)
20–29	32 (32%)	83 (87.36%)	115 (58.97%)
30–39	34 (34%)	7 (7.36%)	41 (21.02%)
40–49	23 (23%)	0 (0)	23 (11.79%)
>50	11 (11%)	1 (1.05%)	12 (6.15%)

Table 2: Seropositivity of *Toxoplasma gondii* and *Toxocara* antibodies in patients with schizophrenia disorder and healthy controls.

	Patients' group *N* (%)	Healthy *N* (%)	Sig	OR	CI_{95}
Toxoplasma gondii	34/100 (34%)	45/95 (47.36%)	0.08	0.57	0.32–1.02
Toxocara	14/100 (14%)	4/95 (4.3%)	0.02	0.27	0.08–0.8

Table 3: The distribution of *Toxoplasma gondii* and *Toxocara* antibodies in patients with different subtypes of schizophrenia disorder.

Subtypes of schizophrenia	*T. gondii* *N* (%)	*P* value	*Toxocara* *N* (%)	*P* value
Paranoid type	24/67 (35.82%)		10/64 (1.56%)	
Catatonic type	3/7 (42.85%)		1/7 (14.28%)	
Residual type	1/3 (33.3%)	0.9	0/3 (0)	0.5
Undifferentiated type	6/18 (33.3%)		2/18 (11.11%)	
Disorganized type	0/5 (0%)		1/5 (20%)	

TABLE 4: The distribution of *Toxoplasma gondii* and *Toxocara* antibodies in patients with schizophrenia based on clinical course of treatment.

	Clinical course	*N* (%)	*P* value	OR	CI_{95}
Toxoplasma gondii	First episode	13/30 (43.33%)	0.1	2.08	0.84–5.12
	Recurrent episodes	18/67 (26.86%)			
Toxocara	First episode	8/30 (26.66%)	0.06	0.22	0.06–0.75
	Recurrent episodes	5/30 (16.66%)			

TABLE 5: The seroprevalence of anti-*T. gondii* IgG antibodies in patients with schizophrenia disorder based on gender.

	Patients' group				
	N (%)		Sig	OR	CI
	Male	Female			
Toxoplasma gondii	16/65 (24.61%)	18/35 (51.42%)	0.009	0.3	0.12–0.73
Toxocara	8/65 (12.30%)	6/35 (17.14%)	0.5	1.47	0.46–4.65

The seroprevalence of *T. gondii* infection in patients living in urban and rural areas was 21.05% and 16.66%, respectively, (nonsignificant, $P = 0.7$). Seroprevalence of *Toxocara* also was not different between patients living in urban and rural areas (Table 6).

The participants were divided into 5 groups based on their age (<20, 20–29, 30–39, 40–49, and >50 years). The seroprevalence of *T. gondii* infection in the five age groups were 0%, 32.25%, 40%, 26.08%, and 36.36%, respectively, in patients; in healthy individuals the seroprevalence was 0%, 44.57%, 71.42%, 0%, and 100%, respectively, (nonsignificant between or within age subgroups, $P > 0.05$, Table 7). For *Toxocara* seroprevalence, there were no differences between or within age subgroups ($P > 0.05$, Table 8). Anti-*Toxocara* antibodies were significantly more prevalent in men with schizophrenia disorder (12.30%) than in healthy men (1.92%) ($P = 0.03$), but there was no difference in women ($P = 0.1$).

4. Discussion

The present study was conducted to investigate associations between schizophrenia disorder and parasitic infections, toxocariasis and toxoplasmosis. Because of poor hygiene, the prevalence of *Toxocara* spp. is higher in most localities of Iran than any elsewhere in the world. Sharif et al. in northern Iran, Arbabi and Hooshyar in central Iran, Sadjjadi et al. in southern Iran, and Khademvatan et al. in Southwest Iran reported 44%, 13.3%, 52.8%, and 45%, respectively, [6, 38–40]. With prevalence of approximately 50% in Iran, toxoplasmosis continues to be a public health problem [41]. The present study is the first to report toxocariasis in patients with schizophrenia in the Iranian population. The association between *Toxoplasma gondii* and schizophrenia also has received little attention in Iran.

The results of the present study show that there were significant differences between patients with schizophrenia disorder and healthy controls in seropositivity of *Toxocara*. We replicate the findings of the study conducted by Kaplan et al. [11] and El-Sayed and Ismail [12] that found that *Toxocara* spp. infection is related to schizophrenia disorder. Similarly, Alvarado-Esquivel [13] also reported that *Toxocara* infection is more frequent in patients with schizophrenia.

These results may be related to the fact that patients with schizophrenia have inadequate hygiene and self-care skills, and they have a greater tendency to eat inappropriate things [12]. Considering the correlation between lifestyle and *Toxocara* infection, and that *Toxocara* spp. is common in areas with low hygiene [11], abnormal behaviors and poor personal hygiene observed in patients with schizophrenia expose them to toxocariasis.

We considered gender differences in seroprevalence of *Toxocara* spp. infection. Although anti-toxocariasis IgG antibodies were significantly more prevalent in men with schizophrenia than in healthy men, no difference was found in seroprevalence of *Toxocara* infection between patients and healthy women. This may be related to the role of gender in the experience of illness, treatment, and recovery of schizophrenia disorder. Women with schizophrenia disorder have better global outcomes than men [42]; hence, it is less probable that women with schizophrenia are exposed to toxocariasis.

In the present study, there were no differences in the prevalence of *Toxoplasma* IgG seropositivity between patients with schizophrenia and healthy subjects. The finding is consistent with the result of the study conducted by Saraei-Sahnesaraei et al. [36] and Xiao et al. [37]. However, these results are in contrast to intervention studies [43, 44] and some direct studies [25–31, 34, 35] that support the link between toxoplasmosis and schizophrenia disorder.

The reason for the difference in these findings may relate to the various genotypes of *T. gondii* that vary in prevalence geographically [36] and have distinct neuropathogenic potential [34, 35]. It also may be due to the timing and route of infection, varying degrees of pathogenicity among infecting organisms, or heterogeneous etiology of schizophrenia disorder [45].

There are a number of challenges to these types of epidemiological studies, including the relative insensitivity of some serological assays [46], arbitrary cutoff selection, classification by percentile ranges, grouping results as low, intermediate, or high, and analyzing antibody levels as a

Table 6: The distribution of *Toxoplasma gondii* and *Toxocara* antibodies in patients with schizophrenia disorder based on their residential area.

	Patients' group				
	N (%)		Sig	OR	CI
	Urban	Rural			
Toxoplasma gondii	16/76 (21.05%)	4/24 (16.66%)	0.7	1.36	0.39–4.7
Toxocara	6/76 (7.89%)	3/24 (12.5%)	0.3	1.7	0.37–7.6

Table 7: The distribution of latent toxoplasmosis according to the age in patients with schizophrenia disorder and healthy controls.

	Patients' group *N* (%)	Healthy *N* (%)	Sig	OR	CI_{95}
Age (years)					
<20	0 (0%)	0/4 (0%)			
20–29	10/32 (32.25%)	37/83 (44.57%)	0.1	2.9	0.68–12.51
30–39	14/34 (41.17%)	5/7 (71.42%)	0.1	0.2	0.04–1.5
40–49	6/23 (26.08%)	0/0 (0%)			
>50	4/11 (36.36%)	1/1 (100%)	0.4	0.3	0.1–0.7

Table 8: The distribution of toxocariasis according to the age in patients with schizophrenia disorder and healthy controls.

	Patients' group *N* (%)	Healthy *N* (%)	Sig	OR	CI_{95}
Age (years)					
<20	0 (0%)	0 (0%)			
20–29	4/32 (12.5%)	3/83 (4.81%)	0.1	2.9	0.68–12.5
30–39	6/34 (17.14%)	1/7 (14.28%)	0.6	1.2	0.12–12.2
40–49	2/23 (8.69%)	0/0 (0%)			
>50	2/11 (18.18%)	0/1 (0%)	0.8	0.81	0.61–1.08

continuous rather than dichotomous or categorical variable [27].

In addition, for the purpose of respecting patients' rights, only those who are able and willing to complete the informed consent form are able to participate in the studies. Previous research suggests that clinical symptoms of infected schizophrenic patients are more severe than those of noninfected patients [47], therefore reducing the probability of incorporating infected schizophrenic patients into studies.

In terms of gender difference, we found differences between male and female patients with schizophrenia disorder ($P = 0.009$). Similar results, that is, higher seropositivity in schizophrenic women than in schizophrenic men, were also reported by Dickerson et al. [48].

The present finding is in contrast with the studies conducted by Alvarado-Esquivel et al. [49], Yuksel [50], and Xiao et al. [37], which demonstrated that seroprevalence of anti-*T. gondii* IgG is not different between men and women with schizophrenia disorder. On the other hand, Lindová et al. [51] reported higher seropositivity in male than in female schizophrenic patients.

Higher burdens in women may be explained on the basis of animal studies. Spleens of male mice produce higher level of interferon-gamma (IFN) in the early stages of *Toxoplasma* infection than those of female mice. High levels of IFN and tumor necrosis factor-alpha help male mice to respond to *T. gondii* infection more rapidly and to control the parasite multiplication [52].

Regarding the residential area, some previous studies found that the risks for *Toxocara* and *Toxoplasma* infections are higher in rural areas than in urban areas [50, 53–55]. Our study failed to show any differences between residential areas in the prevalence of infections, consistent with some other reports [12, 37].

Finally we did not find any significant differences in prevalence of *toxoplasmosis* and *toxocariasis* infections across various age subgroups, subtypes of schizophrenia, or between patients with first-episode schizophrenia disorder and those with recurrent episode schizophrenia.

The screening for *Toxocara* spp. antibodies depends on ELISA and Western blotting, which are the most common methods for immunodiagnosis of toxocariasis. Western blotting is more sensitive and specific than other available tests for diagnosing toxocariasis, capable of detecting low levels of *Toxocara* antibodies [56].

5. Conclusion

In conclusion, our research suggests that patients with schizophrenia disorder are at an elevated risk for *Toxocara* spp. infection. Moreover, contamination with *T. gondii* should be considered as one of the risk factors for schizophrenia disorder in women.

Conflict of Interests

The authors declare that there is no conflict of interests regarding the publication of this paper.

Acknowledgments

This study was funded by Grant no. OG-90120 from Health Research Institute, Infectious and Tropical Diseases Research Center, Ahvaz Jundishapur University of Medical Sciences and approved by the Ethical Committee (no.: ETH-658). The authors appreciate the support of the staff of the Protozoology Laboratory at Ahvaz Jundishapur University of Medical Sciences.

References

[1] L. Medeiros-Ferreira, J. E. Obiols, J. Navarro-Pastor, and A. Zuniga-Lagares, "Metabolic syndrome and health-related quality of life in patients with schizophrenia," *Actas Españolas de Psiquiatría*, vol. 41, no. 1, pp. 17–26, 2013.

[2] L. Cortese, R. Bressan, D. Castle, and S. Mosolov, "Management of Schizophrenia: clinical experience with asenapine," *Journal of Psychopharmacology*, vol. 27, no. 4, pp. 14–22, 2013.

[3] N. Grano, M. Karjalainen, EdlundV et al., "Health-related quality of life among adolescents: a comparison between subjects at risk for psychosis and other help seekers," *Early Intervention in Psychiatry*, 2013.

[4] E. Prandovszky, E. Gaskell, H. Martin, J. P. Dubey, J. P. Webster, and G. A. McConkey, "The neurotropic parasite *Toxoplasma gondii* increases dopamine metabolism," *PLoS ONE*, vol. 6, no. 9, Article ID e23866, 2011.

[5] P. Congdon and P. Lloyd, "*Toxocara* infection in the United States: the relevance of poverty, geography and demography as risk factors, and implications for estimating county prevalence," *International Journal of Public Health*, vol. 56, no. 1, pp. 15–24, 2011.

[6] S. Khademvatan, F. Rahim, M. Tavalla, R. Abdizadeh, and M. Hashemitabar, "PCR-based molecular characterization of *Toxocara* spp. using feces of stray cats: a study from Southwest Iran," *PLoS ONE*, vol. 8, no. 6, Article ID e65293, 2013.

[7] E. Pinelli, T. Herremans, M. G. Harms, D. Hoek, and L. M. Kortbeek, "*Toxocara* and ascaris seropositivity among patients suspected of visceral and ocular larva migrans in the Netherlands: trends from 1998 to 2009," *European Journal of Clinical Microbiology and Infectious Diseases*, vol. 30, no. 7, pp. 873–879, 2011.

[8] J. Gawor, A. Borecka, H. Zarnowska, M. Marczyńska, and S. Dobosz, "Environmental and personal risk factors for toxocariasis in children with diagnosed disease in urban and rural areas of central Poland," *Veterinary Parasitology*, vol. 155, no. 3-4, pp. 217–222, 2008.

[9] G. Quattrocchi, A. Nicoletti, B. Marin, E. Bruno, M. Druet-Cabanac et al., "Toxocariasis and epilepsy: systematic review and meta-analysis," *PLoS Neglected Tropical Diseases*, vol. 6, Article ID e1775, 2012.

[10] H. Smith, C. Holland, M. Taylor, J.-F. Magnaval, P. Schantz, and R. Maizels, "How common is human toxocariasis? Towards standardizing our knowledge," *Trends in Parasitology*, vol. 25, no. 4, pp. 182–188, 2009.

[11] M. Kaplan, A. Kalkan, S. Kuk, K. Demirdag, M. Ozden, and S. S. Kilic, "*Toxocara* seroprevalence in schizophrenic patients in Turkey," *Yonsei Medical Journal*, vol. 49, no. 2, pp. 224–229, 2008.

[12] N. M. El-Sayed and K. A. Ismail, "Relationship between Toxocara canis infection and schizophrenia," *Rawal Medical Journal*, vol. 37, no. 2, pp. 155–161, 2012.

[13] C. Alvarado-Esquivel, "*Toxocara* infection in psychiatric inpatients: a case control Seroprevalence study," *PLoS ONE*, vol. 8, no. 4, Article ID e62606, 2013.

[14] Y. Suzuki, "Host resistance in the brain against *Toxoplasma gondii*," *Journal of Infectious Diseases*, vol. 185, no. 1, pp. S58–S65, 2002.

[15] J. P. Dubey, "*Toxoplasma gondii* infections in chickens (Gallus domesticus): Prevalence, clinical disease, diagnosis and public health significance," *Zoonoses and Public Health*, vol. 57, no. 1, pp. 60–73, 2010.

[16] D. C. Herrmann, N. Pantchev, G. Vrhovec et al., "Atypical *Toxoplasma gondii* genotypes identified in oocysts shed by cats in Germany," *International Journal for Parasitology*, vol. 40, no. 3, pp. 285–292, 2010.

[17] J. P. Dubey and J. L. Jones, "*Toxoplasma gondii* infection in humans and animals in the United States," *International Journal for Parasitology*, vol. 38, no. 11, pp. 1257–1278, 2008.

[18] C. M. Miller, N. R. Boulter, R. J. Ikin, and N. C. Smith, "The immunobiology of the innate response to *Toxoplasma gondii*," *International Journal for Parasitology*, vol. 39, no. 1, pp. 23–39, 2009.

[19] E. Kristina and M. A. Fittipaldi, "*Toxoplasma gondii* as an etiological agent of schizophrenia essay," Presented in Partial Fulfillment of the Requirements of the Degree of Master of Arts at Hofstra University, 2008.

[20] J. Flegr, Š. Zitkovä, P. Kodym, and D. Frynta, "Induction of changes in human behaviour by the parasitic protozoan *Toxoplasma gondii*," *Parasitology*, vol. 113, no. 1, pp. 49–54, 1996.

[21] J. Flegr and J. Havlíček, "Changes in the personality profile of young women with latent toxoplasmosis," *Folia Parasitologica*, vol. 46, no. 1, pp. 22–28, 1999.

[22] J. Flegr, P. Kodym, and V. Tolarová, "Correlation of duration of latent *Toxoplasma gondii* infection with personality changes in women," *Biological Psychology*, vol. 53, no. 1, pp. 57–68, 2000.

[23] M. Novotná, J. Hanusova, J. Klose et al., "Probable neuroimmunological link between Toxoplasma and cytomegalovirus infections and personality changes in the human host," *BMC Infectious Diseases*, vol. 5, article 54, 2005.

[24] S. Khademvatan, S. Izadi-Mazidi, N. Khajeddin, and J. Saki, "Effect of toxoplasmosis on personality profiles of Iranian men and women," *South African Journal of Science*, vol. 109, no. 1-2, pp. 1–4, 2013.

[25] S. S. Mahmoud and M. S. Hasan, "Seroprevalence of *Toxoplasmosis gondii* among Schizophrenic patients," *Yemen Journal For Medical Science*, vol. 1, no. 3, pp. 1–7, 2009.

[26] P. Yuksel, B. Kocazeybek, N. Alpay, C. Babur, and R. Bayer, "Establishing the role of toxoplasmosis in the ethiopathogenesis of Schizophrenia," in *Proceedings of the 13th International Congress on Infectious Disease Abstracts*, 2008.

[27] D. W. Niebuhr, A. M. Millikan, D. N. Cowan, R. Yolken, Y. Li, and N. S. Weber, "Selected infectious agents and risk of schizophrenia among U.S. military personnel," *The American Journal of Psychiatry*, vol. 165, no. 1, pp. 99–106, 2008.

[28] D. Hinze-Selch, W. Däubener, L. Eggert, S. Erdag, R. Stoltenberg, and S. Wilms, "A controlled prospective study of *Toxoplasma gondii* infection in individuals with schizophrenia: beyond seroprevalence," *Schizophrenia Bulletin*, vol. 33, pp. 782–788, 2007.

[29] P. B. Mortensen, B. Nørgaard-Pedersen, B. L. Waltoft et al., "*Toxoplasma gondii* as a risk factor for early-onset schizophrenia: analysis of filter paper blood samples obtained at birth," *Biological Psychiatry*, vol. 61, no. 5, pp. 688–693, 2007.

[30] Z. Cetinkaya, S. Yazar, O. Gecici, and M. N. Namli, "Anti-*Toxoplasma gondii* antibodies in patients with schizophrenia—preliminary findings in a Turkish sample," *Schizophrenia Bulletin*, vol. 33, no. 3, pp. 789–791, 2007.

[31] A. S. Brown, C. A. Schaefer, C. P. Quesenberry Jr., L. Liu, V. P. Babulas, and E. S. Susser, "Maternal exposure to toxoplasmosis and risk of schizophrenia in adult offspring," *The American Journal of Psychiatry*, vol. 162, no. 4, pp. 767–773, 2005.

[32] J. Horacek, J. Flegr, J. Tintera et al., "Latent toxoplasmosis reduces gray matter density in schizophrenia but not in controls: voxel-based-morphometry (VBM) study," *The World Journal of Biological Psychiatry*, vol. 13, pp. 501–509, 2012.

[33] A. Daryani, M. Sharif, S. H. Hosseini, S. A. Karimi, and S. Gholami, "Serological survey of *Toxoplasma gondii* in schizophrenia patients referred to Psychiatric Hospital, Sari City, Iran," *Tropical Biomedicine*, vol. 27, no. 3, pp. 476–482, 2010.

[34] H. Hamidinejat, M. Ghorbanpoor, H. Hosseini et al., "*Toxoplasma gondii* infection in first-episode and inpatient individuals with schizophrenia," *International Journal of Infectious Diseases*, vol. 14, pp. e978–e981, 2010.

[35] M. Sharif, M. Nasrolahei, S. Ziapour et al., "*Toxocara cati* infections in stray cats in northern Iran," *Journal of Helminthology*, vol. 81, pp. 63–66, 2007.

[36] M. Saraei-Sahnesaraei, F. Shamloo, H. Jahani Hashemi, F. Khabbaz, and S. Alizadeh, "Relation between *Toxoplasma gondii* infections and Schizophrenia," *Iranian Journal of Psychiatry and Clinical Psychology*, vol. 15, no. 1, pp. 3–9, 2009.

[37] Y. Xiao, J. Yin, N. Jiang et al., "Seroepidemiology of human *Toxoplasma gondii* infection in China," *BMC Infectious Diseases*, vol. 10, article 4, 2010.

[38] M. Sharif, M. Nasrolahei, S. P. Ziapour et al., "*Toxocara* cati infections in stray cats in northern Iran," *Journal of Helminthology*, vol. 81, no. 1, pp. 63–66, 2007.

[39] M. Arbabi and H. Hooshyar, "Gastrointestinal parasites of stray cats in Kashan, Iran," *Tropical Biomedicine*, vol. 26, no. 1, pp. 16–22, 2009.

[40] S. M. Sadjjadi, A. Oryan, A. R. Jalai, and D. Mehrabani, "Prevalence and intensity of infestation with *Toxocara* cati in stray cats in Shiraz, Iran," *Veterinarski Arhiv*, vol. 71, no. 3, pp. 149–157, 2001.

[41] M. Assmar, A. Amirkhani, N. Piazak, A. Hovanesian, A. Kooloobandi, and R. Etessami, "Toxoplasmosis in Iran, results of a seroepidemiological investigation," *Bulletin de la Societe de Pathologie Exotique*, vol. 90, no. 1, pp. 19–21, 1997.

[42] M. Sajatovic, J. H. Jenkins, M. E. Strauss, Z. A. Butt, and E. Carpenter, "Gender identity and implications for recovery among men and women with schizophrenia," *Psychiatric Services*, vol. 56, no. 1, pp. 96–98, 2005.

[43] J. P. Webster, P. H. L. Lamberton, C. A. Donnelly, and E. F. Torrey, "Parasites as causative agents of human affective disorders? The impact of anti-psychotic, mood-stabilizer and anti-parasite medication on *Toxoplasma gondii*'s ability to alter host behaviour," *Proceedings of the Royal Society B*, vol. 273, no. 1589, pp. 1023–1030, 2006.

[44] L. Jones-Brando, E. F. Torrey, and R. Yolken, "Drugs used in the treatment of schizophrenia and bipolar disorder inhibit the replication of *Toxoplasma gondii*," *Schizophrenia Research*, vol. 62, no. 3, pp. 237–244, 2003.

[45] R. H. Yolken, F. B. Dickerson, and E. Fuller Torrey, "Toxoplasma and schizophrenia," *Parasite Immunology*, vol. 31, no. 11, pp. 706–715, 2009.

[46] E. F. Torrey, J. J. Bartko, Z.-R. Lun, and R. H. Yolken, "Antibodies to *Toxoplasma gondii* in patients with schizophrenia: a meta-analysis," *Schizophrenia Bulletin*, vol. 33, no. 3, pp. 729–736, 2007.

[47] J. Flegr, "How and why Toxoplasma makes us crazy," *Trends in Parasitology*, vol. 29, no. 4, pp. 155–163, 2013.

[48] F. Dickerson, J. Boronow, C. Stallings, A. Origoni, and R. Yolken, "*Toxoplasma gondii* in individuals with schizophrenia: association with clinical and demographic factors and with mortality," *Schizophrenia Bulletin*, vol. 33, no. 3, pp. 737–740, 2007.

[49] C. Alvarado-Esquivel, A. Sifuentes-Alvarez, S. G. Narro-Duarte et al., "Seroepidemiology of *Toxoplasma gondii* infection in pregnant women in a public hospital in northern Mexico," *BMC Infectious Diseases*, vol. 6, article e113, 2006.

[50] P. Yuksel, N. Alpay, C. Babur et al., "The role of latent toxoplasmosis in the aetiopathogenesis of schizophrenia—the risk factor or an indication of a contact with cat?" *Folia Parasitologica*, vol. 57, no. 2, pp. 121–128, 2010.

[51] J. Lindová, M. Novotná, J. Havlíček et al., "Gender differences in behavioral changes induced by latent toxoplasmosis," *International Journal for Parasitology*, vol. 36, no. 14, pp. 1485–1492, 2006.

[52] J. Prandota, "Neuropathological changes and clinical features of autism spectrum disorder participants are similar to that reported in congenital and chronic cerebral toxoplasmosis in humans and mice," *Research in Autism Spectrum Disorders*, vol. 4, no. 2, pp. 103–118, 2010.

[53] N. Doğan, E. C. Dinleyici, O. Bor, S. O. Töz, and Y. Ozbel, "Seroepidemiological survey for *Toxocara* canis infection in the northwestern part of Turkey," *Turkiye Parazitoloji Dergisi*, vol. 31, no. 4, pp. 288–291, 2007.

[54] A. Deutz, K. Fuchs, H. Auer, U. Kerbl, H. Aspöck, and J. Köfer, "*Toxocara*-infestations in Austria: a study on the risk of infection of farmers, slaughterhouse staff, hunters and veterinarians," *Parasitology Research*, vol. 97, no. 5, pp. 390–394, 2005.

[55] G. Rubinsky-Elefant, C. E. Hirata, J. H. Yamamoto, and M. U. Ferreira, "Human toxocariasis: diagnosis, worldwide seroprevalences and clinical expression of the systemic and ocular forms," *Annals of Tropical Medicine and Parasitology*, vol. 104, no. 1, pp. 3–23, 2010.

[56] M. Zibaei, F. Firoozeh, P. Bahrami, and S. M. Sajjadi, "Investigation of anti-*Toxocara* antibodies in epileptic patients and comparison of two methods: ELISA and Western blotting," *Epilepsy Research and Treatment*, vol. 2013, Article ID 156815, 5 pages, 2013.

17

Not All Distraction Is Bad: Working Memory Vulnerability to Implicit Socioemotional Distraction Correlates with Negative Symptoms and Functional Impairment in Psychosis

Quintino R. Mano,[1,2,3] Gregory G. Brown,[1,2,3] Heline Mirzakhanian,[1,2,3] Khalima Bolden,[1,2,3] Kristen S. Cadenhead,[1,2,3] and Gregory A. Light[1,2,3]

[1] *San Diego Veterans Affairs Healthcare System, San Diego, CA 92161, USA*
[2] *VISN-22 Mental Illness, Research, Education and Clinical Center (MIRECC), VA San Diego Healthcare System, San Diego, CA 92161, USA*
[3] *Department of Psychiatry, University of California, San Diego, School of Medicine, San Diego, CA, USA*

Correspondence should be addressed to Gregory G. Brown; gbrown@ucsd.edu

Academic Editor: Steven J. Siegel

This study investigated implicit socioemotional modulation of working memory (WM) in the context of symptom severity and functional status in individuals with psychosis ($N = 21$). A delayed match-to-sample task was modified wherein task-irrelevant facial distracters were presented early and briefly during the rehearsal of pseudoword memoranda that varied incrementally in load size (1, 2, or 3 syllables). Facial distracters displayed happy, sad, or emotionally neutral expressions. Implicit socioemotional modulation of WM was indexed by subtracting task accuracy on nonfacial geometrical distraction trials from facial distraction trials. Results indicated that the amount of implicit socioemotional modulation of *high* WM load accuracy was significantly associated with negative symptoms ($r = 0.63$, $P < 0.01$), role functioning ($r = -0.50$, $P < 0.05$), social functioning ($r = -0.55$, $P < 0.01$), and global assessment of functioning ($r = -0.53$, $P < 0.05$). Specifically, *greater* attentional distraction of *high* WM load was associated with *less* severe symptoms and functional impairment. This study demonstrates the importance of the WM-socioemotional interface in influencing clinical and psychosocial functional status in psychosis.

1. Introduction

Attentional impairments are commonly observed in psychosis [1]. A classic view of attentional distraction is that it reflects cognitive impairment, that is, reduced ability to accurately maintain information in the presence of task-irrelevant stimuli. Yet, there are real-world situations wherein attentional distraction is adaptive. Consider a dyadic social encounter wherein the communicatee's changing facial expressions appropriately disrupt the communicator's thoughts. Here, attentional distraction adaptively permits the communicator to modulate ongoing cognition and attend to changing facial expressions in the communicatee. In other words, effective and reciprocal social encounters are those that demonstrate flexibility whereby communicators are sensitive to the facial expressions of the communicatee and are capable of modulating ongoing thoughts to attend to the communicatee. The present study aimed to capture the adaptability of this everyday challenge and gather proof of concept evidence by examining implicit socioemotional modulation of working memory (WM) in relation to symptom severity and functional status in individuals with psychosis. We reasoned that individuals with relatively severe psychosis have a WM system that is less sensitive to the moment-to-moment modulation of socioemotional stimuli. Though individuals with psychosis have general cognitive impairments, the WM construct was initially targeted because it maps onto ongoing cognitive processes and its interaction with socioemotional modulation.

We utilized a WM paradigm [2] that assesses WM in the context of implicit facial distraction. In the original study, Mano and colleagues [2] found that task-irrelevant socioemotional stimuli disrupted WM in the intermediate load condition (i.e., 2 syllables) but not in the low or high WM load conditions (1 Syllable and 3 syllables, resp.). Such, implicit facial distraction was important to study because although individuals with psychosis demonstrate impairments in explicitly identifying facial emotions [3], many also demonstrate relatively intact implicit facial emotion processing [4–6], even for "emotionally neutral faces" [7, 8]. Load size was manipulated to determine whether associations among implicit facial disruption of WM, symptom severity, and functional status are load dependent. The present delayed match-to-sample task is in standard use to measure the rehearsal and maintenance aspect of WM and is commonly used to assess WM in the psychosis research literature [9].

Viewing implicit socioemotional modulation of WM as adaptive in certain real-world circumstances, we hypothesized that symptom severity and functional status in psychosis are related to attentional distraction of WM by task-irrelevant faces. Specifically, *greater* symptom severity and functional impairment would be associated with relatively *less* implicit facial disruption of WM.

2. Experimental Procedures

2.1. Participants. Twenty-one (7 female; mean age = 23 ± 9; mean years of education = 12 ± 2) individuals are diagnosed with schizophrenia, schizophreniform disorder, psychosis NOS, schizoaffective disorder, or an affective psychosis that was confirmed using the SCID-I [10]. Among these participants, 17 were in their first-episode of psychosis and four with chronic schizophrenia. All were right handed. Exclusion criteria were (a) neurologic disorders, (b) substance abuse in the past 1 month if it is the first episode, (c) substance abuse in the past 6 months if it is chronic schizophrenia, (d) lifetime history of substance dependence, (e) history of head injury with loss of consciousness greater than five minutes and/or posttraumatic amnesia, (f) cognitive impairment, and (g) medical illnesses associated with cognitive impairment.

2.2. Measures of Symptom Severity and Functional Outcome. Symptom severity was scored on the scales for the assessment of positive symptoms (SAPS [11]) and negative symptoms (SANS [12]). Functional status was assessed with the global functioning: social (GF: social [13]) and global functioning: role (GF: role [14]) scales, as well as the global assessment functioning (GAF) scale [15].

2.3. WM Paradigm. The WM paradigm, developed by Mano and colleagues [2], employed a 3 × 2 design with the within-subjects factors including *load size* (1 versus 2 versus 3 syllables) and *distraction* (faces (happy, sad, and emotionally neutral) versus nonfacial geometrical oval figure). Stimuli included (1) pronounceable nonwords, (2) human faces (Radboud Faces Database [16]), and a (3) nonfacial geometrical control. Each trial began with a cross (e.g., "+") presented at central fixation for 1000 ms and was comprised of three sequential phases. In the first phase (encoding), participants were given one, two, or three syllables to subvocally read and memorize (2-second phase duration). Unbeknownst to participants, distracters were briefly presented (33 ms) immediately after the pseudoword presentation phase. Distracters were task-irrelevant and presented at fixation. A non-facial neutral backward mask immediately replaced distracters and filled the duration of the rehearsal phase. (Participants were told the backward mask was a rehearsal indicator.) During the second phase (rehearsal), participants were instructed to mentally rehearse the syllables presented in the first phase, with the rehearsal interval duration varying among 8–16 seconds in two-second increments. The third phase (recognition) consisted of a recognition test in which two sets of pseudowords were presented and the participant was instructed to indicate (using the keyboard number pad with dominant right hand) which set was from the first phase (4-second phase duration). The total duration of the computerized task lasted approximately 40 minutes, with two breaks given after every 36 trials. Stimulus presentation and behavioral recordings were controlled using E-Prime (Psychology Software Tools, Inc., Pittsburgh, PA). Accuracy and speed were stressed. Dependent variables were response latencies and percentage correct.

2.4. Posttask Facial Affect Recognition Test. Following completion of the task, participants were asked in an open-ended manner whether they "noticed anything in the task." If a participant did not freely report detecting a face in the task, then they were given a debriefing statement. If participants reported detecting a face during the task, then they were given the facial affect recognition test prior to presentation of the debriefing statement. This test consisted of pictures of facial expressions representing each of the eight emotional expressions (angry, contemptuous, disgusted, fearful, happy, neutral, sad, and surprised) in the Radboud Faces Database [16]. Participants were instructed to circle three emotions potentially seen in the task to assess awareness of emotional expressions of facial distracters.

2.5. Data Analysis. Outliers were identified and removed at the individual level such that response latencies ±2.5 SD away from each participant's mean were removed from analyses. The primary aim was to assess associations among implicit socioemotional modulation of WM, symptom severity, and functional status. As such, contrast variables were created that demonstrate the effects of facial distractors on WM performance at each load condition (e.g., 1, 2, and 3 syllables). Effects of facial distractors on each load condition were collapsed across valence type (happy, sad, and emotionally neutral) and contrasted with the effect of geometrical distraction, producing contrast variables for each load condition. For example, 1-syllable WM accuracy in the context of happy, sad, and neutral facial distractors was

TABLE 1: Correlations among task variables (percent-correct), symptom severity, and functional outcome (n = 21).

Task variables	SANS	SAPS	Role	Social	GAF
Overall task	−.27	−.24	**.54*****	.20	.29
Overall 1-syllable	.23	−.17	**.53***	.34	.36
Overall 2-syllable	−.10	−.18	**.46***	.16	.20
Overall 3-syllable	−.28	−.27	**.50***	.14	.28
1-syllable/facial distraction *minus* 1-syllable/geometrical distraction	−.11	−.13	.12	.18	.15
2-syllable/facial distraction *minus* 2-syllable/geometrical distraction	−.14	−.08	.12	−.08	.21
3-syllable/facial distraction *minus* 3-syllable/geometrical distraction	**.63****	.35	**−.50***	**−.55****	**−.53***
3-syllable/*happy* facial distraction *minus* 3-syllable/geometrical distraction	**.59****	.27	**−.54***	−.39	**−.53***
3-syllable/*neutral* facial distraction *minus* 3-syllable/geometrical distraction	**.60****	.28	**−.50***	**−.61****	**−.46***
3-syllable/*sad* facial distraction *minus* 3-syllable/geometrical distraction	**.49***	.40	−.30	**−.45***	−.42

SANS: scale for the assessment of negative symptoms; SAPS: scale for the assessment of positive symptoms; role: global functioning: role; social: global functioning: social; GAF: global assessment of functioning.
*$P \leq 0.05$; **$P \leq 0.01$.

averaged and then subtracted from 1-syllable WM accuracy in the context of geometrical distraction. This calculation produced a "1-syllable/facial distraction accuracy *minus* 1-syllable/geometrical distraction accuracy" variable, a calculation that was repeated for the 2 and 3 syllable conditions. Effects of facial distracters were collapsed across valence type (happy, sad, and neutral) because sensitivity to emotional and emotionally neutral faces is common in psychosis [4–8]. Notably, individual differences in WM capacity were controlled with contrast variables because capacity is represented on both sides of the contrast. Pearson correlations assessed associations among contrast variables, symptom severity, and functional status. Finally, a 3 (WM load) × 2 (Distraction) repeated-measures ANOVAs tested for main effects and factorial interaction, performed separately for accuracy and response latency data.

3. Results and Discussion

Overall accuracy ranged from 68% to 100% (M = 88%; SD = 10%)—well above the 50% chance-level. Correlations among contrast variables and measures of negative symptom severity and functional status were statistically significant (Table 1) but only in the highest WM load condition (see Figure 1). The direction of the correlations in the highest WM load condition was such that patients showing the greatest disruption of WM performance due to facial distraction also experienced the least severe negative symptoms and the most intact functioning (Figure 1).

Load had a significant effect on accuracy ($F[2,19]$= 23.079, $P < 0.001$; MSE = 0.01; η^2_p = 0.536) indicating that responses were most accurate for the 1-syllable condition (M = 94%; SD = 6%), intermediately accurate for the 2-syllable condition (M = 90%; SD = 11%), and least accurate for the 3-syllable condition (M = 80%; SD = 15%). In contrast, no significant main effect of distraction ($F[2,19]$= 0.906, P = 0.35; MSE = 0.008; η^2_p = 0.043) or load-by-distraction interaction ($F[2,19]$= 1.394, P = 0.260; MSE = .01; η^2_p = 0.065) was detected. Although the interaction failed to reach statistical significance, the partial eta-squared was of moderate strength and the interaction for response latencies was significant ($F[1,20]$= 3.676, P = 0.034; MSE = 20, 022.396; η^2_p = 0.155). Figure 2 displays the curvilinear relationship between WM load and socioemotional modulation for accuracy and response latencies.

All participants reported detecting a face during the task. Fifty-eight percent of the participants reported that they saw a happy face, 91% reported that they saw a neutral face, and 16% reported that they saw a sad face.

Results of the present study demonstrate that greater distraction of WM by task-irrelevant faces was associated with less severe symptoms and with more intact global mental-health functioning. These associations were load dependent and were observed only in the high WM load condition. How might these findings be explained? One account begins with the thesis that, because of their biological significance, faces are especially potent attractors of attention in the primate visual system [17]. Additionally, more normal facial processing is correlated with better social functioning in psychosis [18]. By implication, psychotic patients with intact face processing may be more distracted by irrelevant facial stimuli than psychotic patients with impaired facial processing and yet should function better.

Moreover, functional brain imaging studies have shown that not only that task-irrelevant emotional distraction can

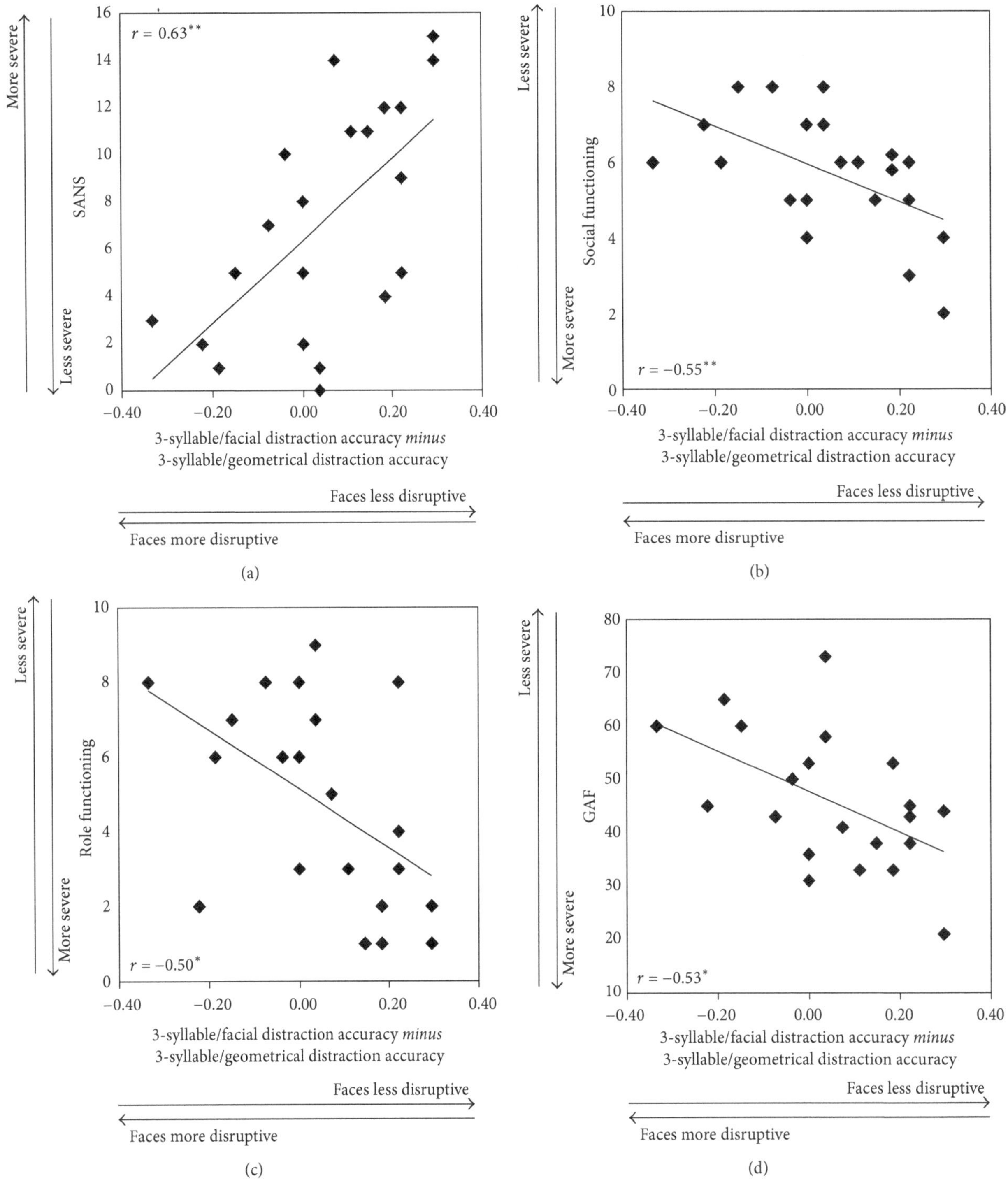

FIGURE 1: Correlations among contrast variables in the high working memory load condition (3 syllables) and measures of negative symptom severity and functional outcome.

impair working memory, but also that disruptive emotional stimuli can activate limbic system sites while reducing activity in the dorsolateral prefrontal cortex [19, 20]. We have previously argued that as the effects associated with affective brain system responses become conscious, they compete with cognitive resources that otherwise would be dedicated to WM activity [21]. When WM load is small, resources may be shared without disrupting WM functioning. As WM load increases, the disruptive effects of facial distraction on WM performance appear until WM load approaches capacity, at which point high WM load processing maximizes capacity and deprives facial stimuli processing resources to cause

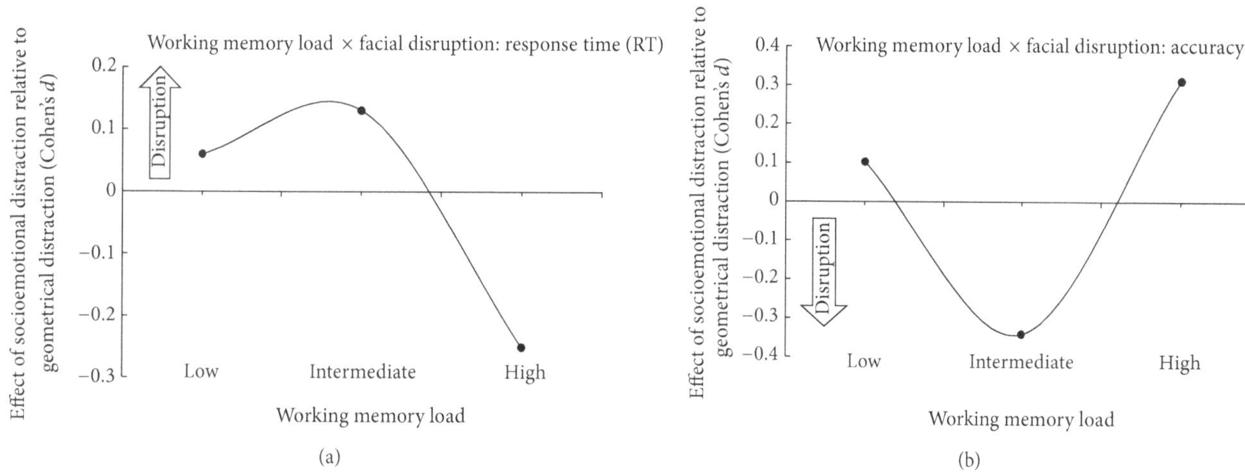

FIGURE 2: Modulation effects of all facial distracters are displayed relative to nonfacial geometric distracters. The zero axis value represents working memory performance in the context of nonfacial geometrical distracters. In (a) depicting response latencies relative to nonfacial geometrical distracters, positive effect sizes connote behavioral disruption while negative effect sizes connote behavioral facilitation. In (b) depicting accuracy relative to nonfacial geometrical distracters, positive effect sizes connote behavioral facilitation while negative effect sizes connote behavioral disruption.

disruption [2, 21]. This interactive process, particularly at the high WM load level, may be uniquely related to psychosocial functioning in disorders of psychosis. Though speculative, it is conceivable that some aspects of socioemotional processing are relatively impaired in psychosis because individuals with psychosis are engaged in high WM load processing during social encounters [21].

4. Conclusions

In a sample of individuals with psychosis, the amount of implicit socioemotional modulation of high WM load accuracy was significantly associated with negative symptoms, role functioning, social functioning, and global assessment of functioning. Specifically, greater attentional distraction of high WM load was associated with less severe symptoms and functional impairment. This study demonstrates the importance of the WM-socioemotional interface in influencing clinical and psychosocial functional status in psychosis.

Conflict of Interests

The authors declare that there is no conflict of interests regarding the publication of this paper.

Acknowledgements

The authors would like to thank Marlena Pela, Joyce Sprock, Nasra Haroun, M.D., Tracy Alderman, Ph.D., and Isabel Domingues, M.D., for their tireless work, as well as dedicated research assistants (Clara Robles, Jason Nunag, and Daniel Roman). This research was supported by the Department of Veteran Affairs Office of Academic Affiliations Advanced Fellowship Program in Mental Illness Research and Clinical Center (MIRECC) (Q.R.M., G.G.B., B.S.M.) and the National Institutes of Health- (NIH-) supported Grants R01 MH60720, U01 MH082022, K24 MH76191 (Kristen S. Cadenhead and Heline Mirzakhanian), and R01 MH079777. Funding sources had no further role in the writing of this paper or decision to submit for publication.

References

[1] M. Fioravanti, O. Carlone, B. Vitale, M. E. Cinti, and L. Clare, "A meta-analysis of cognitive deficits in adults with a diagnosis of schizophrenia," *Neuropsychology Review*, vol. 15, no. 2, pp. 73–95, 2005.

[2] Q. R. Mano, G. G. Brown, K. Bolden, R. Aupperle, M. P. Paulus, and M. B. Stein, "Curvilinear relationship between phonological working memory load and social-emotional modulation," *Cognition & Emotion*, vol. 27, no. 2, pp. 283–304, 2013.

[3] K. Marwick and J. Hall, "Social cognition in schizophrenia: a review of face processing," *British Medical Bulletin*, vol. 88, no. 1, pp. 43–58, 2008.

[4] R. E. Gur, C. McGrath, R. M. Chan et al., "An fMRI study of facial emotion processing in patients with schizophrenia," *The American Journal of Psychiatry*, vol. 159, no. 12, pp. 1992–1999, 2002.

[5] A. V. Rauch, M. Reker, P. Ohrmann et al., "Increased amygdala activation during automatic processing of facial emotion in schizophrenia," *Psychiatry Research*, vol. 182, no. 3, pp. 200–206, 2010.

[6] M. van 't Wout, A. Aleman, R. P. C. Kessels, W. Cahn, E. H. F. de Haan, and R. S. Kahn, "Exploring the nature of facial affect processing deficits in schizophrenia," *Psychiatry Research*, vol. 150, no. 3, pp. 227–235, 2007.

[7] J. Hall, H. C. Whalley, J. W. McKirdy et al., "Overactivation of fear systems to neutral faces in schizophrenia," *Biological Psychiatry*, vol. 64, no. 1, pp. 70–73, 2008.

[8] D. J. Holt, L. Kunkel, A. P. Weiss et al., "Increased medial temporal lobe activation during the passive viewing of emotional

and neutral facial expressions in schizophrenia," *Schizophrenia Research*, vol. 82, no. 2-3, pp. 153–162, 2006.

[9] J. Lee and S. Park, "Working memory impairments in schizophrenia: a meta-analysis," *Journal of Abnormal Psychology*, vol. 114, no. 4, pp. 599–611, 2005.

[10] M. B. First, R. L. Spitzer, M. Gibbon, and G. B. W. Williams, *Structured Clinical Interview for DSM-IV Axis I Disorders (SCID-I, Research Version)*, Biometric Research Department, New York, NY, USA, 1996.

[11] N. C. Andreasen, *The Scale for the Assessment of Negative Symptoms (SANS)*, The University of Iowa, Iowa City, Iowa, USA, 1983.

[12] N. C. Andreasen, *The Scale for the Assessment of Positive Symptoms (SAPS)*, The University of Iowa, Iowa City, Iowa, USA, 1984.

[13] A. M. Auther, C. W. Smith, and B. A. Cornblatt, *Global Functioning: Social Scale (GF: Social)*, Zucker-Hillside Hospital, Glen Oaks, NY, USA, 2006.

[14] T. A. Niedam, C. E. Bearden, J. K. Johnson, and T. D. Cannon, *Global Functioning: Role Scale (GF: Role)*, University of California, Los Angeles, Calif, USA, 2006.

[15] R. C. W. Hall, "Global assessment of functioning: a modified scale," *Psychosomatics*, vol. 36, no. 3, pp. 267–275, 1995.

[16] O. Langner, R. Dotsch, G. Bijlstra, D. H. J. Wigboldus, S. T. Hawk, and A. van Knippenberg, "Presentation and validation of the radboud faces database," *Cognition & Emotion*, vol. 24, no. 8, pp. 1377–1388, 2010.

[17] R. S. Maior, E. Hori, C. E. Uribe et al., "A role for the superior colliculus in the modulation of threat responsiveness in primates: toward the ontogenesis of the social brain," *Reviews in the Neurosciences*, vol. 23, no. 5-6, pp. 697–706, 2012.

[18] S. M. Couture, D. L. Penn, and D. L. Roberts, "The functional significance of social cognition in schizophrenia: a review," *Schizophrenia Bulletin*, vol. 32, supplement 1, pp. S44–S63, 2006.

[19] F. Dolcos, A. D. Iordan, and S. Dolcos, "Neural correlates of emotion-cognition interactions: a review of evidence from brain imaging investigations," *Journal of Cognitive Psychology*, vol. 23, no. 6, pp. 669–694, 2011.

[20] F. Dolcos, A. D. Iordan, J. Kragel et al., "Neural correlates of opposing effects of emotional distraction on working memory and episodic memory: an event-related FMRI investigation," *Frontiers in Psychology*, vol. 6, no. 4, pp. 1–16, 2013.

[21] Q. R. Mano and G. G. Brown, "Cognition-emotion interactions in schizophrenia: emerging evidence on working memory load and implicit facial-affective processing," *Cognition & Emotion*, vol. 27, no. 5, pp. 875–899, 2013.

18

"Sometimes It's Difficult to Have a Normal Life": Results from a Qualitative Study Exploring Caregiver Burden in Schizophrenia

Adam Gater,[1] Diana Rofail,[2] Chloe Tolley,[1] Chris Marshall,[1] Linda Abetz-Webb,[1] Steven H. Zarit,[3] and Carmen Galani Berardo[4]

[1] *Adelphi Mill, Grimshaw Lane, Bollington, Cheshire SK10 5JB, UK*
[2] *Roche Products Ltd., Hexagon Place, 6 Falcon Way, Welwyn Garden City, Hertfordshire AL7 1TW, UK*
[3] *305 Health & Human Development East, The Pennsylvania State University, University Park, PA 16802, USA*
[4] *F. Hoffmann La-Roche Ltd., Grenzacherstrasse 124, 4070 Basel, Switzerland*

Correspondence should be addressed to Adam Gater; adam.gater@adelphivalues.com

Academic Editor: Robin Emsley

Objectives. As a disease typified by early onset and chronic disease course, caring for a person with schizophrenia may have a significant impact on caregivers' lives. This study aimed to investigate the subjective experiences of caregivers of people with schizophrenia as a means of understanding "caregiver burden" in this population. *Methods.* Face-to-face qualitative interviews were conducted with a diverse sample of 19 US-English speaking caregivers of people with schizophrenia (who were at least moderately ill). Interview transcripts were analyzed using grounded theory methods and findings used to inform the development of a preliminary conceptual model outlining caregivers' experiences. *Results.* Findings support assertions that people with schizophrenia were largely dependent upon caregivers for the provision of care and caregivers subsequently reported lacking time for themselves and their other responsibilities (e.g., family and work). Caregiver burden frequently manifested as detriments in physical (e.g., fatigue, sickness) and emotional well-being (e.g., depression and anxiety). *Conclusions.* Caring for a person with schizophrenia has a significant impact on the lives of informal (unpaid) caregivers and alleviating caregiver burden is critical for managing individual and societal costs. Future research should concentrate on establishing reliable and valid means of assessing burden among caregivers of persons with schizophrenia to inform the development and evaluation of interventions for reducing this burden.

1. Introduction

Over the past 50 years, as evidenced by the closure of mental hospitals and advent of community-based care, there has been transition of care for schizophrenia patients from formal hospital-based healthcare systems to outpatient and community services. The financial burden (in terms of direct and indirect costs) of community-dwelling patients with schizophrenia is high with estimated annual costs in the US of $23 billion [1].

It is estimated that 50–90% of people with chronic psychiatric illness live with their families or friends [2, 3] and informal caregivers (i.e., *"a person who has significant responsibility for managing the well-being of a person diagnosed with schizophrenia in an unpaid capacity"*) [4] provide an important service by reducing need for formal care and burden upon healthcare systems [5]. This is true not just of schizophrenia but also of other medical conditions such as stroke [6], cancer [7] and dementia [8], with estimates in 2011 suggesting that the economic value of all informal caregivers' unpaid contributions in the US was $450 billion, having increased from $375 billion in 2007 [9, 10].

Caregiving responsibilities can place a burden on caregivers' daily lives, physical health, and emotional well-being [11–37]. High levels of caregiver burden can have considerable consequences for patients and wider society as a whole as well as for caregivers themselves. For instance, should the impact on the caregiver become too great, then there could be consequences on the delivery of care to patients, an increase in unmet needs of overburdened caregivers [38], and an increasing reliance on formal, paid assistance [39, 40] resulting in costs to healthcare systems and wider society. In addition, caregiving has significant impact on informal caregivers' own physical and psychological health [13]. Alleviating caregiver burden, therefore, is now recognized as a key outcome for healthcare interventions (pharmacological and psychosocial) designed to manage schizophrenia.

Caregiver burden is a complex construct with two distinct components: "objective burden" which refers to the tangible impact of caregiving on a caregiver's life (e.g., financial loss and time lost from daily activities) and "subjective burden" which refers to the caregiver's perception of burden of care [39]. Objective burden may be assessed by a variety of means but subjective burden can only be known by caregivers themselves and it is important that such reports come directly from caregivers themselves. In order to monitor caregiver burden, there is therefore a need for accurate and reliable self-report measures of the impact of caring for a person with schizophrenia. These measures would be important in understanding the impact on caregivers, identifying those caregivers at risk of significant health, social, and financial impacts, and evaluating the efficacy of interventions designed to reduce, alleviate, or protect against caregiver burden.

Although existing measures of caregiver burden have previously been used in schizophrenia, there is little evidence that the content validity of these measures in this population has been confirmed in line with well-established guidelines for the development and evaluation of self-report measures [41]. Consistent with these guidelines, there is a need to understand representation of caregiver burden from caregivers themselves. Although previous research has highlighted the impact of caring for a person with schizophrenia on all aspects of a caregiver's life [42], no studies have thus far developed a conceptual model, which defines the concepts of interest [43, 44], outlining the subjective experiences of caring for a person with schizophrenia. In addition, prior research has identified a number of factors which may impact the subjective burden experienced by caregivers. For example, there is evidence to suggest that

(i) specific clusters of schizophrenia symptoms may have a differential impact on caregiver burden [11, 45, 46] and high levels of symptomology have a significant impact on caregiver burden [47–50];

(ii) there are differences in the concept of caregiver burden in terms of ethnicity (with white caregivers more likely to report high levels of caregiver burden than African Americans) [42, 51, 52];

(iii) the gender of the person receiving the care (males with schizophrenia are more frequently associated with high levels of caregiver burden) [47, 53] and the person providing the care (female caregivers experiencing higher levels of burden than male caregivers) [11, 54] can influence caregiver burden;

(iv) the caregiver relationship to the person with schizophrenia (e.g., mother-daughter and father-daughter) and living situation (living with person or not) can affect the degree of caregiver burden [55];

(v) age of the person receiving care [56, 57] and age of the caregiver [58] may both have an independent effect on reported rates of caregiver burden (studies suggesting that younger people with schizophrenia and older caregivers experience higher levels of burden);

(vi) educational attainment may predict levels of caregiver burden, with those of lower educational backgrounds experiencing higher levels of caregiver burden [59].

The aims of the present study are to investigate, via qualitative interviews, the subjective experiences of informal caregivers of people with schizophrenia and to develop a preliminary conceptual model outlining the impact of caregiving on their daily lives.

2. Methods

2.1. Study Design. Face-to-face, open-ended, semi-structured, qualitative interviews were performed with 19 English speaking informal caregivers of people with a clinician confirmed diagnosis of schizophrenia in the US. Caregivers were identified for inclusion following referrals from patients of private clinicians. Clinicians first identified people with schizophrenia and determined their eligibility for participation in the study.

People with schizophrenia were aged 18 and above and were required to have been diagnosed according to the Diagnostic and Statistical Manual of Mental Disorders, IV, Third Revision (DSM-IV-TR) criteria, to be at least moderately ill (as defined by a Clinical Global Impression of Severity (CGI-S) score ≥4) and currently to be receiving a marketed atypical or typical antipsychotic. To be eligible for participation, people with schizophrenia were also required to be in receipt of care from an informal caregiver. People with schizophrenia were excluded if they had any other DSM-IV-TR Axis I diagnoses, alcohol, or substance dependence within 12 months or abuse within 3 months (with the exception of nicotine) or if they had dementia, delirium, or other amnestic disorder per DSM-IV-TR. They were also excluded if they had a diagnosis of mental retardation/severe organic brain syndromes/a prior or current general medical condition that may be impairing cognition or other neuropsychiatric functioning.

Once eligibility had been confirmed, the informal caregivers of people with schizophrenia were approached to take part in the study. To be eligible for participation, the caregivers had to be aged at least 18 years of age and currently providing care to the person with schizophrenia for at least 4 hours per week. Caregivers themselves were excluded from the study if they were judged by the recruiting physician to have severe neurological or cognitive deficits or an uncontrolled psychiatric condition that might affect their ability to participate in the interview.

Participants were recruited from three sites in the US to avoid geographical bias: Philadelphia (eastern US), Chicago (central US), and New Orleans (southern US). To ensure recruitment of a representative sample of schizophrenia caregivers, a series of recruitment targets were employed including the following.

(i) Schizophrenia subtype: at least two caregivers of people with each DSM-IV schizophrenia subtype.

(ii) Schizophrenia severity: at least five caregivers of people with schizophrenia that have CGI-S scores of 4, 5, and 6.

(iii) Gender: at least four males and at least four female caregivers of people with schizophrenia.

(iv) Relationship to person with schizophrenia: By gender: at least six gender-matched (e.g., daughter-mother, sister-sister) caregivers and at least six gender mismatched (e.g., daughter-father, husband-wife, son-mother, siblings, friends) caregivers. By living situation: at least 6 family members living with person with schizophrenia.

(v) Age: at least six caregivers under 60 years old and at least six caregivers 60 years and older.

(vi) Education: at least 20% of caregivers with high school as their highest level of education.

2.2. Ethics. The study was conducted in accordance with the Declaration of Helsinki and was approved by Copernicus Group, a centralized Institutional Review Board (IRB) in the US (IRB number: ADE2-12-035). Study procedures ensured that written informed consent was obtained from both people with schizophrenia and their caregivers prior to the collection of any data. Any data collected was anonymously stored in a computer database, maintaining confidentiality in accordance with national data legislation.

2.3. Interview Procedure. Each participant took part in a single one-hour interview. All interviews were conducted by a trained interviewer using a semistructured interview guide. This was informed by consideration of existing literature concerning the impact of caring for someone with schizophrenia or other mental health conditions. Initial questions were open-ended and designed to elicit spontaneous discussion concerning each caregiver's experience of providing care to someone with schizophrenia (e.g., "Tell me about your experience of caring for a person with schizophrenia"). Following these broad questions, more direct questions were used to elicit feedback on particular topics of interest, as identified within the existing research literature (e.g., "In what ways does caring for a person with schizophrenia affect you emotionally?"). Throughout this process, care was taken to avoid the use of leading questions, in order to ensure that caregivers' responses were reflective of their experiences and free from external bias. An enabling exercise was also used to facilitate spontaneous reporting of concepts whereby caregivers were asked to put together a collage representing their experiences of caregiving which they would take to the interview and discuss with the interviewer.

2.4. Analysis. All interviews were audio-taped and transcribed verbatim for the purpose of qualitative analysis. Written interview transcripts were then entered into a qualitative software package (Atlas. Ti) [60] which was used to facilitate the analysis of interview content.

Transcripts were analyzed using a grounded theory approach whereby sections of transcripts from individual participants (i.e., quotes) were assigned codes reflective of underlying concepts [61, 62]. In this approach, the meanings of concepts are discovered via the words and actions of participants from the ground up, rather than from application of a priori theory or understanding [63]. This is particularly useful where, as here, the intention is to build an overall picture of participants' experiences to inform development of a preliminary conceptual model. Analysis was performed by two primary researchers and the code list, which was driven by patient quotes, was regularly reviewed and agreed among the wider research team.

There exist no definitive guidelines regarding recommended sample sizes for qualitative studies and available guidance actually states that the number of participants is not as critical as interview quality, with sample size depending on the completeness of information obtained from the analysis of interview transcripts [41]. That the concepts elicited by caregivers had been fully explored during the interviews was assessed by confirmation of conceptual saturation, defined as the point at which no new relevant or important information emerges with the collection of more data [41, 61, 64]. During analysis, spontaneously reported concepts were therefore differentiated from those which caregivers discussed when prompted, allowing for assessment of conceptual saturation. Recent investigations suggest conceptual saturation is typically achieved in sample sizes of 12-13 [64, 65]. Although the primary purpose of qualitative research is not to assess concept frequency, a count of the number of caregivers who mentioned a given concept at least once during an interview was recorded during the process of analysis in order to provide an indicator of the relative importance of each concept within the study sample.

3. Results

3.1. Demographic and Clinical Characteristics. Although it is recognized that future qualitative research involving people with schizophrenia may increasingly focus on positive and negative symptoms as a means of differentiation, the current study ensured that a diverse sample of people with schizophrenia and their caregivers was recruited. The average age of the people with schizophrenia was 51.8 years (21–82) and 12 (63%) of the sample were females. People with schizophrenia had been diagnosed for an average of 16 years and were diagnosed with paranoid (n = 10, 53%), disorganized (n = 4, 21%), undifferentiated (n = 2, 11%), catatonic (n = 2, 11%), and paranoid plus disorganized (n = 1, 5%) DSM-IV-TR subtypes of schizophrenia. People had varying severities of schizophrenia but as per the inclusion criteria were at least moderately ill, with 14 people with schizophrenia (74%) having a CGI-S score of 4-5 and 5 (26%) having a CGI-S score of 6-7 [47–50].

The average age of caregivers was 51.6 years and caregivers were predominantly female (79%), which is consistent with previous research in samples of people with schizophrenia

[24, 66]. The sample of caregivers included representation of Black/African American, White, and Hispanic/Latino caregivers and, of the total sample, 63% of the caregiver-person with schizophrenia dyads were gender matched. Summaries of the demographic characteristics for the people with schizophrenia and their caregivers recruited into the study are provided in Tables 1 and 2 respectively. Relevant clinical characteristics for the people with schizophrenia are also included in Table 1.

3.2. Enabling Exercise. Creative collage tasks can be useful enabling exercises to encourage elicitation of relevant concepts from participants in qualitative research [67]. Prior to the interview, caregivers were asked to create a collage representing their experiences of caring for a person with schizophrenia, which was to be used to facilitate discussions during the interview. All 19 caregivers completed this exercise. Individual collages all made reference to multiple concepts, many of which are discussed below. Select examples of collages prepared by caregivers alongside feedback from caregivers during the interview are provided in Figures 1, 2, and 3.

3.3. The Experience of Caring for a Person with Schizophrenia

3.3.1. Summary of Interview Findings. Findings from interviews with caregivers in this study suggest that "caregiver burden" can be understood in terms of 6 key dimensions: emotional well-being, caregiver concerns, physical impact, impact on daily activities, financial demands, and impact on relationships. Furthermore, study participants also reported that caring for a person with schizophrenia can have a positive impact on their lives.

Based on feedback from caregivers, a preliminary conceptual model was developed to outline and visualize the experiences of caregivers of people with schizophrenia, see Figure 4.

To confirm conceptual saturation in this population, a process of comparative analysis was used, in which concepts emerging from interviews 1–7 (Round 1) were compared to those emerging from interviews 8–13 (Round 2) and then 14–19 (Round 3). Very little new information emerged as data collection neared completion; 32/34 concepts (94%) relating to caregiver burden were elicited during the first 7 interviews, with only one new concept elicited during both Round 2 and Round 3 (financial dependence on caregiver). Findings therefore suggest that conceptual saturation in the present sample was achieved. The concepts most frequently reported by participants concerned the impact of caregiving on the caregivers' emotional state (i.e., feeling "emotional", $n = 14$), the inconsistent and unpredictable nature of the person's schizophrenia ($n = 12$), the negative impact of caregiving on caregivers' relationships with other family members and friends ($n = 11$), and the impact of caregiving on caregivers' ability to work ($n = 10$).

3.3.2. Emotional Impact. The most frequently reported impact of caring for a person with schizophrenia was feeling "emotional" which was reported by 14 (74%) of the caregivers. In addition, caregivers reported the specific emotions they experienced as a result of their role and incorporated a number of these into the enabling exercise. Caring for a person with schizophrenia was described as demanding by caregivers, leading them to feel overwhelmed ($n = 6$). Caregivers also reported that the role made them feel sad ($n = 8$). Feelings of sadness related to the caregivers themselves, the person with schizophrenia, or the feeling that they could not help the person with schizophrenia (e.g., by convincing

Table 1: Persons with schizophrenia and demographic and clinical characteristics ($n = 19$).

Demographic characteristic	Person with schizophrenia ($n = 19$)
Age	
Mean (range)	51.84 (21–82)
Gender *n* (%)	
Male	7 (37)
Female	12 (63)
Ethnicity *n* (%)	
Black/African American	12 (63)
Hispanic/Spanish American/Latin (of any race)	1 (5)
White/Caucasian	6 (32)
Years since diagnosis	
Mean (range)	16 (3–42)
Schizophrenia subtype *n* (%)	
Paranoid	10 (53)
Disorganised	4 (21)
Undifferentiated	2 (11)
Catatonic	2 (11)
Paranoid, disorganized	1 (5)
Schizophrenia severity *n* (%)	
CGI-S score 4	9 (47)
CGI-S score 5	5 (26)
CGI-S score 6	5 (26)
Medication *n* (%)	
Typical antipsychotics	
Haloperidol	5 (26)
Chlorpromazine	3 (16)
Atypical antipsychotics	11 (58)
Aripiprazole	4 (21)
Risperidone	5 (26)
Olanzapine	3 (16)
Quetiapine	0 (0)
Olanzapine/fluoxetine	1 (5)
Ziprasidone	2 (11)
Other	6 (32)
People with schizophrenia on both typical and atypical treatments	5 (26)

Table 2: Caregiver demographic characteristics (n = 19).

Demographic characteristic	Caregivers (n = 19)
Age	
Mean (range)	51.63 (28–69)
Gender n (%)	
Male	4 (21)
Female	15 (79)
Ethnicity n (%)	
Black/African American	11 (58)
Hispanic/Spanish American/Latin (of any race)	2 (11)
White/Caucasian	6 (32)
Relationship with person with schizophrenia n (%)	
Parent	6 (32)
Partner/spouse	2 (11)
Sibling	6 (32)
Son/daughter	3 (16)
Other (nephew, aunt)	2 (11)
Education n (%)	
High school diploma	7 (37)
College or university degree	5 (26)
Graduate or professional degree	5 (26)
Some years of college	2 (11)
Work status n (%)	
Working full or part time	12 (63)
Full time homemaker	3 (16)
Not working	1 (5)
Retired	2 (11)
Other	1 (5)
Coresidence n (%)	
Yes	15 (78.9%)
No	4 (21.1%)
Years spent caring for person with schizophrenia n (%)	
Mean (range)	10.24 (1–32)
Hours per week spent caring for person with schizophrenia n (%)	
<20	1 (5)
21–40	7 (37)
40+	11 (58)
Range	14–168
Mean	86.33
Gender match n (%)	
Yes	
Female	10 (53)
Male	2 (11)
No	7 (37)

them that delusions were not real). Caregivers said that some emotions were experienced as a result of the person with schizophrenia's behavior; these included frustration (n = 9), embarrassment (n = 3), anger (n = 3), and stress (n = 2).

The emotions experienced by caregivers were often changeable and unpredictable *"Emotionally, it's a roller-coaster"* (318-M-55-P), and when discussed in further details, caregivers reported that the unpredictable nature of the person with schizophrenia's behavior was often the reason for them feeling stressed, anxious, and worried (n = 12). Caregivers often used analogies to describe their changeable emotions, sometimes as part of their enabling exercise: *"White-water rafting. It's like - that's how I feel. Like, I'm going up and down with the whole deal. Yeah. You know, like bumps"* (106-F-52-D). Caregivers also used analogies to describe the unpredictability of the person with schizophrenia's behavior: *"I feel like I'm underwater - and he's the shark all the time. I never know whether or not he's a friendly shark, or he is going to bite me. And I'm not in a cage, so I'm really, literally, feeling as though, you know, its danger lurking all the time."* (105-F-46-P).

3.3.3. Caregiver Concerns. Caregivers reported a number of specific concerns relating to their role; they were afraid of what the future holds in terms of the person with schizophrenia's care (n = 4), worried about the person with schizophrenia having an "episode" (n = 5), and worried that the person with schizophrenia's symptoms would get worse (n = 3).

3.3.4. Impact on Daily Activities. The main impact of caring for a person with schizophrenia on participants' daily activities was the lack of time, both for themselves (n = 8) and for their other responsibilities (n = 8): *"Um, I do not have much of a life anymore. So between running around for the kids and caring for my mother, there's not much time for anything else."* (103-F-38-P). Caregivers spoke about having to cancel plans (n = 1) and not being able to spend time with other family members (n = 4). They also felt that they had lost control of their lives which now centered around the person with schizophrenia (n = 2): *"In the know means you have to always be - have knowledge about the situation - the medication - her life, where she is going, what doctor appointments. You cannot just - just forget about anything."* (104-F-48-D).

Caregivers felt that people with schizophrenia were dependent on them for help with numerous aspects of their lives (n = 5). They were relied upon to take the person with schizophrenia to appointments (n = 3), remind the person with schizophrenia about their personal hygiene (n = 2), take medication (n = 6), and even to eat (n = 1). They found their role difficult (n = 3) and felt uncertain about the best way to fulfill it (n = 3). One caregiver said that he felt he was not able to care for the person with schizophrenia as well as he would have liked: *"So the challenge is we're not specific in that aspect. It's myself, lady friend - sometimes my son, brother. There's a neighbor. But there is not that specificity, you know, therapist on - on, uh, site. People that can deal with it. Uh, even maintenance people."* (102-M-40-C). Many caregivers

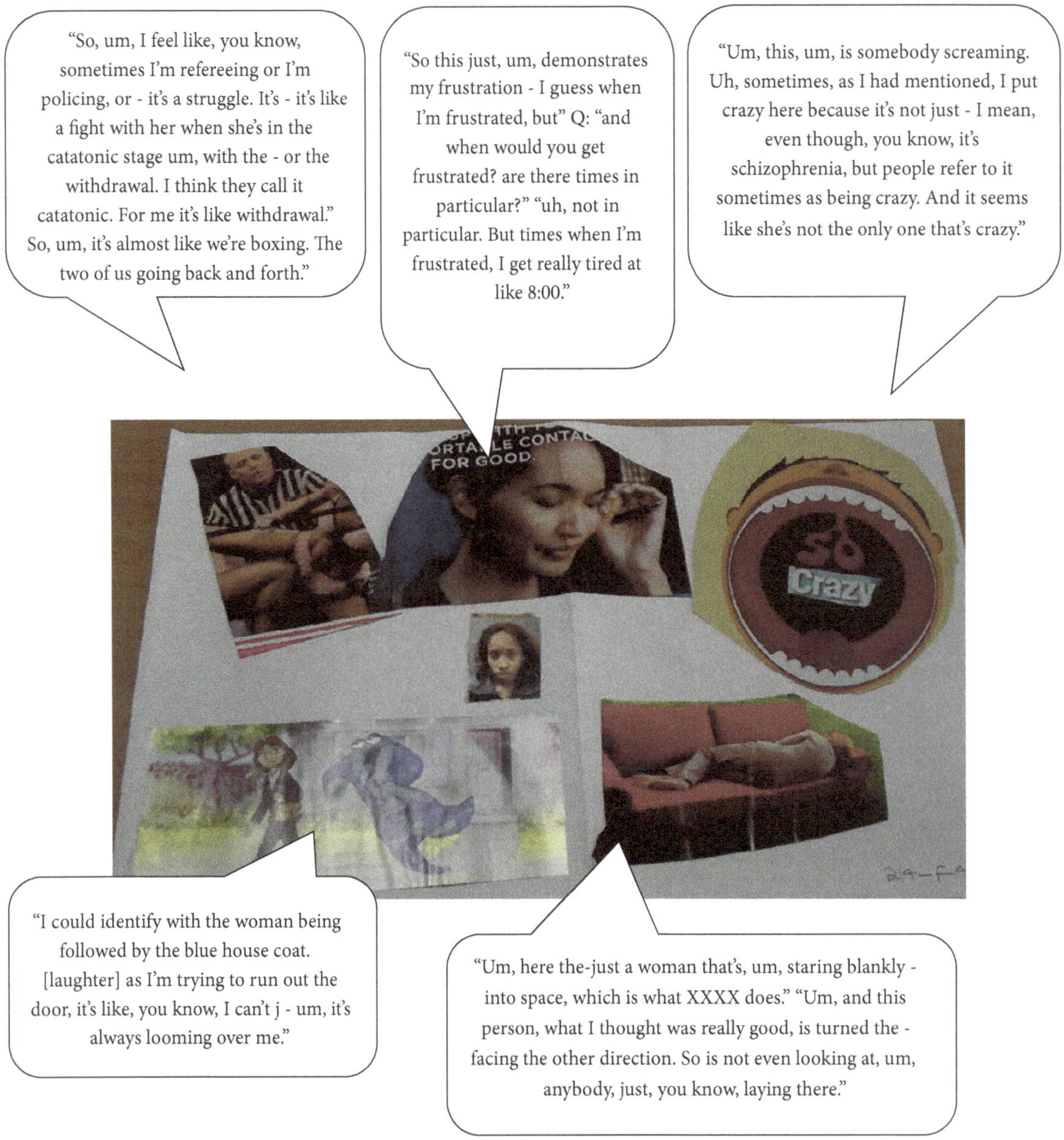
"So, um, I feel like, you know, sometimes I'm refereeing or I'm policing, or - it's a struggle. It's - it's like a fight with her when she's in the catatonic stage um, with the - or the withdrawal. I think they call it catatonic. For me it's like withdrawal." So, um, it's almost like we're boxing. The two of us going back and forth."
"So this just, um, demonstrates my frustration - I guess when I'm frustrated, but" Q: "and when would you get frustrated? are there times in particular?" "uh, not in particular. But times when I'm frustrated, I get really tired at like 8:00."
"Um, this, um, is somebody screaming. Uh, sometimes, as I had mentioned, I put crazy here because it's not just - I mean, even though, you know, it's schizophrenia, but people refer to it sometimes as being crazy. And it seems like she's not the only one that's crazy."
FOR GOOD.
So
Crazy
"I could identify with the woman being followed by the blue house coat. [laughter] as I'm trying to run out the door, it's like, you know, I can't j - um, it's always looming over me."
"Um, here the-just a woman that's, um, staring blankly - into space, which is what XXXX does." "Um, and this person, what I thought was really good, is turned the - facing the other direction. So is not even looking at, um, anybody, just, you know, laying there."

FIGURE 1: Caregiver ID: 214-F-48-C.

included their caregiving responsibilities into the enabling exercise, such as ensuring the person with schizophrenia took their medicine ($n = 9$) and having to take them to the doctors ($n = 2$).

Despite caregivers often having large families, they sometimes felt alone in caring for the person with schizophrenia ($n = 3$) and other family members and friends would not help out as much as the caregiver would have liked: *"I'm the only one that - that - that does it now. That actually cares. Because of - because of that disease - it has pushed my siblings, relatives away because they just do not know how to handle it, per se."* (318-M-55-P).

3.3.5. Physical Impact. Caring for a person with schizophrenia affected caregivers' physical health ($n = 9$) as it left them feeling tired ($n = 5$), worn out ($n = 2$), drained ($n = 3$), and stressed ($n = 2$). Interestingly, the only physical impacts to emerge from the enabling exercise were tiredness and stress. In some cases the additional burden of being a caregiver exacerbated their existing problems: *"Um, so yeah, it did affect me physically. And I remember one time the doctor, the gastroenterologist, said to me if you do not divorce him, your stomach will never be OK."* (109-F-69-P). In addition to this, some caregivers talked about disturbed sleep due to the person with schizophrenia's behavior and having to continue their caregiving role through the night ($n = 2$). *"If she's already in an episode - I might not be able to sleep thoroughly. I might have to stay up with her for hours - on end at times."* (212-M-39-P).

Caregivers also felt that the emotional impacts of worry, anxiety, and stress affected them physically ($n = 3$). The physical demands of caregiving meant one caregiver felt

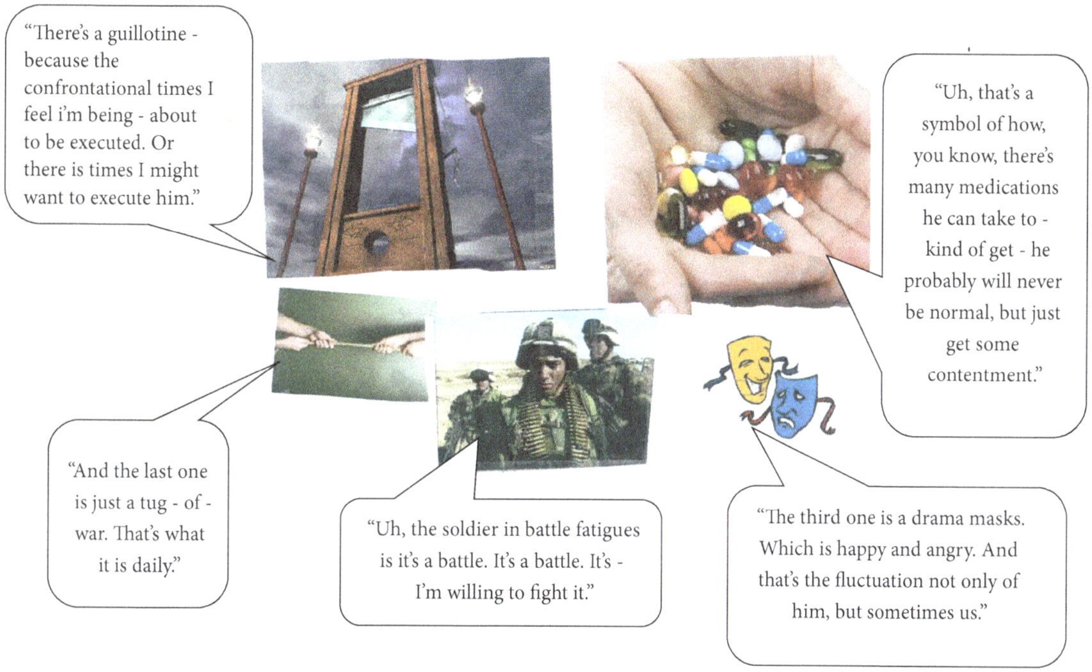

Figure 2: Caregiver ID: 102-M-40-C.

she wouldn't be able to continue caring for the person with schizophrenia for much longer.

3.3.6. Financial Impact/Impact on Employment. The person with schizophrenia was often described as being dependent on the caregiver for financial support ($n = 6$) and one of the main financial demands for caregivers was the cost of medication ($n = 3$). *"Well, financially, because, um, sometimes we need people to, uh, to stay with her, to watch her, you know, medical bills for certain things at times."* (212-M-39-P).

As a result of this financial dependence, some caregivers said that they did not have enough money to care for the person with schizophrenia in addition to the rest of their expenses ($n = 6$). They saw the money spent on caregiving as a sacrifice ($n = 1$) and were spending their own savings ($n = 2$). A contributing factor to the financial difficulties faced by caregivers was the impact of their role on their work ($n = 10$). Caregivers either had to give up work ($n = 3$), change the way that they worked, or change their profession ($n = 3$). Of those caregivers that remained at work, their role still interfered with their working life as they would get disturbed at work by the person with schizophrenia, or suffered from a lack of sleep ($n = 3$). For caregivers who had given up work, it sometimes meant that others had to increase their work load to compensate ($n = 1$). *"I cannot go to work. So financially, it has put a burden. My husband had to take a - second job because - to - to supplement my income and it still is not supplementing it."* (103-F-38-P).

3.3.7. Impact on Relationships with Others. The caregivers' relationship with the person with schizophrenia often had an impact on their relationships with other family members and friends in a negative way ($n = 11$). Caregivers saw less of their children than they would have liked ($n = 3$) and noticed strain in their marriage ($n = 2$). *"It affects me where I do not have as much time. Like, my - both of my kids are athletes, so it's not like I have as much time to do their games."* (106-F-52-D).

Outside of family life, caregiver social life was also affected ($n = 7$); caregivers had to give up their previous social life ($n = 2$) and felt they had to stay in or near the house ($n = 2$). In addition to this, they felt uncomfortable about having friends over to see them ($n = 2$) because they did not want their friends to witness the person with schizophrenia's behavior. *"Um, well, it's kind of affected my social life a lot. Um, I do not have friends that come over too much anymore since she's been living with me now."* (211-F-59-D).

3.3.8. Impact on Relationship with Person with Schizophrenia. In the enabling exercise, some caregivers described their role as a fight or battle with the person with schizophrenia ($n = 4$): *"I mean, it's just a battle sometimes to get her to get dressed, take a shower, take her medicine, to eat. It's just a battle."* (211-F-59-D). However others said that they worked with the person with schizophrenia as a team ($n = 3$): *"I chose this one because it takes teamwork to - to climb this mountain. And without teamwork, you know, they - they - they - they wouldn't have been successful. So that's what I find, that he and I, we are a team. We are a team."* (315-F-59-D). Caregivers also described trying to understand what the person with schizophrenia is going through as a puzzle or maze ($n = 2$): *"I try to s - you know, try to feel what she's feeling. So - and you know, if I cannot - I cannot understand it, I cannot get it, it's a maze to me."* (212-M-39-P).

3.3.9. Positive Impacts. Despite the high levels of burden associated with caring for a person with schizophrenia, 17

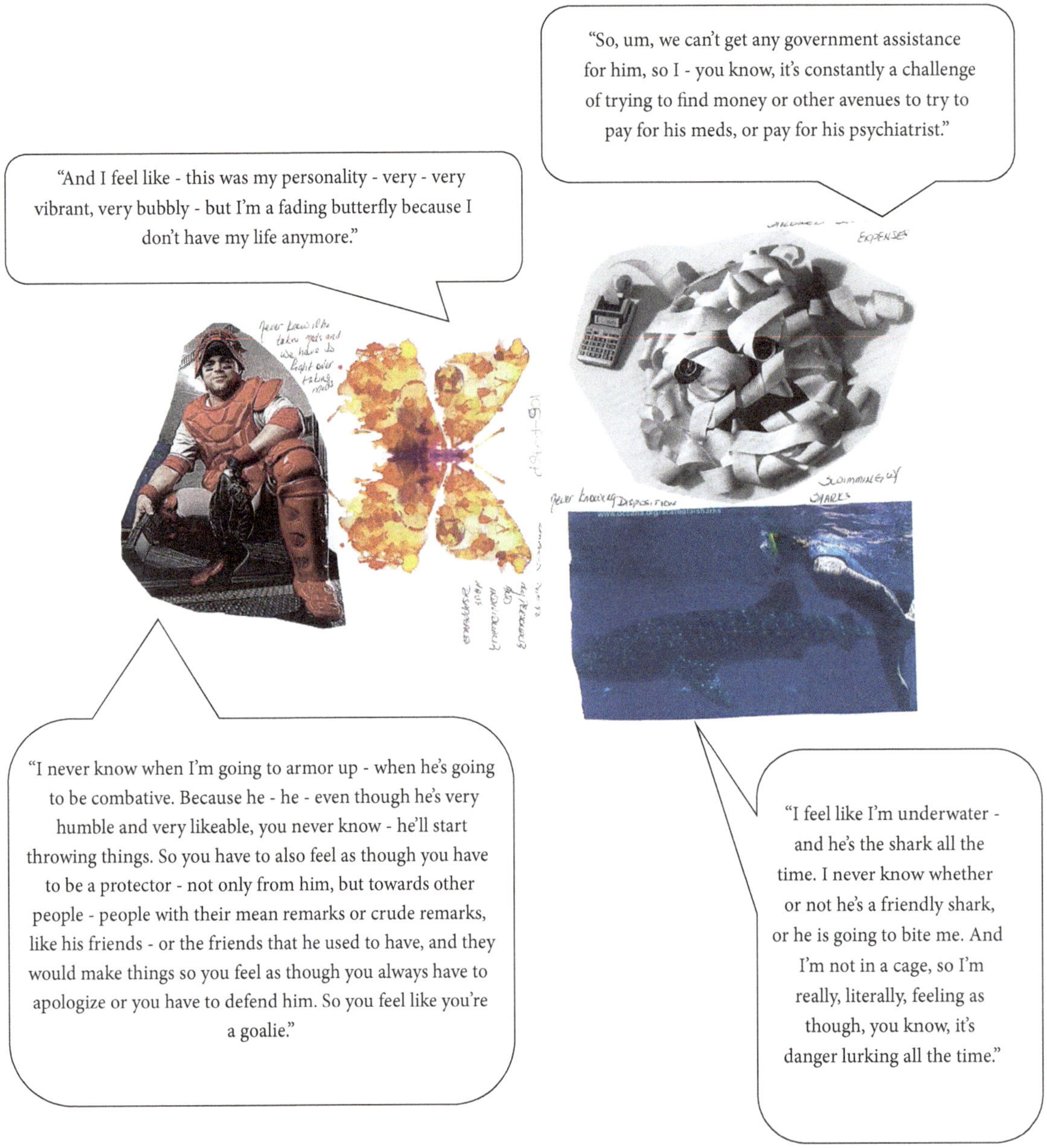

FIGURE 3: Caregiver ID: 105-F-46-P.

caregivers also spoke about the positive aspects of their role. The most commonly reported benefit was the love that the caregiver shared with the person with schizophrenia ($n = 9$): *"Right. And then I have a heart because I love her. And I probably love her even more now."* (104-F-48-D).

Other benefits included being able to care for the person with schizophrenia and notice problems ($n = 3$), ensuring the person with schizophrenia was safe and being cared for ($n = 3$), and understanding what the person with schizophrenia was going through ($n = 6$). Caregivers also felt they had a higher level of patience ($n = 9$), were a "better person" ($n = 1$), had grown as a person ($n = 2$), and felt reward and satisfaction ($n = 4$): *"Uh, the benefits? Patience. The patience and the love you have you know. Those are the most important."* (108-M-50-D); *"- but I think, for me, like I said, it's - it's helped me develop more as a person."* (213-F-38-P).

Some caregivers also said that they enjoyed having the person with schizophrenia at home, had fun with them, and saw them as a companion.

4. Discussion

Caring for a person with schizophrenia was found to have significant implications for caregivers' perceived physical and emotional well-being and these findings are consistent with those from prior qualitative investigations in informal caregivers of schizophrenia patients [14–37]. Thus, findings from

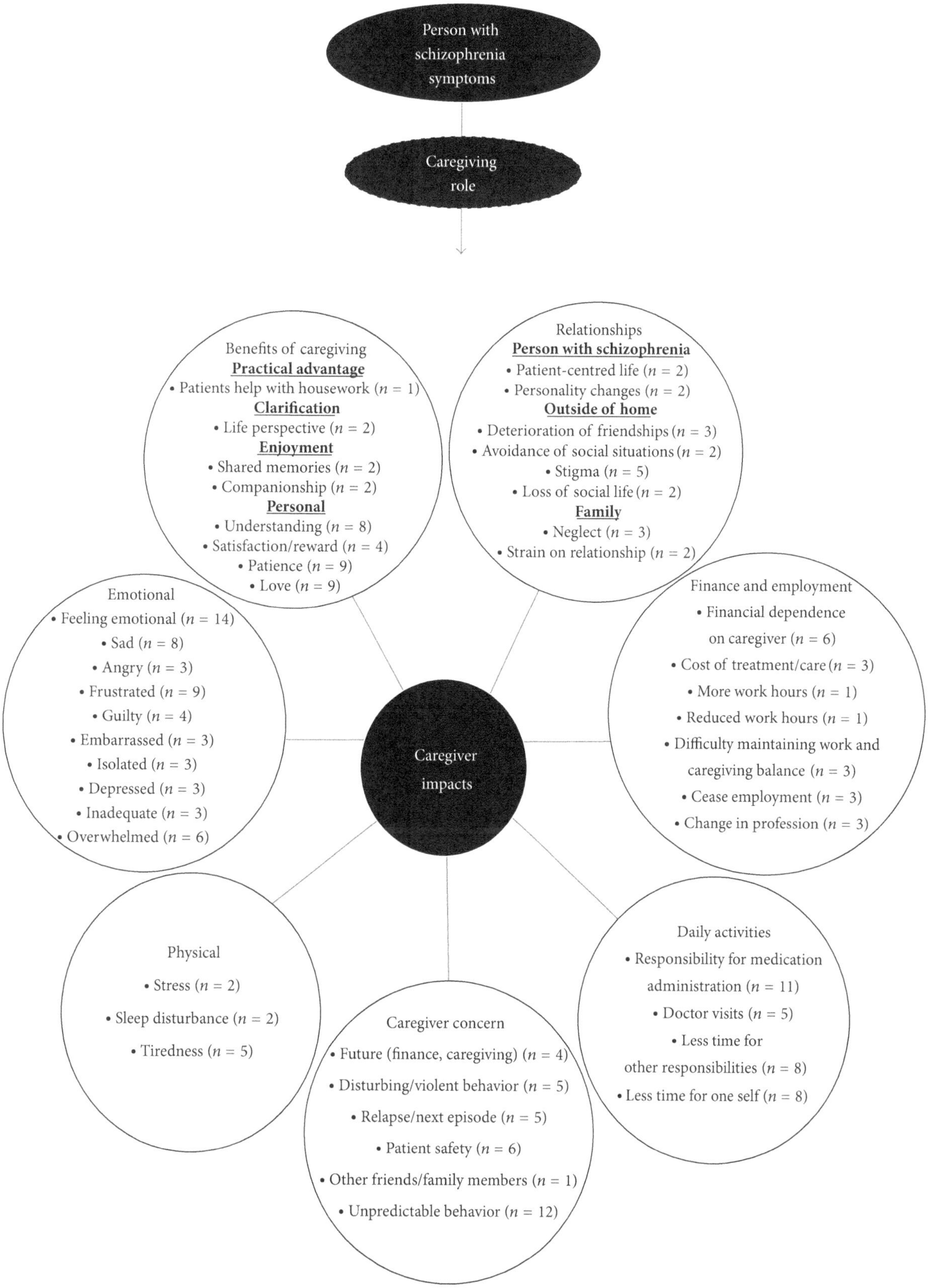

Figure 4: Preliminary conceptual model of caregiver experiences of providing care for a person with schizophrenia. Note: numbers refer to the number of caregivers who discussed each concept and for whom this concept was relevant. This preliminary conceptual model does not seek to convey the strength, direction, or nature of relationships between concepts and domains. This is to be the subject of future research.

the current study serve to highlight the burden and unmet needs among caregivers of persons with schizophrenia.

The preliminary conceptual model which was developed to outline the experiences of caregivers of people with schizophrenia, as informed by qualitative findings, demonstrates that the caregiving role has a significant impact on numerous facets of caregivers' lives. In addition to identifying potential measurement concepts, such models may also inform decisions regarding how best to measure these concepts in research studies and help to contextualise findings from studies in this area [43]. A limitation of this preliminary model is that, in seeking to provide a rich and comprehensive understanding of the concepts of relevance to caregivers of people with schizophrenia using qualitative evidence, we were not able to confirm the influence of moderating factors and draw generalizable conclusions regarding interrelationships between concepts. Qualitative research is often used in psychiatry to provide a broader and more thorough understanding of the patient or caregiver experience; however, statistically confirmed, quantitative methods are required to investigate concepts and their interrelationships in more details [68]. Future research, including larger quantitative studies, may be used to validate the model and could provide further insight into how concepts relate to each other and how moderating variables affect the strength and direction of these relationships.

A diverse sample of caregivers of people with schizophrenia was interviewed as part of this study. This included caregivers of people with different subtypes of schizophrenia as determined by the DSM-IV. While this subtype classification has since been discontinued in the DSM-V, this criterion (alongside targets for clinically defined severity) offers assurances that the views of caregivers of a clinically diverse population were considered.

4.1. Implications. These findings reiterate the need for strategies to reduce caregiver burden in informal caregivers of persons with schizophrenia. This is in accordance with recent health initiatives, which highlight the need to prioritize the mitigation of caregiver burden and implement strategies into real-world practice (e.g., Centers for Disease Control and Prevention) [69].

Feedback from study participants indicates that caregiver burden may vary according to certain caregiver and patient characteristics; for example, feedback from participants suggested that the concept of caregiver "burden" was less relevant among Black-African American caregivers than among White caregivers. This appeared to be largely due to a strong focus on faith and religion: *"You have to take these things. If you have a belief in God, you have to take that system - and employ it in this situation... Whatever God you serve"* (318-M-55-P). Similarly, differences according to the age of the caregiver and relationship to the person with schizophrenia were noted. Such findings are consistent with previous investigations among schizophrenia caregivers which found that a number of external factors contribute to the level of caregiver burden experienced and therefore highlight the potential need for individually tailored interventions [11, 42, 45–53, 59, 70]. Findings, however, should be interpreted with caution due to the small sample sizes in the current study. Further exploration of differences among subsets of caregivers of people with schizophrenia within larger quantitative studies should be an avenue for future research.

These findings highlight the need for assessment of the impact on caregivers, in addition to patient-centered outcomes, in both clinical practice and clinical research. In clinical practice, routine assessment of impact on caregivers could serve to identify those caregivers most at risk of ill health as a result of providing care for a person with schizophrenia. Such information could be used to inform of the development and evaluation of individually tailored solutions designed to alleviate caregiver burden. This study suggests that caregiver burden is closely linked to symptom manifestation in the person with schizophrenia: Q: *"- are there any that impact you more or less than others?"* 109-F-69-P: *"Yeah. When he gets abusive to me."* Assessments of caregiver burden as an exploratory endpoint in clinical trials could therefore potentially serve as an additional means of evaluating improvement in person with schizophrenia functionality (e.g., independence) and the development and evaluation of interventions (e.g., support networks).

Although such outcomes are unlikely to support product labeling claims and indications for novel pharmacological therapies, this information is important for communicating the wider benefit of treatments to patients/caregivers, payers, and prescribers. Health Technology Assessment (HTA) agencies increasingly require that patient relevant endpoints such as global and functional outcomes (readiness for discharge and readiness for work), quality of life, patient satisfaction, family burden, and resource utilization should be included in schizophrenia trials. The National Institute for Health and Care Excellence (NICE) HTA Guidance for schizophrenia, for example [71], emphasizes the need for assessment of caregiver burden and provision of adequate support to caregivers; highlighting that information regarding caregiver burden potentially has an important role to play in pricing and reimbursement decisions. Caregiver burden, therefore, may serve as a key indicator of treatment value, particularly in markets (e.g., UK) where decisions must be made regarding the most efficient allocation of finite healthcare resources.

4.1.1. Current Challenges Associated with the Assessment of Caregiver Burden. There are a number of self-report instruments available to measure caregiver burden; however, none has been evaluated in accordance with current guidance for self-report measures [72]. It is important that any instrument assessing burden among caregivers of persons with schizophrenia assesses those particular issues of relevance and importance to such caregivers and demonstrates reliability and validity of assessment of caregiver burden in this population. Combined with existing qualitative research, findings from the current study could serve to inform modifications to existing measures or development of new measures of caregiver burden in persons with schizophrenia. Assessing quality of life in caregivers of people with schizophrenia could also inform assessment of utility which may have a direct influence of the cost-effectiveness analysis for schizophrenia interventions. This is increasingly important as HTA agencies seek to consider information concerning societal burden when making decisions regarding access to new therapies.

5. Conclusions

Caring for a person with schizophrenia places significant impact on caregivers' lives, manifesting emotionally, physically, financially, in daily activities, and in relationships. This burden may vary according to numerous individual factors. Findings highlight the need for valid and reliable means of assessing burden among caregivers of persons with schizophrenia so as to inform of the development and evaluation of interventions (e.g., support networks) for reducing caregiver burden.

Conflict of Interests

F. Hoffmann-La Roche Ltd. has commissioned Adelphi Values, a health outcomes agency. AG, LA, CM, and CT have no other competing interests to declare. DR and CB are both employees of F. Hoffmann-La Roche Ltd. Dr. Zarit is Distinguished Professor at Penn State University and has no competing interests.

Authors' Contribution

Diana Rofail and Carmen Berardo conceived the study. Diana Rofail, Carmen Berardo, Adam Gater, and Linda Abetz participated in the study design and provided scientific oversight for the conduct and analysis of interviews. Chloe Tolley and Chris Marshall conducted the interviews and primary data analysis. Professor Zarit and all authors were involved in the interpretation of research findings and developed the paper.

References

[1] P. R. Desai, K. A. Lawson, J. C. Barner, and K. L. Rascati, "Estimating the direct and indirect costs for community-dwelling patients with schizophrenia," *Journal of Pharmaceutical Health Services Research*, vol. 4, no. 4, pp. 187–194, 2013.

[2] W. Rössler, H. J. Salize, G. Cucchiaro, I. Reinhard, and C. Kernig, "Does the place of treatment influence the quality of life of schizophrenics?" *Acta Psychiatrica Scandinavica*, vol. 100, no. 2, pp. 142–148, 1999.

[3] T. Honkonen, S. Saarinen, and R. K. R. Salokangas, "Deinstitutionalization and schizophrenia in Finland II: discharged patients and their psychosocial functioning," *Schizophrenia Bulletin*, vol. 25, no. 3, pp. 543–551, 1999.

[4] Nevada Revised Statutes (NRS) 453A.080, 2012, http://definitions.uslegal.com/c/caregiver.

[5] P. S. Arno, C. Levine, and M. M. Memmott, "The economic value of informal caregiving," *Health Affairs*, vol. 18, no. 2, pp. 182–188, 1999.

[6] K. Salter, L. Zettler, N. Foley, and R. Teasell, "Impact of caring for individuals with stroke on perceived physical health of informal caregivers," *Disability & Rehabilitation*, vol. 32, no. 4, pp. 273–281, 2010.

[7] B. H. P. Osse, M. J. F. J. Vernooij-Dassen, E. Schadé, and R. P. T. M. Grol, "Problems experienced by the informal caregivers of cancer patients and their needs for support," *Cancer Nursing*, vol. 29, no. 5, pp. 378–388, 2006.

[8] P. G. Serrano-Aguilar, J. Lopez-Bastida, and V. Yanes-Lopez, "Impact on health-related quality of life and perceived burden of informal caregivers of individuals with Alzheimer's disease," *Neuroepidemiology*, vol. 27, no. 3, pp. 136–142, 2006.

[9] M. J. Gibson and A. Houser, "Valuing the invaluable: a new look at the economic value of family caregiving," *Issue Brief*, no. 82, pp. 1-12, 2007.

[10] L. Feinberg and S. C. Reinhard, *Valuing the Invaluable: 2011 Update the Growing Contributions and Costs of Family Caregiving*, 2011.

[11] D. G. Dyck, R. Short, and P. P. Vitaliano, "Predictors of burden and infectious illness in schizophrenia caregivers," *Psychosomatic Medicine*, vol. 61, no. 4, pp. 411–419, 1999.

[12] P. P. Vitaliano, J. Zhang, and J. M. Scanlan, "Is caregiving hazardous to one's physical health? A meta-analysis," *Psychological Bulletin*, vol. 129, no. 6, pp. 946–972, 2003.

[13] M. Pinquart and S. Sörensen, "Differences between caregivers and noncaregivers in psychological health and physical health: a meta-analysis," *Psychology and Aging*, vol. 18, no. 2, pp. 250–267, 2003.

[14] M. Birchwood and R. Cochrane, "Families coping with schizophrenia: coping styles, their origins and correlates," *Psychological Medicine*, vol. 20, no. 4, pp. 857–865, 1990.

[15] L. Y. Bogren, "Expressed emotion, family burden, and quality of life in parents with schizophrenic children," *Nordic Journal of Psychiatry*, vol. 51, no. 4, pp. 229–233, 1997.

[16] L. Chaffey and E. Fossey, "Caring and daily life: occupational experiences of women living with sons diagnosed with schizophrenia," *Australian Occupational Therapy Journal*, vol. 51, no. 4, pp. 199–207, 2004.

[17] F.-P. Chen and J. S. Greenberg, "A positive aspect of caregiving: the influence of social support on caregiving gains for family members of relatives with schizophrenia," *Community Mental Health Journal*, vol. 40, no. 5, pp. 423–435, 2004.

[18] C. A. Chesla, "Parents' caring practices with schizophrenic offspring," *Qualitative Health Research*, vol. 1, no. 446, 468 pages, 1991.

[19] J. Coldwell, S. Meddings, and P. M. Camic, "How people with psychosis positively contribute to their family: a grounded theory analysis," *Journal of Family Therapy*, vol. 33, no. 3, pp. 353–371, 2011.

[20] R. M. Friedrich, S. Lively, L. Rubenstein, and K. Buckwalter, "The Friedrich-Lively instrument to assess the impact of schizophrenia on siblings (FLIISS): part I—instrument construction," *Journal of Nursing Measurement*, vol. 10, no. 3, pp. 219–230, 2002.

[21] L. M. Gerace, D. Camilleri, and L. Ayres, "Sibling perspectives on schizophrenia and the family," *Schizophrenia Bulletin*, vol. 19, no. 3, pp. 637–647, 1993.

[22] P. B. Howard, "The experience of fathers of adult children with schizophrenia," *Issues in Mental Health Nursing*, vol. 19, no. 4, pp. 399–413, 1998.

[23] J. Jungbauer and M. C. Angermeyer, "Living with a schizophrenic patient: a comparative study of burden as it affects parents and spouses," *Psychiatry*, vol. 65, no. 2, pp. 110–123, 2002.

[24] J. Jungbauer, B. Wittmund, S. Dietrich, and M. C. Angermeyer, "Subjective burden over 12 months in parents of patients with

schizophrenia," *Archives of Psychiatric Nursing*, vol. 17, no. 3, pp. 126–134, 2003.

[25] J. Jungbauer, K. Stelling, S. Dietrich, and M. C. Angermeyer, "Schizophrenia: problems of separation in families," *Journal of Advanced Nursing*, vol. 47, no. 6, pp. 605–613, 2004.

[26] J. Jungbauer, B. Wittmund, S. Dietrich, and M. C. Angermeyer, "The disregarded caregivers: subjective burden in spouses of schizophrenia patients," *Schizophrenia Bulletin*, vol. 30, no. 3, pp. 665–675, 2004.

[27] D. L. Macinnes and J. P. Watson, "The differences in perceived burdens between forensic and non-forensic caregivers of individuals suffering from schizophrenia," *Journal of Mental Health*, vol. 11, no. 4, pp. 375–388, 2002.

[28] P. J. Milliken, "Disenfranchised mothers: caring for an adult child with schizophrenia," *Health Care for Woman International*, vol. 22, no. 1-2, pp. 149–166, 2001.

[29] H. Potasznik and G. Nelson, "Stress and social support: the burden experienced by the family of a mentally ill person," *American Journal of Community Psychology*, vol. 12, no. 5, pp. 589–607, 1984.

[30] T. Rudge and K. Morse, "Did anything change? Caregivers and schizophrenia after medication changes," *Journal of Psychiatric and Mental Health Nursing*, vol. 11, no. 1, pp. 3–11, 2004.

[31] K. A. Ryan, "Mothers of adult children with schizophrenia: an ethnographic study," *Schizophrenia Research*, vol. 11, no. 1, pp. 21–31, 1993.

[32] R. Schmid, T. Schielein, H. Binder, G. Hajak, and H. Spiessl, "The forgotten caregivers: siblings of schizophrenic patients," *International Journal of Psychiatry in Clinical Practice*, vol. 13, no. 4, pp. 326–337, 2009.

[33] G. Stålberg, H. Ekerwald, and C. M. Hultman, "At issue: siblings of patients with schizophrenia: sibling bond, coping patterns, and fear of possible schizophrenia heredity," *Schizophrenia Bulletin*, vol. 30, no. 2, pp. 445–458, 2004.

[34] I. Tuck, P. Du Mont, G. Evans, and J. Shupe, "The experience of caring for an adult child with schizophrenia," *Archives of Psychiatric Nursing*, vol. 11, no. 3, pp. 118–125, 1997.

[35] J. Wancata, M. Krautgartner, J. Berner et al., "The "Carers' needs assessment for Schizophrenia". An instrument to assess the needs of relatives caring for schizophrenia patients," *Social Psychiatry and Psychiatric Epidemiology*, vol. 41, no. 3, pp. 221–229, 2006.

[36] H. R. Winefield and E. J. Harvey, "Needs of family caregivers in chronic schizophrenia," *Schizophrenia Bulletin*, vol. 20, no. 3, pp. 557–566, 1994.

[37] C. H. Stein and V. A. Wemmerus, "Searching for a normal life: personal accounts of adults with schizophrenia, their parents and well-siblings," *American Journal of Community Psychology*, vol. 29, no. 5, pp. 725–746, 2001.

[38] J. A. Clausen and M. R. Yarrow, "The impact of mental illness on the family," *Journal of Social Issues*, vol. 11, no. 4, pp. 3–64, 1955.

[39] J. Hoenig and M. W. Hamilton, "The schizophrenic patient in the community and his effect on the household," *International Journal of Social Psychiatry*, vol. 12, no. 3, pp. 165–176, 1966.

[40] R. C. Dillehay and M. R. Sandys, "Caregivers for Alzheimer's patients: what we are learning from research," *International Journal of Aging and Human Development*, vol. 30, no. 4, pp. 263–285, 1990.

[41] FDA, *Guidance for Industry. Patient Reported Outcomes Measures: Use in Medical Product Development to Support Labeling Claims*, 2009.

[42] A. G. Awad and L. N. P. Voruganti, "The burden of schizophrenia on caregivers: a review," *Pharmacoeconomics*, vol. 26, no. 2, pp. 149–162, 2008.

[43] D. L. Patrick, L. B. Burke, C. J. Gwaltney et al., "Content validity—establishing and reporting the evidence in newly developed patient-reported outcomes (PRO) instruments for medical product evaluation: ISPOR PRO good research practices task force report: part 1—eliciting concepts for a new PRO instrument," *Value in Health*, vol. 14, no. 8, pp. 967–977, 2011.

[44] M. L. Rothman, P. Beltran, J. C. Cappelleri, J. Lipscomb, B. Teschendorf, and J. A. Sloan, "Patient-reported outcomes: conceptual issues," *Value in Health*, vol. 10, supplement 2, pp. S66–S75, 2007.

[45] D. Kimhy, S. Harlap, S. Fennig et al., "Maternal household crowding during pregnancy and the offspring's risk of schizophrenia," *Schizophrenia Research*, vol. 86, no. 1–3, pp. 23–29, 2006.

[46] L. Magliano, A. Fiorillo, C. Malangone et al., "Family burden in schizophrenia: effects of socio-environmental and clinical variables and family intervention," *Epidemiologia e Psichiatria Sociale*, vol. 7, no. 3, pp. 178–187, 1998.

[47] O. Mors, L. V. Sorensen, and M. L. Therkildsen, "Distress in the relatives of psychiatric patients admitted for the first time," *Acta Psychiatrica Scandinavica*, vol. 85, no. 5, pp. 337–344, 1992.

[48] J. E. D. Wolthaus, P. M. A. J. Dingemans, A. H. Schene et al., "Caregiver burden in recent-onset schizophrenia and spectrum disorders: the influence of symptoms and personality traits," *Journal of Nervous and Mental Disease*, vol. 190, no. 4, pp. 241–247, 2002.

[49] H. L. Provencher and K. T. Mueser, "Positive and negative symptom behaviors and caregiver burden in the relatives of persons with schizophrenia," *Schizophrenia Research*, vol. 26, no. 1, pp. 71–80, 1997.

[50] C. Webb, M. Pfeiffer, K. T. Mueser et al., "Burden and well-being of caregivers for the severely mentally ill: the role of coping style and social support," *Schizophrenia Research*, vol. 34, no. 3, pp. 169–180, 1998.

[51] P. J. Guarnaccia and P. Parra, "Ethnicity, social status, and families' experiences of caring for a mentally ill family member," *Community Mental Health Journal*, vol. 32, no. 3, pp. 243–260, 1996.

[52] I. S. Rosenfarb, A. S. Bellack, and N. Aziz, "A sociocultural stress, appraisal, and coping model of subjective burden and family attitudes toward patients with schizophrenia," *Journal of Abnormal Psychology*, vol. 115, no. 1, pp. 157–165, 2006.

[53] M. Scazufca and E. Kuipers, "Links between expressed emotion and burden of care in relatives of patients with schizophrenia," *British Journal of Psychiatry*, vol. 168, pp. 580–587, 1996.

[54] J. Wancata, M. Freidl, M. Krautgartner et al., "Gender aspects of parents' needs of schizophrenia patients," *Social Psychiatry and Psychiatric Epidemiology*, vol. 43, no. 12, pp. 968–974, 2008.

[55] R. Schulz and P. R. Sherwood, "Physical and mental health effects of family caregiving," *Journal of Social Work Education*, vol. 44, pp. 105–113, 2008.

[56] M. G. Mcdonell, R. A. Short, C. M. Berry, and D. G. Dyck, "Burden in schizophrenia caregivers: impact of family psychoeducation and awareness of patient suicidality," *Family Process*, vol. 42, no. 1, pp. 91–104, 2003.

[57] S. Srivastava, "Perception of burden by caregivers of patients with schizophrenia," *Indian Journal of Psychiatry*, vol. 47, no. 3, pp. 148–152, 2005.

[58] W.-T. Chien, S. W. C. Chan, and J. Morrissey, "The perceived burden among Chinese family caregivers of people with schizophrenia," *Journal of Clinical Nursing*, vol. 16, no. 6, pp. 1151–1161, 2007.

[59] J. Li, C. E. Lambert, and V. A. Lambert, "Predictors of family caregivers' burden and quality of life when providing care for a family member with schizophrenia in the People's Republic of China," *Nursing & Health Sciences*, vol. 9, no. 3, pp. 192–198, 2007.

[60] *Atlas.ti Software Version 7*, ATLAS.ti Scientific Software Development GmbH, Berlin, Germany, 2013.

[61] B. G. Glaser and A. L. Strauss, *The Discovery of Grounded Theory: Strategies for Qualitative Research*, Aldine de Gruyter, 1967.

[62] G. A. Bowen, "Grounded theory and sensitizing concepts," *International Journal of Qualitative Methods*, vol. 5, no. 3, pp. 12–23, 2006.

[63] K. E. Lasch, P. Marquis, M. Vigneux et al., "PRO development: rigorous qualitative research as the crucial foundation," *Quality of Life Research*, vol. 19, no. 8, pp. 1087–1096, 2010.

[64] G. Guest, A. Bunce, and L. Johnson, "How many interviews are enough? An experiment with data saturation and variability," *Field Methods*, vol. 18, pp. 59–82, 2006.

[65] J. J. Francis, M. Johnston, C. Robertson et al., "What is an adequate sample size? Operationalising data saturation for theory-based interview studies," *Psychology and Health*, vol. 25, no. 10, pp. 1229–1245, 2010.

[66] C. Roick, D. Heider, P. E. Bebbington et al., "Burden on caregivers of people with schizophrenia: comparison between Germany and Britain," *British Journal of Psychiatry*, vol. 190, pp. 333–338, 2007.

[67] L. Butler-Kisber and T. Poldma, "The power of visual approaches in qualitative inquiry: the use of collage making and oncept mapping in experiential research," *Journal of Research Practice*, vol. 6, no. 2, article M18, 2010.

[68] M. Razafsha, H. Behforuzi, H. Azari et al., "Qualitative versus quantitative methods in psychiatric research," *Methods in Molecular Biology*, vol. 829, pp. 49–62, 2012.

[69] CDC, *Assuring Healthy Caregivers*, 2012, http://www.cdc.gov/aging/pdf/caregiving_monograph.pdf.

[70] D. A. Perlick, R. A. Rosenheck, R. Kaczynski, M. S. Swartz, J. M. Cañive, and J. A. Lieberman, "Components and correlates of family burden in schizophrenia," *Psychiatric Services*, vol. 57, no. 8, pp. 1117–1125, 2006.

[71] NICE Clinical Guideline 82, *Schizophrenia: Core Interventions in the Treatment and Management of Schizophrenia in Adults in Primary and Secondary Care*, 2009.

[72] J. F. Deeken, K. L. Taylor, P. Mangan, K. R. Yabroff, and J. M. Ingham, "Care for the caregivers: a review of self-report instruments developed to measure the burden, needs, and quality of life of informal caregivers," *Journal of Pain and Symptom Management*, vol. 26, no. 4, pp. 922–953, 2003.

19

Polyphenols from Berries of *Aronia melanocarpa* Reduce the Plasma Lipid Peroxidation Induced by Ziprasidone

Anna Dietrich-Muszalska,[1] Justyna Kopka,[1] and Bogdan Kontek[2]

[1] *Department of Biological Psychiatry, The Chair of Experimental and Clinical Physiology, Medical University of Lodz, 6/8 Mazowiecka Street, 92-215 Lodz, Poland*
[2] *Department of General Biochemistry, Faculty of Biology and Environmental Protection, University of Lodz, 90-236 Lodz, Poland*

Correspondence should be addressed to Anna Dietrich-Muszalska; tzn_lodz@post.pl

Academic Editor: Robin Emsley

Background. Oxidative stress in schizophrenia may be caused partially by the treatment of patients with antipsychotics. The aim of the study was to establish the effects of polyphenol compounds derived from berries of *Aronia melanocarpa* (Aronox) on the plasma lipid peroxidation induced by ziprasidone *in vitro*. *Methods.* Lipid peroxidation was measured by the level of thiobarbituric acid reactive species (TBARS). The samples of plasma from healthy subjects were incubated with ziprasidone (40 ng/ml; 139 ng/ml; and 250 ng/ml) alone and with Aronox (5 ug/ml; 50 ug/ml). *Results.* We observed a statistically significant increase of TBARS level after incubation of plasma with ziprasidone (40 ng/ml; 139 ng/ml; and 250 ng/ml) (after 24 h incubation: $P = 7.0\times 10^{-4}$, $P = 1.6\times 10^{-3}$, and $P = 2.7\times 10^{-3}$, resp.) and Aronox lipid peroxidation caused by ziprasidone was significantly reduced. After 24-hour incubation of plasma with ziprasidone (40 ng/ml; 139 ng/ml; and 250 ng/ml) in the presence of 50 ug/ml Aronox, the level of TBARS was significantly decreased: $P = 6.5\times 10^{-8}$, $P = 7.0\times 10^{-6}$, and $P = 3.0\times 10^{-5}$, respectively. *Conclusion.* Aronox causes a distinct reduction of lipid peroxidation induced by ziprasidone.

1. Introduction

Oxidative stress plays an important role in schizophrenia and other psychiatric disorders. Schizophrenia is a chronic psychiatric disorder that affects at young age many cultures around the world. The aetiology of schizophrenia remains elusive, although several hypotheses have been suggested including abnormalities in cell membrane phospholipids metabolism or its alteration and dysfunction of cell membranes. Oxidative stress plays an important role in the pathophysiology of schizophrenia [1–9].

In schizophrenic patients, dysregulation of reactive oxygen species (ROS) generation and metabolism, as detected by abnormal activities of critical antioxidant enzymes and other indicators such as lipid peroxidation in plasma, red blood cells, blood platelets, and cerebrospinal fluid, are observed [3, 10–12]. It is well known that oxidative stress with peroxidation of polyunsaturated fatty acids (PUFA) in the membrane can lead to the abnormalities that have been observed in schizophrenia [11, 13, 14]. Oxidative stress occurs when the production of ROS exceeds the natural antioxidant defence mechanisms, causing damage to macromolecules such as DNA, proteins, and lipids. Antioxidant defence mechanisms remove the free radicals to prevent oxidative damage to biomolecules. The antioxidant system comprises of different types of functional components such as enzymatic (superoxide dismutase, catalase, glutathione peroxidase, glutathione reductase, and glutathione S-transferase) and nonenzymatic antioxidants. The nonenzymatic antioxidants include reduced glutathione, vitamin C, vitamin E (α tocopherol), uric acid, and various exogenous antioxidants including polyphenols. Antioxidants are substances that due to reduction of oxidative stress may prevent potentially disease-producing cell damage. The oxidative stress and oxidative injury in schizophrenia may be dependent partly on antipsychotics used and on dietary supplementation of antioxidants such as vitamins, carotenoids, polyphenol compounds, or EPUFAs that can correct membrane phospholipids. Some polyphenolic compounds extracted from berries of *Aronia melanocarpa* and used as Aronox (Agropharm/Adamed) have been reported to be protective agents in patients with breast cancer *in vitro* [15].

Lipid peroxidation is considered an important marker of oxidative stress and was found to be higher after treatment of patients with first generation antipsychotics (FGAs) [16]. Studies on rats indicate that treatment with both FGAs and second generation antipsychotics (SGAs) for <14 days does not alter the antioxidant defence enzymes and levels of lipid peroxides [17, 18]. Meta-analysis of oxidative stress-mediated damage showed a significant increase in TBARS levels in schizophrenia patients compared to healthy controls [19]. Moreover, increased levels of TBARS were reported in plasma/serum of neuroleptic-free patients with schizophrenia compared to normal controls [20]. Antipsychotics treatment was found to increase TBARS levels in plasma [21] and CSF [22–24] in chronic schizophrenic patients. The research on animal models suggests that antioxidant supplementations have beneficial effects and may prolong life of patients [17]. Some observations also suggest that antioxidant supplementations may prolong the human life, whereas other studies demonstrate neutral or even harmful effects [25–28]. In schizophrenia, the antioxidant defence system is altered, and activities of antioxidant enzymes are also changed [3, 9, 29]. Moreover, earlier studies showed that in schizophrenic patients reduced status of plasma total antioxidant capacity was observed [8, 30]. In schizophrenia, oxidative stress manifested by increased lipid peroxidation may be also induced by treatment with antipsychotic drugs [31, 32]. Our earlier results showed that treatment with antipsychotics such as haloperidol and ziprasidone caused an increase in lipid peroxidation measured by TBARS level in plasma [33, 34] whereas the second-generation antipsychotics such as olanzapine and risperidone *in vitro* did not cause plasma lipid peroxidation [30, 35]. Decrease of lipid peroxidation induced by amisulpride, clozapine, or quetiapine was also observed [33, 34, 36]. Lohr et al. [22] in the 1990s found that oxidative stress contributed to the toxicity of haloperidol, which activated a sequence of cellular processes leading even to cell death; the production of ROS was an integral part of this cascade. An experimental study in animals showed elevated level of lipid peroxidation and oxidative neuronal injury caused by haloperidol [37].

It is known that the exogenous plant antioxidants present in human diet, such as resveratrol, quercetin, and other polyphenols, may protect against oxidative stress [38, 39]. Since the direct estimation of reactive oxygen species generation *in vivo* is difficult, a common approach to measure oxidative stress *in vivo* and *in vitro* is to determine lipid peroxidation by means of commonly used assay with thiobarbituric acid (TBA). Therefore the aim of this study was to establish *in vitro* the action of ziprasidone (SGA) on lipid peroxidation in human plasma measured by the level of TBARS and determine the effect of polyphenols derived from berries of *Aronia melanocarpa* (Aronox) on this process. Ziprasidone (5-[2-(4-[1,2-benzisothiazol-3-yl]-1-piperazinyl)ethyl]-6-chloro-1,3-dihydro-2H-indol-2-one) was used *in vitro* at final concentrations corresponding to doses used for treatment of acute episode of schizophrenia [40, 41].

2. Materials and Methods

2.1. Materials. Ziprasidone (active substance) was obtained from Pfizer Inc. (USA) and Aronox (polyphenols) from Agropharm/Adamed (Poland). All other reagents were of analytical grade and were provided by commercial suppliers. Stock solution of ziprasidone and Aronox were made in 0.001% dimethylsulfoxide (DMSO).

2.2. Inclusion Criteria of Volunteers. Blood samples were taken from 30 healthy volunteers (15 males and 15 females) aged between 25 and 27 years (average: 25.9; SD = 1.7 years) without psychiatric, neurological, or somatic disorders and history of head injuries, allergy, and lipid or carbohydrate metabolism disorders, untreated with drugs. Healthy subjects did not use addictive substances and antioxidant supplementation and lived in similar socioeconomic conditions, and their diet was balanced (meat and vegetables). Subjects with significant medical illness were excluded. There were no smokers. The psychiatric examination MINI (Mini-International Neuropsychiatric Interview) [42], neurological and somatic examinations, and total cholesterol, LDL, HDL, triglycerides, and glucose concentrations were performed.

All volunteers included in the study had been informed about aims of the study and methods implemented and they expressed their written informed consent for participation in this study. The protocol was passed by the Committee for Research on Human Subjects of the Medical University of Lodz (number RNN/899/2000).

2.3. Isolation and Incubation of Plasma with Ziprasidone and Aronox. Human blood from healthy volunteers was collected into sodium citrate (5 mmol/l at final concentration) and immediately centrifuged (3000 × g, 15 min) to get plasma. Ziprasidone solutions were added to the samples of plasma (0.5 mL) to get the final concentration of 40 ng/mL; 139 ng/mL; and 250 ng/mL. For each experiment the control samples (without the drug) were prepared. The plasma samples with ziprasidone (final concentration 40 ng/mL; 139 ng/mL; 250 ng/mL) and the control samples were incubated for 1 and 24 h at 37°C. To measure the effects of plant polyphenols derived from Aronox, the samples of plasma were preincubated for 5 min at 37°C with Aronox solutions in 0,001% DMSO (final concentrations: 5 ug/mL; 50 ug/mL) and then ziprasidone was added. After 1 h or 24 h incubation (37°C) the levels of TBARS were measured.

2.4. Estimation of Thiobarbituric Acid Reactive Substances (TBARS) in Plasma. Samples of plasma after 1 or 24 h incubation with ziprasidone alone and/or Aronox were stopped by cooling the samples in an ice bath. Samples of plasma were transferred to an equal volume of 20% (v/v) cold trichloroacetic acid in 0.6 M HCl and centrifuged at 1200 × g for 15 min. One volume of clear supernatant was mixed with 0.2 volume of 0.12 M thiobarbituric acid in 0.26 M Tris, pH 7.0, and immersed in a boiling water bath for 15 min. The absorbance was measured in the SEMCO spectrophotometer at 535 nm, according to the Rice-Evans method [43] modified by Wachowicz et al. [44]. The TBARS expressed in μmol/l were calculated based on the absorbance value, using the molar extinction coefficient for TBARS ($\varepsilon = 1.56 \times 10^5\ M^{-1} \times cm^{-1}$). All estimations were performed twice, including control samples, where spontaneous lipid peroxidation, without the influence of the drug on plasma, was measured.

2.5. Statistical Analyses. All the values in this study were expressed as mean ± SEM. In order to eliminate uncertain data, Grubbs' test was performed. The statistical analysis of difference between the control plasma (without drug) and plasma treated with ziprasidone or ziprasidone and *Aronia melanocarpa* (Aronox) was done with a paired Student's t-test using StatSoft Inc. "Statistica" v. 6.0.

3. Results

Our results show that polyphenols from *Aronia melanocarpa* have an inhibitory effect on lipid peroxidation in plasma measured as TBARS level (Figures 1 and 2). We observed the dose-dependent increased level of TBARS after the incubation of plasma for 1 and 24 hours with ziprasidone (final concentrations: 40 ng/mL; 139 ng/mL; and 250 ng/mL) (Figure 2) compared to control samples without drug (1 h: 0.712 ± 0.04 umol/l; 24 h: 1.564 ± 0.06 umol/l, resp.) expressed as 100% (1 h: $P = 9.4 \times 10^{-3}$; $P = 1.3 \times 10^{-3}$; $P = 4.4 \times 10^{-6}$, resp.) (Figure 2(a)) after (24 h: $P = 7.0 \times 10^{-4}$, $P = 1.6 \times 10^{-3}$, $P = 2.7 \times 10^{-3}$, resp.) (Figure 2(b)). The polyphenol extract (final concentrations: 5 ug/mL, 50 ug/mL) caused distinct reduction of TBARS level. The effects are presented in Figure 1. We showed that used concentrations of polyphenols from *Aronia melanocarpa* (Aronox) had inhibitory effects on the increase of TBARS level in plasma induced by ziprasidone. After 1- and 24-hour incubation of plasma with extract from *Aronia melanocarpa* (50 ug/mL), the TBARS level was reduced by about 65% ($P = 3.4 \times 10^{-6}$) and by 82% ($P = 6.8 \times 10^{-9}$), respectively (Figure 1). The reduction of TBARS level in plasma treated with ziprasidone (40 ng/mL, 139 ng/mL, and 250 ng/mL) at the presence of Aronox (50 ug/mL) is presented in Figure 2. After 1 h the TBARS levels were reduced by about 51% ($P = 7.3 \times 10^{-4}$), 42% ($P > 0.05$), and 38% ($P > 0.05$), respectively (Figure 2(a)). After 24 h the TBARS levels was reduced by about 85% ($P = 6.5 \times 10^{-8}$), 80% ($P = 7.0 \times 10^{-6}$), and 79% ($P = 3.0 \times 10^{-5}$), respectively (Figure 2(b)). The reduction of TBARS level in plasma treated with ziprasidone (40 ng/mL, 139 ng/mL, and 250 ng/mL) at the presence of Aronox (5 ug/mL) after 1 h was about 4%, 10%, and 15%, respectively ($P > 0.05$), and after 24 h the TBARS levels were reduced by about 34% ($P = 6.2 \times 10^{-3}$), 32% ($P = 1.0 \times 10^{-3}$), and 28% (4.9×10^{-2}), respectively. The reduction of TBARS level was dependent on the concentration of Aronox (Figure 1).

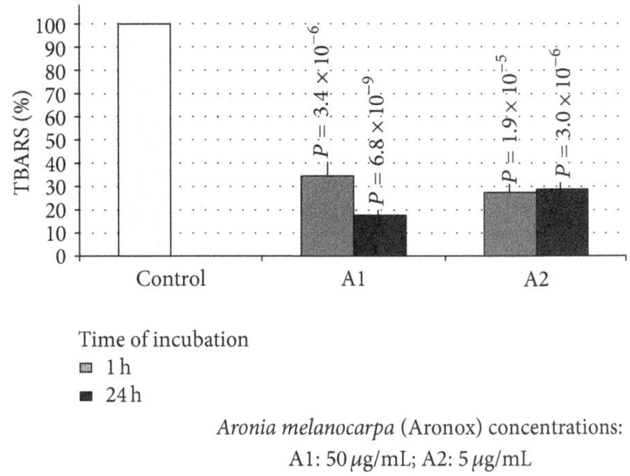

FIGURE 1: The inhibitory effect of compounds derived from *Aronia melanocarpa* on lipid peroxidation in plasma. Plasma was incubated with 5 μg/mL; 50 μg/mL of Aronox solution for 1 and 24 hours at 37°C. The level of TBARS in control plasma (1 h: 0.712 ± 0.04 μmol/l; 24 h: 1.564 ± 0.06 μmol/l) was expressed as 100%.

4. Discussion

During oxidative stress in biological systems the most readily accessible reaction partner is the biological membrane, in particular the polyunsaturated fatty acids of the membrane phospholipids. Once the reaction generates a lipid radical, a radical chain reaction occurs, leading to the formation of a variety of lipid peroxidation products which react with thiobarbituric acid and form TBARS. TBARS are very sensitive markers of this process. Oxidative stress-mediated injury is a part of the primary illness for many disorders including schizophrenia and it can be exacerbated by certain neuroleptics [45, 46]. Several studies indicated that the occurrence of movement disorders, including extrapyramidal symptoms in patients with psychotic disorders treated by classic neuroleptics, was associated with their oxidative stress [32]. In the cerebrospinal fluid of patients treated with antipsychotics, the concentration of TBARS was found to be increased [23], especially in patients with drug-induced movement disorders [22]. In schizophrenic patients with symptoms of tardive dyskinesia the lipid peroxidation in plasma was found to be increased [21]. Our earlier studies by using various specific biomarkers of oxidative stress revealed that in peripheral blood platelets or plasma from schizophrenic patients (in an acute period of psychosis) increased lipid peroxidation [3, 30] and oxidative/nitrative modifications of proteins [47, 48] occurred. According to other authors the antipsychotic treatment (especially FGAs) exhibits prooxidative effects [22, 32], whereas SGAs may exhibit antioxidative effects [32, 35]. Our earlier results indicate that SGAs, including clozapine, quetiapine, and olanzapine (at the concentrations proposed for therapeutic use in schizophrenic patients [49],

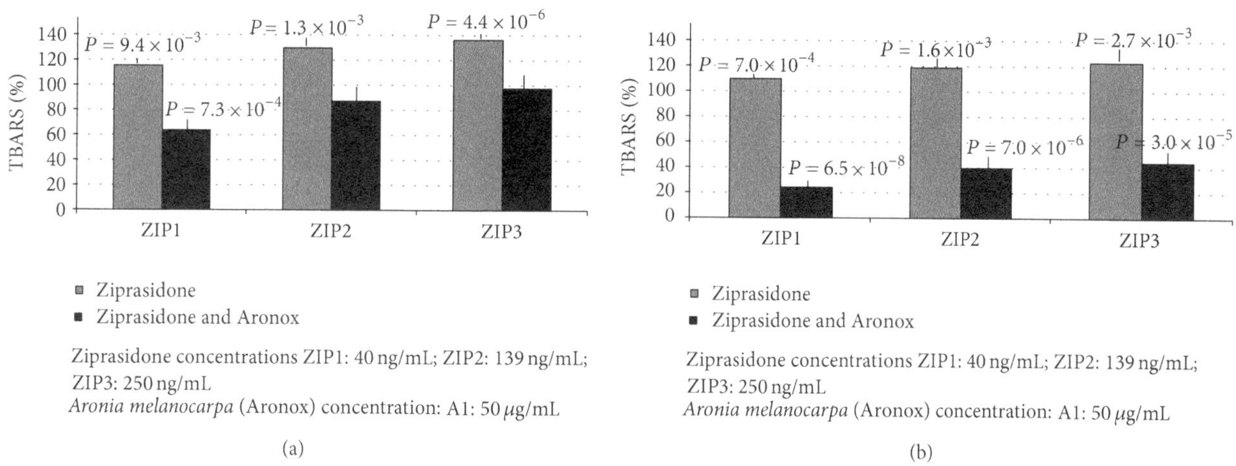

FIGURE 2: (a) The effects of ziprasidone alone (gray columns) and ziprasidone at the presence of 50 μg/mL Aronox (black columns) on the lipid peroxidation (TBARS) in plasma after 1 h incubation. TBARS level in control plasma (without ziprasidone and Aronox) was expressed as 100%. The level of TBARS in control plasma (1 h: 0.712 ± 0.04 μmol/l). (b) The effects of 24 h incubation of plasma with ziprasidone and ziprasidone with Aronox (50 μg/mL) on the level of lipid peroxidation measured as TBARS. The TBARS level in control plasma (without ziprasidone and Aronox) was expressed as 100%. The level of TBARS in control plasma (24 h: 1.564 ± 0.06 μmol/l).

did not induce plasma lipid peroxidation *in vitro* [33, 34]. Risperidone, even at very high concentrations, did not induce oxidative stress in plasma or in blood platelets [35].

The results presented in this study confirmed our earlier observation that ziprasidone induces lipid peroxidation in plasma [34]. Epidemiological and clinical study evidence suggests that a diet rich in fruits and vegetables decreases the risk of premature mortality from major clinical conditions, including heart disease and cancer. Recently, much attention has focused on possible role of diet in the prevention of chronic diseases [25, 50, 51]. In the present *in vitro* study, we assessed the effects of polyphenols present in *Aronia* extract on TBARS level in plasma treated with ziprasidone. The extract from *Aronia melanocarpa (Rosaceae)* containing anthocyanidins, phenolic acids, and quercetine glycosides may play an important protective role against lipid peroxidation. Phenolic compounds found naturally in fruits, nuts, flowers, seeds, and bark of different plants are an integral part of human diet.

They exhibit a wide range of biological effects, including antiplatelet, anti-inflammatory, anticancer, antimutagenic, and antifungal properties [51–53]. They are potent antioxidants and scavengers of reactive oxygen species and metal chelators. Some polyphenols like quercetin reverse haloperidol-induced catalepsy during schizophrenia or other affective disorders [54]. Here, we have shown for the first time that polyphenols present in *Aronia melanocarpa* extract *in vitro* distinctly reduced lipid peroxidation of plasma treated with ziprasidone. We conclude that natural products present in extract of *Aronia melanocarpa* may have some promising effects *in vivo* because they are strong antioxidants in the tested models *in vitro*. It seems that polyphenols from *Aronia melanocarpa* can be also useful as protecting factors against antipsychotic drugs used during schizophrenia. The life style of schizophrenic patients with low consumption of fruits and vegetables and treatment with prooxidative drugs leads to increased oxidative stress. Therefore the supplementation with antioxidants such as Aronox rich in polyphenols with antioxidant properties may have beneficial effects on the improved outcome of illness.

Plasma total antioxidant status (TAS) was significantly lower in schizophrenia subjects than in normal controls. Recently, reduced levels of plasma TAS have been shown in first-episode drug-naive patients with schizophrenia [55]. Individual plasma antioxidants, albumin, bilirubin [8, 56], and uric acid [8] were also found to be lower in schizophrenia subjects. Moreover, decreases of total and reduced GSH levels in plasma together with altered antioxidant enzyme activities have been reported in drug-naive first-episode patients with schizophrenia when compared with healthy control subjects [57].

In schizophrenia subjects, the mean values of serum MDA (malonyldialdehyde) levels were found significantly higher than that in the healthy individuals [10, 58]. Similar results were also observed in the blood of chronic schizophrenic patients compared to normal controls [59, 60]. Moreover, elevated serum TBARS were also found in different phases of bipolar disorder and in schizophrenia [61]. It seems that oxidative stress due to higher lipid peroxidation might play a critical role in pathogenesis of schizophrenia at very early course of illness.

Although antipsychotic drugs are the first choice of treatment for schizophrenia, their long-term treatment is known to produce adverse effects and may be responsible for increased lipid peroxidation and oxidative damage. Oxidative stress induced by antipsychotics may be counteracted by antioxidant enzymes and exogenous antioxidants. Therefore, it is essential to develop adjunctive or alternative treatment strategy to augment antipsychotic actions and improve the quality of life for schizophrenia patients. Some clinical, preclinical, and epidemiological studies suggest that many of antioxidant compounds present in fruits and vegetables, especially polyphenols, possess neuroprotective and anti-inflammatory activities, to greater or lesser extent, and could be considered as important adjunctive therapy for schizophrenia [36, 54]. We suggest that Aronox containing few important polyphenolic antioxidants might be used for the therapeutic purpose in this disorder; however more studies are required. Carefully monitored clinical trials in the future will provide more information regarding the effects of extract from *Aronia melanocarpa* in patients treated with antipsychotics.

Conflict of Interests

The authors have no conflict of interests with any commercial or other association in connection with the submitted paper.

Acknowledgments

This work was supported by Grant 502-03/1-155-02/502-14-106 from Medical University of Lodz, Poland, and by Grant dec. no. 2011/01/B/NZ4/04903 from National Centre of Science.

References

[1] H.-G. Bernstein, B. Bogerts, and G. Keilhoff, "The many faces of nitric oxide in schizophrenia: a review," *Schizophrenia Research*, vol. 78, no. 1, pp. 69–86, 2005.

[2] A. Dietrich-Muszalska and B. Olas, "Isoprostenes as indicators of oxidative stress in schizophrenia," *World Journal of Biological Psychiatry*, vol. 10, no. 1, pp. 27–33, 2009.

[3] A. Dietrich-Muszalska, B. Olas, and J. Rabe-Jablonska, "Oxidative stress in blood platelets from schizophrenic patients," *Platelets*, vol. 16, no. 7, pp. 386–391, 2005.

[4] H.-C. Li, Q.-Z. Chen, Y. Ma, and J.-F. Zhou, "Imbalanced free radicals and antioxidant defense systems in schizophrenia: a comparative study," *Journal of Zhejiang University Science B*, vol. 7, no. 12, pp. 981–986, 2006.

[5] R. D. Reddy and J. K. Yao, "Free radical pathology in schizophrenia: a review," *Prostaglandins Leukotrienes and Essential Fatty Acids*, vol. 55, no. 1-2, pp. 33–43, 1996.

[6] N. Srivastava, M. K. Barthwal, P. K. Dalal et al., "Nitrite content and antioxidant enzyme levels in the blood of schizophrenia patients," *Psychopharmacology*, vol. 158, no. 2, pp. 140–145, 2001.

[7] J. K. Yao and M. S. Keshavan, "Antioxidants, redox signaling, and pathophysiology in schizophrenia: an integrative view," *Antioxidants and Redox Signaling*, vol. 15, no. 7, pp. 2011–2035, 2011.

[8] J. K. Yao, R. Reddy, L. G. Mcelhinny, and D. P. van Kammen, "Reduced status of plasma total antioxidant capacity in schizophrenia," *Schizophrenia Research*, vol. 32, no. 1, pp. 1–8, 1998.

[9] J. K. Yao, R. D. Reddy, L.G. Mcelhinny, and D. P. van Kammen, "Oxidative damage and schizophrenia: an overview of the evidence and its therapeutic implications," *CNS Drugs*, vol. 15, no. 4, pp. 287–310, 2001.

[10] N. G. Gomes, M. G. Campos, J. M. Orfão, and C. A. Ribeiro, "Plants with neurobiological activity as potential targets for drug discovery," *Progress in Neuro-Psychopharmacology and Biological Psychiatry*, vol. 33, no. 8, pp. 1372–1389, 2009.

[11] D. F. Horrobin, "Schizophrenia as a membrane lipid disorder which is expressed throughout the body," *Prostaglandins Leukotrienes and Essential Fatty Acids*, vol. 55, no. 1-2, pp. 3–7, 1996.

[12] D. P. van Kammen, J. K. Yao, and K. Goetz, "Polyunsaturated fatty acids, prostaglandins, and schizophrenia," *Annals of the New York Academy of Sciences*, vol. 559, pp. 411–423, 1989.

[13] D. F. Horrobin, M. S. Manku, H. Hillman, A. Iain, and M. Glen, "Fatty acid levels in the brains of schizophrenics and normal controls," *Biological Psychiatry*, vol. 30, no. 8, pp. 795–805, 1991.

[14] J. K. Yao, S. Leonard, and R. D. Reddy, "Membrane phospholipid abnormalities in postmortem brains from schizophrenic patients," *Schizophrenia Research*, vol. 42, no. 1, pp. 7–17, 2000.

[15] M. Kunz, C. S. Gama, A. C. Andreazza et al., "Elevated serum superoxide dismutase and thiobarbituric acid reactive substances in different phases of bipolar disorder and in schizophrenia," *Progress in Neuro-Psychopharmacology and Biological Psychiatry*, vol. 32, no. 7, pp. 1677–1681, 2008.

[16] M. Kedzierska, B. Olas, B. Wachowicz et al., "An extract from berries of *Aronia melanocarpa* modulates the generation of superoxide anion radicals in blood platelets from breast cancer patients," *Planta Medica*, vol. 75, no. 13, pp. 1405–1409, 2009.

[17] V. Parikh, M. M. Khan, and S. P. Mahadik, "Differential effects of antipsychotics on expression of antioxidant enzymes and membrane lipid peroxidation in rat brain," *Journal of Psychiatric Research*, vol. 37, no. 1, pp. 43–51, 2003.

[18] A. Pillai, V. Parikh, A. V. Terry Jr., and S. P. Mahadik, "Long-term antipsychotic treatments and crossover studies in rats: differential effects of typical and atypical agents on the expression of antioxidant enzymes and membrane lipid peroxidation in rat brain," *Journal of Psychiatric Research*, vol. 41, no. 5, pp. 372–386, 2007.

[19] M. Zhang, Z. Zhao, L. He, and C. Wan, "A meta-analysis of oxidative stress markers in schizophrenia," *Science China Life Sciences*, vol. 53, no. 1, pp. 112–124, 2010.

[20] A. O. Skinner, S. P. Mahadik, and D. L. Garver, "Thiobarbituric acid reactive substances in the cerebrospinal fluid in schizophrenia," *Schizophrenia Research*, vol. 76, no. 1, pp. 83–87, 2005.

[21] M. Peet, J. Laugharne, N. Rangarajan, and G. P. Reynolds, "Tardive dyskinesia, lipid peroxidation, and sustained amelioration with vitamin E treatment," *International Clinical Psychopharmacology*, vol. 8, no. 3, pp. 151–153, 1993.

[22] J. B. Lohr, R. Kuczenski, H. S. Bracha, M. Moir, and D. V. Jeste, "Increased indices of free radical activity in the cerebrospinal fluid of patients with tardive dyskinesia," *Biological Psychiatry*, vol. 28, no. 6, pp. 535–539, 1990.

[23] H. S. Pall, A. C. Williams, D. R. Blake, and J. Lunec, "Evidence of enhanced lipid peroxidation in the cerebrospinal fluid of patients taking phenothiazines," *The Lancet*, vol. 2, no. 8559, pp. 596–599, 1987.

[24] G. Tsai, D. C. Goff, R. W. Chang, J. Flood, L. Baer, and J. T. Coyle, "Markers of glutamatergic neurotransmission and oxidative stress associated with tardive dyskinesia," *The American Journal of Psychiatry*, vol. 155, no. 9, pp. 1207–1213, 1998.

[25] G. Bjelakovic, D. Nikolova, L. L. Gluud, R. G. Simonetti, and C. Gluud, "Antioxidant supplements for prevention of mortality in healthy participants and patients with various diseases," *Cochrane Database of Systematic Reviews*, vol. 3, Article ID CD007176, 2012.

[26] G. Bjelakovic, D. Nikolova, and C. H. Gluud, "Meta-regression analyses, meta-analyses, and trial sequential analyses of the

effects of supplementation with beta-carotene, vitamin A, and vitamin E singly or in different combinations on all-cause mortality: do we have evidence for lack of harm?" *PLoS ONE*, vol. 8, no. 9, Article ID e74558, 2013.

[27] S. Eilat-Adar, T. Sinai, C. Yosefy, and Y. Henkin, "Nutritional recommendations for cardiovascular disease prevention review," *Nutrients*, vol. 5, no. 9, pp. 3646–3683, 2013.

[28] L. Hooper, P. A. Kroon, E. B. Rimm et al., "Flavonoids, flavonoid-rich foods, and cardiovascular risk: a meta-analysis of randomized controlled trials," *The American Journal of Clinical Nutrition*, vol. 88, no. 1, pp. 38–50, 2008.

[29] R. Reddy, M. P. Sahebarao, S. Mukherjee, and J. N. Murthy, "Enzymes of the antioxidant defense system in chronic schizophrenic patients," *Biological Psychiatry*, vol. 30, no. 4, pp. 409–412, 1991.

[30] A. Dietrich-Muszalska and B. Kontek, "Lipid peroxidation in patients with schizophrenia," *Psychiatry and Clinical Neurosciences*, vol. 64, no. 5, pp. 469–475, 2010.

[31] C. S. Gama, M. Salvador, A. C. Andreazza, F. Kapczinski, and P. Silva Belmonte-de-Abreu, "Elevated serum superoxide dismutase and thiobarbituric acid reactive substances in schizophrenia: a study of patients treated with haloperidol or clozapine," *Progress in Neuro-Psychopharmacology and Biological Psychiatry*, vol. 30, no. 3, pp. 512–515, 2006.

[32] I. Jeding, P. J. Evans, D. Akanmu et al., "Characterization of the potential antioxidant and pro-oxidant actions of some neuroleptic drugs," *Biochemical Pharmacology*, vol. 49, no. 3, pp. 359–365, 1995.

[33] A. Dietrich-Muszalska, B. Kontek, and J. Rabe-Jabłońska, "Quetiapine, olanzapine and haloperidol affect human plasma lipid peroxidation *in vitro*," *Neuropsychobiology*, vol. 63, no. 4, pp. 197–201, 2011.

[34] A. Dietrich-Muszalska, J. Kopka, and A. Kwiatkowska, "The effects of ziprasidone, clozapine and haloperidol on lipid peroxidation in human plasma (*in vitro*): comparison," *Neurochemical Research*, vol. 38, no. 7, pp. 1490–1495, 2013.

[35] A. Dietrich-Muszalska, "Evaluation of the effects of different concentrations of risperidone, corresponding to the drug doses used in treatment of schizophrenic patients, on lipid peroxidation in plasma and blood platelets at *in vitro* studies," *PsychIatria I PsychologIa Kliniczna*, vol. 4, no. 4, pp. 215–223, 2004.

[36] A. Dietrich-Muszalska and B. Olas, "Inhibitory effects of polyphenol compounds on lipid peroxidation caused by antipsychotics (haloperidol and amisulpride) in human plasma *in vitro*," *World Journal of Biological Psychiatry*, vol. 11, no. 2, pp. 276–281, 2010.

[37] Y. Sagara, "Induction of reactive oxygen species in neurons haloperidol," *Journal of Neurochemistry*, vol. 71, no. 3, pp. 1002–1012, 1998.

[38] S. Chung, H. Yao, S. Caito, J.-W. Hwang, G. Arunachalam, and I. Rahman, "Regulation of SIRT1 in cellular functions: role of polyphenols," *Archives of Biochemistry and Biophysics*, vol. 501, no. 1, pp. 79–90, 2010.

[39] B. Olas, M. Kedzierska, B. Wachowicz, A. Stochmal, and W. Oleszek, "Effects of polyphenol-rich extract from berries of *Aronia melanocarpa* on the markers of oxidative stress and blood platelet activation," *Platelets*, vol. 21, no. 4, pp. 274–281, 2010.

[40] A. F. Schatzberg and C. B. Nemeroff, Eds., *The American Psychiatric Publishing Textbook of Psychopharmacology*, American Psychiatric Publishing, Arlington, Va, USA, 2004.

[41] E. Stip, S. Zhornitsky, H. Moteshafi et al., "Ziprasidone for psychotic disorders: a meta-analysis and systematic review of the relationship between pharmacokinetics, pharmacodynamics, and clinical profile," *Clinical Therapeutics*, vol. 33, no. 12, pp. 1853–1867, 2011.

[42] D. V. Sheehan, Y. Lecrubier, K. H. Sheehan et al., "The mini-international neuropsychiatric Interview (M.I.N.I.): the development and validation of a structured diagnostic psychiatric interview for DSM-IV and ICD-10," *Journal of Clinical Psychiatry*, vol. 59, supplement 20, pp. 22–33, 1998.

[43] C. A. Rice-Evans, A. T. Diplock, and M. C. Symons, *Techniques in Free Radical Research*, Elsevier, New York, NY, USA, 1991.

[44] B. Wachowicz and J. Kustron, "Effect of cisplatin on lipid peroxidation in pig blood platelets," *Cytobios*, vol. 70, pp. 41–47, 1992.

[45] S. P. Machadik, S. Mukherjee, R. Scheffer, E. E. Correnti, and J. S. Mahadik, "Elevated plasma lipid peroxides at the onset of nonaffective psychosis," *Biological Psychiatry*, vol. 43, no. 9, pp. 674–679, 1998.

[46] R. G. McCreadie, E. MacDonald, D. Wiles, G. Campbell, and J. R. Paterson, "The nithsdale schizophrenia surveys. XIV: plasma lipid peroxide and serum vitamin E levels in patients with and without tardive dyskinesia, and in normal subjects," *The British Journal of Psychiatry*, vol. 167, no. 5, pp. 610–617, 1995.

[47] A. Dietrich-Muszalska and B. Olas, "Modifications of blood platelet proteins of patients with schizophrenia," *Platelets*, vol. 20, no. 2, pp. 90–96, 2009.

[48] A. Dietrich-Muszalska, B. Olas, R. Głowacki, and E. Bald, "Oxidative/nitrative modifications of plasma proteins and thiols from patients with schizophrenia," *Neuropsychobiology*, vol. 59, no. 1, pp. 1–7, 2009.

[49] D. Taylor, C. Paton, and R. Kerwin, *The South London and Maudsley NHS Trust. Prescribing Guidelines*, Martin Dunitz, Taylor & Francis, London, UK, 7th edition, 2003.

[50] P. S. Naidu and S. K. Kulkarni, "Quercefin, a bioflavonoid, reverses haloperidol-induced catalepsy," *Methods and Findings in Experimental and Clinical Pharmacology*, vol. 26, no. 5, pp. 323–326, 2004.

[51] B. Olas and B. Wachowicz, "Resveratrol, a phenolic antioxidant with effects on blood platelet functions," *Platelets*, vol. 16, no. 5, pp. 251–260, 2005.

[52] M. Bijak, M. Bobrowski, M. Borowiecka, A. Podsędek, J. Golański, and P. Nowak, "Anticoagulant effect of polyphenols-rich extracts from black chokeberry and grape seeds," *Fitoterapia*, vol. 82, no. 6, pp. 811–817, 2011.

[53] M. Naruszewicz and M. Dluzniewski, "Flavonoids from choheberry fruits (*Aronia melanocarpa*) reduce oxidative stress and inflammation in patients with coronary artery disease treated with statins (Short lectures)," *Planta Medica*, vol. 73, 2007.

[54] X. F. Li, Y. L. Zheng, M. H. Xiu, D. C. Chen, T. R. Kosten, and X. Y. Zhang, "Reduced plasma total antioxidant status in first-episode drug-naive patients with schizophrenia," *Progress in Neuro-Psychopharmacology and Biological Psychiatry*, vol. 35, no. 4, pp. 1064–1067, 2011.

[55] J. K. Yao, R. Reddy, and D. P. van Kammen, "Abnormal age-related changes of plasma antioxidant proteins in schizophrenia," *Psychiatry Research*, vol. 97, no. 2-3, pp. 137–151, 2000.

[56] M. Raffa, F. Atig, A. Mhalla, A. Kerkeni, and A. Mechri, "Decreased glutathione levels and impaired antioxidant enzyme activities in drug-naive first-episode schizophrenic patients," *BMC Psychiatry*, vol. 11, article 124, 2011.

[57] S. Grignon and J. M. Chianetta, "Assessment of malondialdehyde levels in schizophrenia: a meta-analysis and some methodological considerations," *Progress in Neuro-Psychopharmacology and Biological Psychiatry*, vol. 31, no. 2, pp. 365–369, 2007.

[58] B. M. Al-Chalabi, I. A. J. Thanoon, and F. A. Ahmed, "Potential effect of olanzapine on total antioxidant status and lipid peroxidation in schizophrenic patients," *Neuropsychobiology*, vol. 59, no. 1, pp. 8–11, 2009.

[59] G. Dadheech, S. Mishra, S. Gautam, and P. Sharma, " Evaluation of antioxidant deficit in schizophrenia," *Indian Journal of Psychiatry*, vol. 50, no. 1, pp. 16–20, 2008.

[60] M. Padurariu, A. Ciobica, I. Dobrin, and C. Stefanescu, "Evaluation of antioxidant enzymes activities and lipid peroxidation in schizophrenic patients treated with typical and atypical antipsychotics," *Neuroscience Letters*, vol. 479, no. 3, pp. 317–320, 2010.

[61] S. Kropp, V. Kern, K. Lange et al., "Oxidative stress during treatment with first- and second-generation antipsychotics," *Journal of Neuropsychiatry and Clinical Neurosciences*, vol. 17, no. 2, pp. 227–231, 2005.

Explaining Attitudes and Adherence to Antipsychotic Medication: The Development of a Process Model

Martin Wiesjahn,[1] Esther Jung,[1] Fabian Lamster,[1] Winfried Rief,[1] and Tania M. Lincoln[2]

[1] *Department of Psychology, Division of Clinical Psychology and Psychotherapy, Philipps-Universität Marburg, 35032 Marburg, Germany*
[2] *Institute of Psychology, Department of Clinical Psychology and Psychotherapy, Universität Hamburg, 20146 Hamburg, Germany*

Correspondence should be addressed to Martin Wiesjahn; martin.wiesjahn@staff.uni-marburg.de

Academic Editor: Patrick W. Corrigan

Although nonadherence to antipsychotic medication poses a threat to outcome of medical treatment, the processes preceding the intake behavior have not been investigated sufficiently. This study tests a process model of medication adherence derived from the Health Belief Model which is based on cost-benefit considerations. The model includes an extensive set of potential predictors for medication attitudes and uses these attitudes as a predictor for medication adherence. We conducted an online study of 84 participants with a self-reported psychotic disorder and performed a path analysis. More insight into the need for treatment, a higher attribution of the symptoms to a mental disorder, experience of less negative side effects, presence of biological causal beliefs, and less endorsement of psychological causal beliefs were significant predictors of more positive attitudes towards medication. The results largely supported the postulated process model. Mental health professionals should consider attitudes towards medication and the identified predictors when they address adherence problems with the patient in a shared and informed decision process.

1. Introduction

A substantial proportion of patients with psychotic disorders do not take their medication as prescribed. Estimations of the frequency of nonadherence to antipsychotic medication range widely depending on the definition of adherence. The nonadherence rate is estimated to be 49.5% based on a definition of adherence as "taking medications as prescribed at least 75% of the time" [1, page 901]. Nonadherence can be problematic as medication withdrawal has been found to be associated with a higher risk of relapse [2], increased hospital admission rates [3], and in turn high costs for the health care system [4]. Research on dopaminergic supersensitivity [5, 6] indicates that in certain cases irregular intake and sudden dose reductions may be worse than taking no medication at all. Moncrieff [5] concludes that in some patients relapse into psychosis "may be a feature of drug withdrawal rather than the re-emergence of an underlying illness" (page 3).

In order to address the risks associated with sudden discontinuation of antipsychotic medication it is essential to understand the processes that lead to negative attitudes towards the medication and to nonadherence. For this purpose it appears promising to evaluate the individual costs and benefits of antipsychotic medication for each individual patient as described in the Health Belief Model (HBM [7, 8]) which was developed to explain general health behavior by evaluative processes. In the course of a shared decision process [9, 10] the clinician needs to inform the patient about potential benefits and unwanted effects of medication and the risk associated with nonadherence. Beyond weighing the pro of likely effectiveness and the con of side effects, the patient's adherence and attitudes towards medication are likely to be affected by previous experiences, social influences, or even symptomatology in itself. Knowing the relevant factors that explain attitudes and adherence can help clinicians to support patients in arriving at an informed decision about the treatment options. Such knowledge might also help to further develop interventions aimed at improving adherence [11, 12] for those patients who are likely to benefit from medication.

Previous research has focused on several factors that might be related to medication attitudes and adherence in patients with psychotic disorders. More positive attitudes about medication and medication adherence have been consistently found to be associated with the "insight" into the presence of a mental disorder [1, 13–16] and with a good relationship to the treating physician [1, 14, 17–19]. In Lacro and colleagues' review [1] most studies did not show an association between self-rated side effects and adherence which the authors attempted to explain with the lack of systematic side effect ratings. In support of this explanation, recent studies in patients with psychotic disorders [20, 21] and in other populations [22] applied standardized assessments of side effects and found them to be consistently related to lower medication adherence. The findings on psychotic symptoms as a predictor for medication attitudes and adherence are heterogeneous. In the review by Lacro et al. [1] half of the studies revealed fewer symptoms to be associated with higher adherence, whereas the other half did not find such a relationship. Positive beliefs about symptoms (e.g., "during psychosis, I had a feeling of importance and power" [20, page 3]) were only recently included in the field of research and the study by Moritz et al. [20] indicated their importance for medication adherence. Social support was associated with better adherence in the studies by Coldham et al. [15] and Dassa et al. [19], whereas Lacro and colleagues' review found mixed results in regard to this relationship [1]. One recent study indicates that the attitudes towards medication held by the immediate social environment of the person can also be a reason for discontinuation of medication [16]. The potential impact of causal beliefs about the disorder on medication attitudes and adherence has not been investigated in people with psychotic disorders so far. However, in an experimental study in a healthy sample, a biological causal model increased the motivation to take medication [23].

Following these findings, the relevance of some predictors, such as insight and alliance, seems to be evident. For others further clarification is needed (e.g., social support, attitudes of the immediate social environment, or causal beliefs). Also, this field of research faces several methodological obstacles which make it difficult to interpret and compare the findings. For one, studies have typically used outcome measures that mix the constructs of adherence, attitudes, and side effects, such as the Drug Attitude Inventory [24]. This is problematic as it confounds adherence as the actual behavior with preceding conditions. To understand the processes involved in medication adherence it would be helpful to differentiate between adherence as the behavioral component, attitudes as the evaluative component, and side effects and other "costs and benefits" of the treatment. The HBM [7, 8] could serve as a conceptual framework for this differentiation. Following the HBM, medication adherence is likely to be influenced by subjective attitudes towards the medication, which in turn depend on cost-benefit considerations [8]. As another limitation previous studies mostly included small subsets of possible predictors [14, 15] rather than considering a comprehensive set of predictors. This makes it difficult to estimate the incremental amount of variance explained by each predictor. Furthermore, many studies included only participants who were in psychiatric inpatient treatment at that time which limits the generalizability of the findings. Also, the risk of biased answers could be higher in inpatient settings because patients might fear negative consequences of reported nonadherence.

The aim of the present study was to increase our understanding of the processes that are involved in the formation of attitudes towards medication and might impact on medication adherence. With a differentiated and systematic assessment of possible predictors, attitudes towards medication, and medication adherence we investigated a process model derived from the HBM. It integrates an extensive set of possible predictors for attitudes towards antipsychotic medication and uses these attitudes to explain the variance in medication adherence (see Figure 1). We included the set of known predictors (different aspects of insight, positive and negative symptoms, side effects, relationship to the treating physician, and social support) as well as less frequently investigated factors (biological and psychological causal beliefs about the disorder, positive and negative beliefs about paranoia, and the attitudes towards medication held by the immediate social environment). We used an online assessment to reduce selection effects and increase the likelihood of unbiased responses.

2. Method

2.1. Procedure. The data was collected using SoSci-Survey (https://www.soscisurvey.de/). We invited members of nonprofit online forums on psychotic disorders in German language to participate. The link was also placed in newsletters and notice boards of self-help groups and in public places such as supermarkets in several German cities (a list of all websites and organizations can be retrieved from the first author). The objective of the study was explained (investigation of attitudes and adherence to antipsychotic medication). Participants had to agree to the terms of participation explained on the first page of the study. The completion of the questionnaire took approximately 30 min. As an incentive, a lottery for five 10€ online gift certificates was performed. We included participants who were 18 years or older, completed the full questionnaire, and reported to have been diagnosed with at least one of the following psychotic disorders: schizophrenia, schizoaffective disorder, delusional disorder, or unspecified psychotic disorder. In order to focus on the long term process of medication attitudes and adherence we excluded individuals who reported to have been diagnosed with a brief psychotic disorder. Furthermore, we included only those participants who reported to take antipsychotic medication in the present or have taken it in the past.

2.2. Measures. To assess the adherence to antipsychotic medication we used the Medication Adherence Questionnaire (MAQ [25]). The 4-item scale is behaviorally formulated and has been shown to predict actual intake behavior [26]. In previous research the MAQ items showed an internal consistency of $\alpha = 0.67$ [26]. Lüllmann and Lincoln [27] developed an authorized German version by translating and blindly retranslating the questionnaire. The participants were

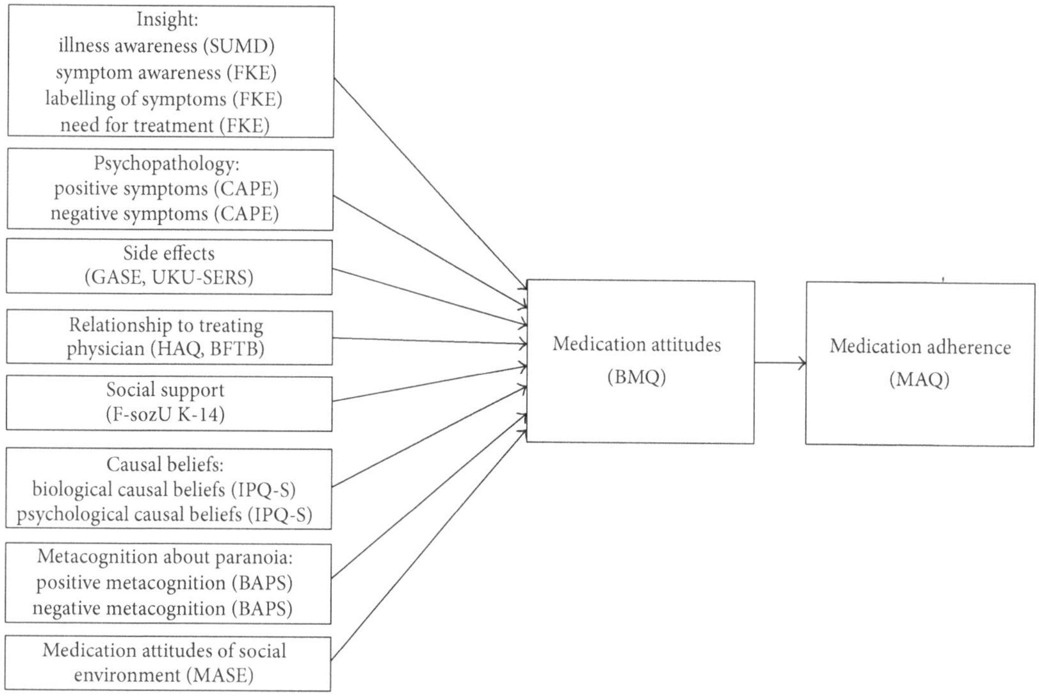

FIGURE 1: Process model to explain the variance in medication adherence with medication attitudes and possible predictors.

asked to refer all questions to antipsychotic medication only. A higher score indicates better adherence.

To assess attitudes towards antipsychotic medication we used the German version [28] of the Beliefs about Medicines Questionnaire (BMQ [29]). The 18-item instrument refers to positive and negative beliefs about medication. In previous research [28] the BMQ showed a three-factor structure with internal consistencies between $\alpha = 0.70$ and 0.85. We instructed the participants to refer all items to antipsychotic medication. In order to estimate overall attitudes towards antipsychotic medication we calculated the mean score. A higher score implies more positive attitudes.

We assessed the general awareness of having a mental disorder with the first item of the Scale to Assess Unawareness of Mental Disorder (SUMD [30]), which is highly correlated with other general insight measures [13]. The SUMD and its German version are well-established and validated [28]. In the original semistructured interview, items are rated by the interviewer following anchoring criteria. For the purpose of this study, we transformed the first item into a self-report multiple choice item with three response options analogous to the original anchors: "I believe that I have a mental disorder," "I am not sure that I have a mental disorder but I can entertain the idea that I might," and "I do not believe that I have a mental disorder." A higher score indicates more general insight.

For a more differentiated assessment of insight we used the FKE (Fragebogen zur Krankheitseinsicht (Questionnaire of Illness Insight [31])). This German instrument includes the subscales symptom awareness (3 items), labeling of symptoms as a mental disorder (3 items), and insight into the need for treatment (4 items). Internal consistencies were acceptable to good in previous research ($\alpha = 0.70 - 0.85$ [31]). In each subscale higher scores indicate more insight.

We assessed psychotic symptoms with the Community Assessment of Psychic Experiences (CAPE [32]). The CAPE consists of 42 items on the three dimensions: positive symptoms, negative symptoms, and depression. The German version has demonstrated good internal consistencies ($\alpha = 0.84 - 0.91$ [33]). In order to assess specific psychotic symptoms we used the subscales positive symptoms (20 items) and negative symptoms (14 items) with higher scores indicating more symptoms. For reasons of economy we omitted the depression subscale.

To assess medication side effects we used the Generic Assessment of Side Effects (GASE) by Rief et al. [34] who found a high internal consistency of the German version ($\alpha = 0.89$). Participants are instructed to rate the intensity of the presented potential side effects on 4-point scales. In our study the participants were asked whether they attribute the phenomena to antipsychotic medication or not. In order to also assess side effects that are more specific for antipsychotic medication (e.g., "increased salivation") we added nine items from the UKU Side Effect Rating Scale (UKU-SERS [35]), which assesses side effects of antipsychotic medication. We used the German version [36] and adapted the rating format to the items of the GASE. For the estimation of side effects we used the sum-score of all GASE and UKU-SERS items that were attributed to antipsychotic medication with a higher score implying more side effects.

We assessed the quality of the alliance between the participant and the treating physician with the validated German version of the Health Alliance Questionnaire (HAQ [37]). We used the 6-item HAQ subscale referring to the patient's satisfaction with the therapeutic relationship ($\alpha = 0.89$ [37]). To assess the relationship in more detail we added items from the BFTB (Bonner Fragebogen für Therapie und Beratung (Bonn Questionnaire for Therapy and Consulting [38])). This German instrument contains three relationship scales based on Roger's conceptualization of alliance [39]. Participants are asked as how empathic and genuine they perceive or perceived their treating physician and how accepted they feel or felt. We used a subset of five items for each of the three subscales, which demonstrated excellent internal consistencies in previous research ($\alpha = 0.90 - 0.91$ [38]). The combined assessment of the alliance consisted of 21 items. Participants were instructed to refer the statements to the current or recent treating physician who prescribed the antipsychotic medication. A higher score implies better alliance.

Social support was assessed with the F-sozU K-14 (Fragebogen zur sozialen Unterstützung, Kurzform (Social Support Questionnaire, Short Version [40])). This 14-item instrument assesses the subjective perception of the availability of social support. The instrument has demonstrated excellent internal consistency in previous research ($\alpha = 0.94$ [40]). A higher score indicates more perceived social support.

We assessed the beliefs about the causes of the disorder with items from the German version [41] of the Illness Perception Questionnaire for Schizophrenia (IPQ-S [42]) which assesses a set of beliefs about schizophrenia. Regarding causal beliefs participants are asked to rate their agreement to potential causes on 5-point scales. We used the 13-item psychological and the 4-item biological factors which have shown good to acceptable internal consistencies in previous research ($\alpha = 0.89 - 0.63$ [23]). We used the mean scores of the subscales with higher values indicating higher agreement.

Positive and negative beliefs about paranoid experiences were assessed with the Beliefs about Paranoia Scale (BAPS [43]) which refers to metacognitive beliefs about paranoia. The authors found good to excellent internal consistencies for the subscales survival beliefs, negative beliefs, and normalizing beliefs ($\alpha = 0.85 - 0.91$). Via translation and blinded retranslation we developed a German version, which was approved by the first author of the scale. For the purpose of this study, we included the subscales negative beliefs and, as an indicator of positive metacognition, survival beliefs. Higher scores indicate higher beliefs. The questionnaire was only administered to those participants who reported to have had paranoid experiences.

In order to assess the attitudes of the immediate social environment towards antipsychotic medication we developed a 6-item instrument called Medication Attitude of the Social Environment (MASE). It assesses the perceived opinion of relevant others ("People who are important for me think that it is right that I take antipsychotics."). The items are to be rated on 5-point scales. In our study the internal consistency of this scale was good ($\alpha = 0.88$). A higher score indicates a more positive attitude.

An overview of the instruments is depicted in Figure 1. Demographic data and clinical history were assessed via self-report.

2.3. Analysis. The data was analyzed with SPSS 21 and AMOS 19. In a first step we investigated the bivariate relationships between the variables. This step involved testing whether the variables were normally distributed (Kolmogorov-Smirnov test) to decide whether to use Pearson's (r) or Spearman's correlations (r_s). Then we calculated correlations between the potential predictors, medication attitudes, and adherence. Additionally, we examined the path model depicted in Figure 1. In the first step we included all possible predictors for medication attitudes into a path analysis (based on a maximum likelihood estimation). Then, we adjusted the path model by reducing the number of predictors in a step by step approach. In each step we excluded the predictor with the lowest path coefficient. Then we reevaluated the path model and excluded the next predictor until only significant predictors were included. Post hoc we tested for possible mediation effects with the Sobel test [44].

3. Results

3.1. Sample Characteristics. Of the 214 people who accepted the terms of participation and started the assessment, 107 completed the full questionnaire. Twenty-one participants were excluded because they did not report to have been diagnosed with one of the psychotic disorders described in the inclusion criteria. Two individuals were excluded because they reported to have never taken antipsychotic medication. The excluded participants did not differ from the included sample with regard to gender, age, or education. The remaining sample included $n = 84$ participants (54.8% female) with a mean age of 38.3 (SD = 9.7). One quarter (23.8%) were married or in a relationship, 66.7% were single, and 9.5% were divorced. Asked for their level of education, 29.8% reported to have completed university, 36.9% high school, 26.2% intermediate secondary school, and 7.1% general secondary school or below. One third (33.3%) were working on the "first labor market," 29.8% were not working because they were considered as "disabled due to disorder," 16.7% were in training, 10.7% were unemployed, 2.4% worked in sheltered workshops, and 7.1% provided no data on employment status.

Regarding diagnoses, 73.8% of the participants indicated to have been diagnosed with schizophrenia, 35.7% with schizoaffective disorder, 8.3% with delusional disorder, and 8.3% with unspecified psychotic disorder. The majority (72.6%) reported one diagnosis, 21.4% two, and 6.0% three or four diagnoses. The mean number of psychotic episodes was 5.8 (SD = 6.8). All participants reported to have received some kind of treatment for their mental health problems; 89.3% were currently in treatment and 10.7% had received treatment in the past. The majority (92.9%) had been admitted to a psychiatric clinic in the past. Most participants (81.0%) were taking antipsychotic medication at the time of data collection and 19% indicated that they had been taking medication in the past but not now.

3.2. Bivariate Relationships between Medication Attitudes and Predictors. The bivariate analyses (see Table 1) showed a positive correlation between medication attitudes and medication adherence ($r_s = 0.30$, $P < 0.01$). We found significant

Table 1: Bivariate correlations between medication attitudes, medication adherence, and possible predictors (n = 84).

	Attitudes	Adherence	Insight				Psychopathology		Side effects	Alliance	Social support	Causal beliefs		Metacognition	
	BMQ	MAQ[a]	SUMD[a]	FKE-SA	FKE-LS	FKE-NT	CAPE-POS[a]	CAPE-NEG	GASE, UKU	HAQ, BFTB	F-sozU K-14	IPQ-S-BIO	IPQ-S-PSY	BAPS-POS[b]	BAPS-NEG[b]
MAQ[a]	0.30**														
SUMD[a]	0.23*	0.22*													
FKE-SA	0.24*	−0.10	0.02												
FKE-LS	0.34**	0.03	0.30**	0.82***											
FKE-NT	0.53***	0.12	0.38***	0.37***	0.45***										
CAPE-POS[a]	0.08	−0.20	−0.13	0.64***	0.51***	0.19									
CAPE-NEG	0.16	−0.22*	0.07	0.43***	0.39***	0.35**	0.57***								
GASE, UKU	−0.36**	−0.20	−0.17	0.25*	0.15	−0.12	0.30**	0.00							
HAQ, BFTB	0.34**	0.00	0.23*	0.11	0.12	0.54***	0.08	0.13	−0.20						
F-sozU K-14	0.00	0.09	−0.08	0.09	0.00	0.25*	−0.08	−0.12	0.20	0.23*					
IPQ-S-BIO	0.43***	0.03	0.40***	0.26*	0.34**	0.42***	0.16	0.29**	−0.08	0.33**	0.02				
IPQ-S-PSY	−0.01	0.01	0.27*	0.23*	0.28*	0.35**	0.32**	0.17	0.10	0.14	0.00	0.22*			
BAPS-POS[b]	0.18	−0.17	0.07	0.37**	0.26*	0.07	0.53***	0.25*	0.40***	−0.01	−0.09	0.07	0.21		
BAPS-NEG[b]	0.31**	−0.03	0.24*	0.49***	0.59***	0.32**	0.48***	0.44***	0.08	0.03	−0.11	0.28*	0.09	0.25*	
MASE	0.38***	−0.03	0.08	0.23*	0.20	0.50***	0.23*	0.22*	−0.05	0.25*	0.31**	0.17	0.11	−0.05	0.23*

[a]Values are Spearman's correlations (nonparametric scales); [b]reduced sample size due to filter question (n = 78); $^{*}P < 0.05$; $^{**}P < 0.01$; $^{***}P < 0.001$; MAQ: Medication Adherence Questionnaire; BMQ: Beliefs about Medicines Questionnaire; SUMD: Scale to Assess Unawareness of Mental Disorder; FKE: Questionnaire of Illness Insight; FKE-SA: Symptom Awareness; FKE-LS: Labeling of Symptoms; FKE-NT: Need for Treatment; CAPE: Community Assessment of Psychic Experience; CAPE-POS: Positive Symptoms; CAPE-NEG: Negative Symptoms; GASE: Generic Assessment of Side Effects; UKU-SERS: UKU Side Effect Rating Scale; HAQ: Health Alliance Questionnaire; BFTB: Bonn Questionnaire for Therapy and Consulting; F-sozU K-14: Social Support Questionnaire; IPQ-S: Illness Perception Questionnaire for Schizophrenia; IPQ-S-BIO: Biological Causal Beliefs; IPQ-S-PSY: Psychological Causal Beliefs; BAPS: Beliefs about Paranoia Scale; BAPS-POS: Positive Metacognition; BAPS-NEG: Negative Metacognition; MASE: Medication Attitudes of Social Environment.

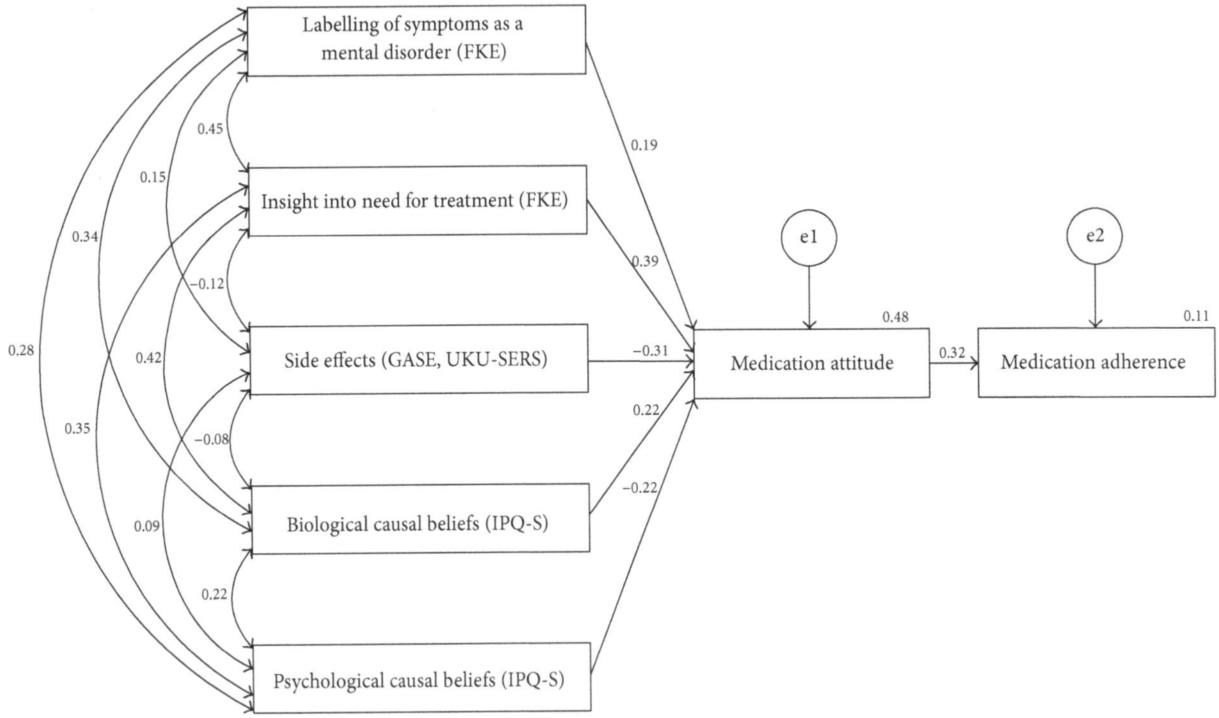

FIGURE 2: Path analysis to explain the variance in medication adherence with medication attitudes and related variables.

positive correlations between attitudes towards medication and the four components of insight (illness awareness, r_s = 0.23, $P < 0.05$; symptom awareness, $r = 0.24$, $P < 0.05$; labeling of symptoms as a mental disorder, $r = 0.34$, $P < 0.01$; and insight into the need for treatment, $r = 0.53$, $P < 0.001$). Also, more positive attitudes towards medication were associated with fewer side effects ($r = -0.36$, $P < 0.01$), a better relationship to the treating physician ($r = 0.34$, $P < 0.01$), higher biological causal beliefs ($r = 0.43$, $P < 0.001$), more negative metacognition about paranoia ($r = 0.31$, $P < 0.01$), and better medication attitudes of the immediate social environment ($r = 0.38$, $P < 0.001$).

3.3. Results from the Path Analysis. We included all 14 possible predictors for medication attitudes in the first step of the path analysis. In nine steps we reduced the number of predictors until only significant predictors remained in the model. The final model (compare Figure 2) contained five predictors for more positive attitudes towards medication: higher scores in the scale labeling the symptoms as a mental disorder ($\beta = 0.19$; $P < 0.05$), more insight into the need for treatment ($\beta = 0.39$; $P < 0.001$), fewer side effects ($\beta = -0.31$; $P < 0.001$), more biological causal beliefs ($\beta = 0.22$; $P < 0.05$), and fewer psychological causal beliefs ($\beta = -0.22$; $P < 0.01$). Forty-eight percent of the variance in medication attitudes and eleven percent of the variance in medication adherence were explained.

We considered several aspects of model fit. The nonsignificant χ^2 ($\chi^2 = 4.29$, df = 5, *n.s.*) is a first indicator for good fit. The Normed Fit Index (NFI) compares the χ^2 of the model to the χ^2 of the independence model. The score of 0.97 is above the cutoff 0.95 indicating a good fit. The Goodness of Fit Index (GFI), which refers to the proportion of variance and covariance explained by the model, has a cut-off score of 0.95 and also indicates a good fit for our data (GFI = 0.99). The Comparative Fit Index (CFI) describes the incremental power of the model in comparison to the independence model. The score of 1.00 was clearly above the cut-off score of 0.95 which also indicates a good fit. The overall fit index RMSEA (Root Mean Square Error of Approximation) compares the proposed model to the saturated model with smaller values indicating a better fit. In our data the RMSEA was set at 0.00 because the χ^2 score was lower than the number of degrees of freedom (df). Although this value indicates a close fit [45], the 90% confidence interval for the RMSEA is relatively wide (from 0.00 to 0.14). This indicates an imprecision of the estimation which might be due to the relatively small sample size [46].

4. Discussion

Our findings largely support the postulated process model, which emphasizes the importance of individual evaluative processes that precede medication intake behavior. According to our path analysis, fewer perceived side effects, a higher attribution of the symptoms to a mental disorder, a greater sense of needing treatment, more endorsement of biological causes of the disorder, and less approval to psychological causes were associated with more positive attitudes towards medication, which in turn partly predicted better adherence.

4.1. Predictors for Attitudes towards Antipsychotic Medication. The association between more positive attitudes towards medication and higher scores in the two facets of insight (labeling the symptoms as a mental disorder and insight into the need for treatment) is in line with previous research [1, 13–16]. However, our results go beyond earlier findings as we assessed various aspects of insight and controlled for intercorrelations between the potential predictors. We identified labeling of the symptoms and insight into need for treatment to be the only aspects of insight that explained an incremental amount of variance in medication attitudes. A possible explanation for the specific importance of these facets is that they evaluate the person's own situation ("It is good for my health to have regular contact to a psychiatrist.") and symptoms ("Because of a mental disorder I have unusual experiences that occur only in my head."). Thus, in order to see the benefits of the medication it seems to be important that the person perceives his or her individual symptoms as being a part of some kind of disorder that needs to be treated.

We assessed side effects in a systematic and extensive manner and found more side effects to be associated with more negative medication attitudes. This is in line with recent research [20–22] and supports the hypothesis that earlier null findings underestimated the relevance of side effects for medication attitudes due to insufficient measurement methods [1].

The relevance of biological causal beliefs to medication attitudes indicates that it is important that the person perceives the treatment as being plausible with regard to the etiology of the disorder. For individuals who believe their disorder to have biological causes it probably "makes sense" and appears to be beneficial to accept a biological treatment, that is, medication.

In contrast, the results of the path analysis suggest that psychological causal beliefs antagonize the establishment of positive medication attitudes. According to this finding a stronger belief in psychological causes might question the perceived benefits of antipsychotic medication. This would partly contradict the results by Lüllmann et al. [23], who found that clinicians should aim at an etiological model that combines psychosocial and biological causes because this combination fosters the success of various kinds of treatment, including medication. However, in our data psychological causal beliefs received a significant path coefficient ($\beta = -0.22$; $P < 0.01$) although the variable was not significantly correlated to medication attitudes in the bivariate analysis ($r = -0.01$, *n.s.*). This indicates a suppression effect; that is, one or more of the other predictors in the path analysis suppress irrelevant variance in the variable and thereby statistically increase its predictive power. We performed post hoc analyses and separately combined psychological causal beliefs with each of the other predictors. Labeling of symptoms was revealed to be the only suppressor variable; that is, psychological causal beliefs can only be incorporated into the model if labeling of symptoms is included. This restricts the distinct importance of the variable and thereby reduces the contradiction to previous findings.

The nonsignificance of the other possible predictors sheds a new light on some of the "usual suspects" [20]. In contrast to earlier research [1, 47] our data revealed no association between psychotic symptoms and medication attitudes. We found no support for the assumption that patients with more positive symptoms have a more negative opinion about medication as was found by Haq et al. [47]. In contrast to Haq et al. [47], however, we assessed symptoms via self-report. Although self-report measures of positive symptoms have been shown to be valid [48] the differences in assessment might nevertheless be responsible for the diverging findings. Insight has been shown to be the most significant predictor of patient-clinician discrepancies in positive symptoms rating with lower insight predicting higher clinician compared to patient ratings [48]. To avoid a confounding impact of insight on the association of symptoms and medication attitudes, future studies might, therefore, need to consider including both patient and observer ratings of positive symptoms.

Although the perceived quality of the relationship to the physician was correlated with medication attitudes in the bivariate analysis the association did not remain significant in the multivariate analysis. This was surprising in the light of consistent previous findings [1, 14, 17–19]. This result could be partially due to a substantial correlation between relationship ratings and insight into the need for treatment ($r = 0.54$, $P < 0.001$). A post hoc Sobel test suggested that the association between the perceived relationship and medication attitudes is mediated by insight into need for treatment ($z = 3.48$, $P < 0.001$). More positive contact to the physician might foster the perception of needing treatment, which in turn increases positive medication attitudes.

In our data social support was not associated with medication attitudes. Previous findings on this relationship are heterogeneous [1, 15, 18, 19], which might be explained by differences in the operationalization of social support. In contrast to our assessment of general social support, the studies who found a significant relationship between medication attitudes and social support [15, 19] used a narrow definition of it as the family being involved in the treatment. Our results suggest that people with all degrees of general social integration can have positive attitudes towards medication.

Analogous to previous research [16] we found a positive bivariate association between attitudes towards medication in the immediate social environment and patients' attitudes. However, this variable did not remain a significant predictor after controlling for other possible predictors. This might be due to a statistical and conceptual overlap between this variable and insight into need for treatment ($r = 0.50$, $P < 0.001$). Results of a post hoc Sobel test suggest that the association between medication attitudes of the immediate social network and the patients' attitudes is mediated by insight into need for treatment ($z = 3.27$, $P < 0.01$). Friends' and family's opinion about the medical treatment could impact on the person's perceived need for treatment in general and thereby influence medication attitudes. Thereby attitudes of the immediate social environment might form a subjective norm as described by Ajzen [49].

Finally, positive metacognition (i.e., survival beliefs) about paranoid experiences was not associated with medication attitudes. With regard to negative metacognition the bivariate analysis revealed participants who perceived their paranoia as more distressing to have more positive medication attitudes. However, this association did not remain significant in the multivariate analysis, which is likely to be due to an overlap between negative metacognitive beliefs and aspects of insight. A post hoc Sobel test indicated that the relationship between negative metacognition and medication attitudes is mediated by insight into need for treatment ($z = 2.51$, $P < 0.05$). A more negative perception of paranoid experiences and their consequences is likely to increase the awareness of needing treatment, which in turn promotes positive medication attitudes.

4.2. Predictors of Adherence. It is noteworthy that our process model explained a substantial amount of the variance in medication attitudes and a significant, albeit small, proportion of the variance in adherence. This can be explained by the general discrepancy between attitudes and behavior that rarely correlate to more than $r = 0.30$ [50]. Another reason might be that we focused on evaluative factors, whereas more practical reasons for nonadherence such as forgetfulness or disorganization were not assessed and should be included in future research.

4.3. Strengths and Limitations. The test of the differentiated process model to explain medication attitudes and adherence addresses a central problem of earlier research and presents a key strength of our study. A further advantage is the comprehensive set of possible predictors, which we assessed systematically. Furthermore, the online assessment probably reduced the danger of biased responses. The dropout rate of 50% corresponds to the average proportion of completed surveys in the online survey system SoSci-Survey [51]. This indicates that it might have been due to the nature of online studies in general, in which distracting factors or absence of personal contact to the researcher tend to lead to reduced engagement of the participants. However, we compared completers and dropouts with regard to demographic variables and found no differences in matters of age, gender, level of education, or diagnoses. This indicates that there was no systematic dropout. Nevertheless, as our sample was not large enough for a crossvalidation, our results need to be replicated with a larger sample to achieve a more precise estimation of the model and to control for possible biases in the sample. A possible selection effect has to be considered because parts of the sample were assessed via online forums and self-help groups. Participation in these forums and groups might have influenced the attitudes. The cross-sectional design limits the conclusions that can be drawn (e.g., the participants and their immediate social environment might influence each other in both directions with regard to their attitudes towards medication). The self-reported diagnoses pose a further limitation as they were not testable. However, several aspects indicate the accuracy of the data. Firstly, there was no incentive for lying as participation in the lottery was also possible for people who had not reported a psychotic diagnosis. Secondly, regarding the proportions of diagnoses our sample is representative of patients with psychotic disorders [52] and recent research indicates that online studies are a fairly reliable way to assess psychotic symptoms [53]. Finally, although we assessed a large number of possible predictors, future research could incorporate even more differentiated constructs such as the person's confidence that the disorder can be treated or further aspects of psychopathology such as depression which has been shown to be associated with adherence in somatic disorders [54].

4.4. Practical Implications. The study draws the attention to an assortment of factors that should be addressed when discussing medication issues with patients. For one, it seems important to assess whether the patient perceives himself or herself to be in need of treatment in general and—if this is not the case—attempt to strengthen the patient's insight into the need for treatment. Following Zygmunt and colleagues' findings [55], it is promising to illustrate that medical, along with psychosocial, treatments could be helpful for the patient to achieve personal goals. At the same time, following West's request for patients' self-determination [9], the clinician should accept a rejection of medical treatment if a patient concludes that medication will not help to achieve personal goals. Additionally, following the results of the mediation analyses the relationship to the treating physician, the immediate social norm and negative metacognition seem to be relevant for the insight into need for treatment. Clinicians should aim at a positive and cooperative relationship to the patient in order to foster the trust into the treatment and to increase the adherence to it. Family members or friends could be included into the discussion in order to promote the benefits of possible medical or psychosocial therapies and thereby establish a common agreement on the treatment. Furthermore, clinicians might consider negative metacognition when discussing the perceived need for treatment. In the case of patients who are not aware of the negative consequences of their symptoms it could be promising to evaluate the personal costs of the symptoms together with the patient and then strengthen the confidence in the treatment to overcome these adverse consequences. In addition, our results suggest that it is beneficial for the establishment of positive medication attitudes if a patient attributes his or her symptoms to a mental disorder. Such an attribution might help to clarify the patient's problems, which is generally part of a successful therapeutic process [56]. Thereby it could strengthen the patient's motivation to adhere to all parts of a treatment plan, including medication. However, such an attribution bears the risk of consolidating a self-perception as being ill. In contrast, normalizing beliefs that describe symptoms as being common experiences are seen as functional and helpful for patients [43]. Therefore, professionals should aim at a balance between clarifying the symptoms and taking them seriously on the one hand and normalizing them on the other hand. Furthermore, our results indicate that integrating biological causal explanations into the personal model of the disorder could be helpful to improve medication attitudes. The clinician could actively strengthen biological explanations or use a Socratic dialogue to introduce them to patients who are likely to benefit from medication. However, taking into account the results by Lüllmann et al. [23], a combination between psychosocial and biological causes should be aspired. Our results also suggest that the clinician should actively assess the side effects of antipsychotic medication that have been experienced or are expected by the patient. The choice of a specific substance should aim at minimizing side effects that are likely to undermine positive medication attitudes and adherence. Furthermore, as described by Rief et al. [57], clinicians need to keep in mind that negative expectations might increase the perception of side effects. The clinician should provide information about possible side effects in a way that reduces this nocebo effect. Among other suggestions Colloca and Miller [58] recommend framing the information "positively" by focusing on the proportion of patients who do not experience the side effect. Furthermore, following Meehan et al. [59], coping strategies for side effects should be strengthened.

In order to remain open minded it can be helpful for clinicians to be aware that antipsychotic medication is not helpful for every patient [60] despite the fact that they are recommended as a standard treatment [61]. In Leucht and colleagues' meta-analysis [62] the effects of antipsychotic medication were consistent but smaller than expected (mean moderate effect size of −0.51) and responder rates were low. The authors concluded that six patients needed to be treated with a second-generation antipsychotic drug in order to achieve a significant improvement for one patient. Furthermore, long term risks are becoming more and more apparent [63, 64]. In contrast, there is encouraging support for a treatment with minimal use of antipsychotic medication (e.g., the Soteria approach [65]) and for psychological interventions, such as CBT, as an alternative to medication [66]. Therefore, if a patient decides against a medical treatment as a result of a shared and informed decision process the clinician should be open to accept this as a rational choice.

Conflict of Interests

The authors declare that there is no conflict of interests regarding the publication of this paper.

References

[1] J. P. Lacro, L. B. Dunn, C. R. Dolder, S. G. Leckband, and D. V. Jeste, "Prevalence of and risk factors for medication nonadherence in patients with schizophrenia: a comprehensive review of recent literature," *Journal of Clinical Psychiatry*, vol. 63, no. 10, pp. 892–909, 2002.

[2] A. C. Viguera, R. J. Baldessarini, J. D. Hegarty, D. P. Van Kammen, and M. Tohen, "Clinical risk following abrupt and gradual withdrawal of maintenance neuroleptic treatment," *Archives of General Psychiatry*, vol. 54, no. 1, pp. 49–55, 1997.

[3] M. Valenstein, L. A. Copeland, F. C. Blow et al., "Pharmacy data identify poorly adherent patients with schizophrenia at increased risk for admission," *Medical Care*, vol. 40, no. 8, pp. 630–639, 2002.

[4] R. Emsley, "The true cost of non-adherence in schizophrenia," *Mind & Brain, the Journal of Psychiatry*, vol. 1, no. 2, pp. 17–22, 2010.

[5] J. Moncrieff, "Does antipsychotic withdrawal provoke psychosis? Review of the literature on rapid onset psychosis (supersensitivity psychosis) and withdrawal-related relapse," *Acta Psychiatrica Scandinavica*, vol. 114, no. 1, pp. 3–13, 2006.

[6] A.-N. Samaha, P. Seeman, J. Stewart, H. Rajabi, and S. Kapur, ""Breakthrough" dopamine supersensitivity during ongoing antipsychotic treatment leads to treatment failure over time," *Journal of Neuroscience*, vol. 27, no. 11, pp. 2979–2986, 2007.

[7] I. M. Rosenstock, "Why people use health services," *The Milbank Memorial Fund quarterly*, vol. 44, no. 3, pp. 94–127, 1966.

[8] C. J. Carpenter, "A meta-analysis of the effectiveness of health belief model variables in predicting behavior," *Health Communication*, vol. 25, no. 8, pp. 661–669, 2010.

[9] C. West, "Powerful choices: peer support and individualized medication self-determination," *Schizophrenia Bulletin*, vol. 37, no. 3, pp. 445–450, 2011.

[10] M. Swarbrick and D. Roe, "Experiences and motives relative to psychiatric medication choice," *Psychiatric Rehabilitation Journal*, vol. 35, no. 1, pp. 45–50, 2011.

[11] X. F. Amador, *I Am Not Sick, I Don't Need Help!*, Vida Press, New York, NY, USA, 10th edition, 2010.

[12] P. J. Weiden and N. Rao, "Teaching medication compliance to psychiatric residents: placing an orphan topic into a training curriculum," *Academic Psychiatry*, vol. 29, no. 2, pp. 203–210, 2005.

[13] T. M. Lincoln, E. Lüllmann, and W. Rief, "Correlates and long-term consequences of poor insight in patients with schizophrenia. A systematic review," *Schizophrenia Bulletin*, vol. 33, no. 6, pp. 1324–1342, 2007.

[14] J. C. Day, R. P. Bentall, C. Roberts et al., "Attitudes toward antipsychotic medication: the impact of clinical variables and relationships with health professionals," *Archives of General Psychiatry*, vol. 62, no. 7, pp. 717–724, 2005.

[15] E. L. Coldham, J. Addington, and D. Addington, "Medication adherence of individuals with a first episode of psychosis," *Acta Psychiatrica Scandinavica*, vol. 106, no. 4, pp. 286–290, 2002.

[16] S. Moritz, M. J. V. Peters, A. Karow, A. Deljkovic, P. Tonn, and D. Naber, "Cure or curse? Ambivalent attitudes towards neuroleptic medication in schizophrenia and non-schizophrenia patients," *Mental Illness*, vol. 1, no. 1, pp. 4–9, 2009.

[17] D. Misdrahi, M. Petit, O. Blanc, F. Bayle, and P.-M. Llorca, "The influence of therapeutic alliance and insight on medication adherence in schizophrenia," *Nordic Journal of Psychiatry*, vol. 66, no. 1, pp. 49–54, 2012.

[18] A. G. Awad, "Antipsychotic medications: compliance and attitudes towards treatment," *Current Opinion in Psychiatry*, vol. 17, no. 2, pp. 75–80, 2004.

[19] D. Dassa, L. Boyer, M. Benoit, S. Bourcet, P. Raymondet, and T. Bottai, "Factors associated with medication non-adherence in patients suffering from schizophrenia: a cross-sectional study in a universal coverage health-care system," *Australian and New Zealand Journal of Psychiatry*, vol. 44, no. 10, pp. 921–928, 2010.

[20] S. Moritz, J. Favrod, C. Andreou et al., *Beyond the Usual Suspects: Positive Attitudes Towards Positive Symptoms is Associated with Medication Noncompliance in Psychosis*, Schizophrenia Bulletin, 2012.

[21] M. DiBonaventura, S. Gabriel, L. Dupclay, S. Gupta, and E. Kim, "A patient perspective of the impact of medication side effects on adherence: results of a cross-sectional nationwide survey of patients with schizophrenia," *BMC Psychiatry*, vol. 12, article 20, 2012.

[22] J. A. Glombiewski, Y. Nestoriuc, W. Rief, H. Glaesmer, and E. Braehler, "Medication adherence in the general population," *PLoS ONE*, vol. 7, no. 12, Article ID e50537, 2012.

[23] E. Lüllmann, S. Berendes, W. Rief, and T. M. Lincoln, "Benefits and harms of providing biological causal models in the treatment of psychosis—an experimental study," *Journal of Behavior Therapy and Experimental Psychiatry*, vol. 42, no. 4, pp. 447–453, 2011.

[24] T. P. Hogan, A. G. Awad, and R. Eastwood, "A self-report scale predictive of drug compliance in schizophrenics: reliability and discriminative validity," *Psychological Medicine*, vol. 13, no. 1, pp. 177–183, 1983.

[25] D. E. Morisky, L. W. Green, and D. M. Levine, "Concurrent and predictive validity of a self-reported measure of medication adherence," *Medical Care*, vol. 24, no. 1, pp. 67–74, 1986.

[26] L. Fialko, P. A. Garety, E. Kuipers et al., "A large-scale validation study of the Medication Adherence Rating Scale (MARS)," *Schizophrenia Research*, vol. 100, no. 1-3, pp. 53–59, 2008.

[27] E. Lüllmann and T. M. Lincoln, *The Medication Adherence Questionnaire (MAQ)—German Version*, Philipps-Universität Marburg, Marburg, Germany, 2008.

[28] E.-M. Beck, R. Vögelin, M. Wirtz, M. Cavelti, S. Kvrgic, and R. Vauth, "Do patients with Schizophrenia distinguish between attitudes toward antipsychotic medication and pharmacotherapy in general? Validation of the beliefs about medication questionnaire," *Journal of Nervous and Mental Disease*, vol. 200, no. 1, pp. 33–43, 2012.

[29] R. Horne, J. Weinman, and M. Hankins, "The beliefs about medicines questionnaire: the development and evaluation of a new method for assessing the cognitive representation of medication," *Psychology and Health*, vol. 14, no. 1, pp. 1–24, 1999.

[30] X. F. Amador, D. H. Strauss, S. A. Yale, M. M. Flaum, J. Endicott, and J. M. Gorman, "Assessment of insight in psychosis," *American Journal of Psychiatry*, vol. 150, no. 6, pp. 873–879, 1993.

[31] L. Dudenbostel, *Psychometric assessment of dimensions of illness insight in schizophrenia [Diploma thesis]*, Osnabrück University, Osnabrück, Germany, 2009.

[32] M. Konings, M. Bak, M. Hanssen, J. Van Os, and L. Krabbendam, "Validity and reliability of the CAPE: a self-report instrument for the measurement of psychotic experiences in the general population," *Acta Psychiatrica Scandinavica*, vol. 114, no. 1, pp. 55–61, 2006.

[33] T. M. Lincoln, N. Peter, M. Schäfer, and S. Moritz, "Impact of stress on paranoia: an experimental investigation of moderators and mediators," *Psychological Medicine*, vol. 39, no. 7, pp. 1129–1139, 2009.

[34] W. Rief, A. J. Barsky, J. A. Glombiewski, Y. Nestoriuc, H. Glaesmer, and E. Braehler, "Assessing general side effects in clinical trials: reference data from the general population," *Pharmacoepidemiology and Drug Safety*, vol. 20, no. 4, pp. 405–415, 2011.

[35] O. Lingjaerde, U. G. Ahlfors, P. Bech, S. J. Dencker, and K. Elgen, "The UKU side effect rating scale. A new comprehensive rating scale for psychotropic drugs and a cross-sectional study of side effects in neuroleptic-treated patients," *Acta Psychiatrica Scandinavica, Supplement*, vol. 334, pp. 1-100, 1987.

[36] M. Hummer, R. Holzmeister, G. Kemmler et al., "Attitudes of patients with schizophrenia toward placebo-controlled clinical trials," *Journal of Clinical Psychiatry*, vol. 64, no. 3, pp. 277–281, 2003.

[37] M. Bassler, B. Potratz, and H. Krauthauser, "The "helping alliance questionnaire" (HAQ) by Luborsky," *Psychotherapeut*, vol. 40, no. 1, pp. 23–32, 1995.

[38] H. Berth and E. Brähler, "Bonn questionnaire for therapy and consulting (BFTB)," *Diagnostica*, vol. 49, no. 4, pp. 191–194, 2003.

[39] C. R. Rogers, *Client-Centered Therapy*, Constable, London, UK, 1976.

[40] T. Fydrich, G. Sommer, S. Tydecks, and E. Brähler, "Social support questionnaire (F-SozU): standardization of short form (K-14)," *Zeitschrift fur Medizinische Psychologie*, vol. 18, no. 1, pp. 43–48, 2009.

[41] L. Pruß, K. H. Wiedl, E. Lüllmann, T. M. Lincoln, and M. Waldorf, "'That doesn't take long... I have it under control'. Illness perceptions, insight, and coping in schizophrenia," Poster presented at 47. Congress of German Society of Psychology (DGPs), Bremen, Germany, 2010.

[42] F. Lobban, C. Barrowclough, and S. Jones, "Assessing cognitive representations of mental health problems. I. The illness perception questionnaire for schizophrenia," *British Journal of Clinical Psychology*, vol. 44, no. 2, pp. 147–162, 2005.

[43] A. P. Morrison, A. I. Gumley, K. Ashcroft et al., "Metacognition and persecutory delusions: tests of a metacognitive model in a clinical population and comparisons with non-patients," *British Journal of Clinical Psychology*, vol. 50, no. 3, pp. 223–233, 2011.

[44] K. J. Preacher and A. F. Hayes, "SPSS and SAS procedures for estimating indirect effects in simple mediation models," *Behavior Research Methods, Instruments, and Computers*, vol. 36, no. 4, pp. 717–731, 2004.

[45] B. G. Tabachnick and L. S. Fidell, *Using Multivariate Statistics*, Pearson/Allyn & Bacon, Boston, Mass, USA, 5th edition, 2007.

[46] B. M. Byrne, *Equation Modeling With AMOS: Basic Concepts, Applications and Programming*, Routledge, New York, NY, USA, 2nd edition, 2010.

[47] F. Haq, C. Behan, N. McGlade et al., "Factors that influence patients' attitudes to antipsychotic medication," *Irish Journal of Psychological Medicine*, vol. 26, no. 1, pp. 6–11, 2009.

[48] T. M. Lincoln, M. Ziegler, E. Lüllmann, M. J. Müller, and W. Rief, "Can delusions be self-assessed? Concordance between self- and observer-rated delusions in schizophrenia," *Psychiatry Research*, vol. 178, no. 2, pp. 249–254, 2010.

[49] I. Ajzen, "The theory of planned behavior," *Organizational Behavior and Human Decision Processes*, vol. 50, no. 2, pp. 179–211, 1991.

[50] A. W. Wicker, "Attitudes versus actions: the relationship of verbal and overt behavioral responses to attitude objects.," *Journal of Social Issues*, vol. 25, no. 4, pp. 41–78, 1969.

[51] D. J. Leiner, oFb in Zahlen [oFb in numbers] 2012, https://www.soscisurvey.de/index.php?page=info.

[52] S. Leucht, J. Fritze, M. H. Lanczik, L. Vauth, and H. M. Olbrich, "Schizophrenia and other psychotic disorders," in *Mental Disorders: Clinic and Therapy*, M. Berger, Ed., pp. 411–490, Elsevier, Urban & Fischer, München, Germany, 3rd edition, 2009.

[53] S. Moritz, N. van Quaquebeke, T. M. Lincoln, U. Köther, and C. Andreou, "Can we trust the internet to measure psychotic symptoms?" *Schizophrenia Research and Treatment*, vol. 2013, Article ID 457010, 5 pages, 2013.

[54] J. L. Grenard, B. A. Munjas, J. L. Adams et al., "Depression and medication adherence in the treatment of chronic diseases in the United States: a meta-analysis," *Journal of General Internal Medicine*, vol. 26, no. 10, pp. 1175–1182, 2011.

[55] A. Zygmunt, M. Olfson, C. A. Boyer, and D. Mechanic, "Interventions to improve medication adherence in schizophrenia," *American Journal of Psychiatry*, vol. 159, no. 10, pp. 1653–1664, 2002.

[56] K. Grawe, R. Donati, and F. Bernauer, *Psychotherapy in Transition: From Religion to Profession*, Hogrefe, Göttingen, Germany, 1994.

[57] W. Rief, J. Avorn, and A. J. Barsky, "Medication-attributed adverse effects in placebo groups: implications for assessment of adverse effects," *Archives of Internal Medicine*, vol. 166, no. 2, pp. 155–160, 2006.

[58] L. Colloca and F. G. Miller, "The nocebo effect and its relevance for clinical practice," *Psychosomatic Medicine*, vol. 73, no. 7, pp. 598–603, 2011.

[59] T. Meehan, T. Stedman, and J. Wallace, "Consumer strategies for coping with antipsychotic medication side effects," *Australasian Psychiatry*, vol. 19, no. 1, pp. 74–77, 2011.

[60] R. Whitaker, "The case against antipsychotic drugs: a 50-year record of doing more harm than good," *Medical Hypotheses*, vol. 62, no. 1, pp. 5–13, 2004.

[61] J. Kreyenbuhl, R. W. Buchanan, F. B. Dickerson, and L. B. Dixon, "The schizophrenia patient outcomes research team (PORT): updated treatment recommendations 2009," *Schizophrenia Bulletin*, vol. 36, no. 1, pp. 94–103, 2010.

[62] S. Leucht, D. Arbter, R. R. Engel, W. Kissling, and J. M. Davis, "How effective are second-generation antipsychotic drugs? A meta-analysis of placebo-controlled trials," *Molecular Psychiatry*, vol. 14, no. 4, pp. 429–447, 2009.

[63] C. U. Correll and E. M. Schenk, "Tardive dyskinesia and new antipsychotics," *Current Opinion in Psychiatry*, vol. 21, no. 2, pp. 151–156, 2008.

[64] B.-C. Ho, N. C. Andreasen, S. Ziebell, R. Pierson, and V. Magnotta, "Long-term antipsychotic treatment and brain volumes: a longitudinal study of first-episode schizophrenia," *Archives of General Psychiatry*, vol. 68, no. 2, pp. 128–137, 2011.

[65] J. R. Bola and L. R. Mosher, "Treatment of acute psychosis without neuroleptics: two-year outcomes from the Soteria project," *Journal of Nervous and Mental Disease*, vol. 191, no. 4, pp. 219–229, 2003.

[66] A. P. Morrison, P. Hutton, M. Wardle et al., "Cognitive therapy for people with a schizophrenia spectrum diagnosis not taking antipsychotic medication: an exploratory trial," *Psychological Medicine*, vol. 42, no. 5, pp. 1049–1056, 2012.

21

Eating Disorders in Schizophrenia: Implications for Research and Management

Youssef Kouidrat,[1,2] Ali Amad,[3] Jean-Daniel Lalau,[1] and Gwenole Loas[4]

[1] *Department of Endocrinology, University of Picardie-Jules Verne, CHU d'Amiens, Amiens, France*
[2] *Department of Nutrition, Hôpital maritime, Assistance Publique-Hôpitaux de Paris (AP-HP), 62600 Berck, France*
[3] *Psychiatry Department and SCA-lab, PSYchiC team, Université de Lille, 59100 Lille, France*
[4] *Department of Psychiatry, Erasme Hospital, ULB, 1070 Brussels, Belgium*

Correspondence should be addressed to Youssef Kouidrat; youssef.kouidrat@gmail.com

Academic Editor: Luis San

Objective. Despite evidence from case series, the comorbidity of eating disorders (EDs) with schizophrenia is poorly understood. This review aimed to assess the epidemiological and clinical characteristics of EDs in schizophrenia patients and to examine whether the management of EDs can be improved. *Methods.* A qualitative review of the published literature was performed using the following terms: "schizophrenia" in association with "eating disorders," "anorexia nervosa," "bulimia nervosa," "binge eating disorder," or "night eating syndrome." *Results.* According to our literature review, there is a high prevalence of comorbidity between schizophrenia and EDs. EDs may occur together with or independent of psychotic symptoms in these patients. Binge eating disorders and night eating syndromes are frequently found in patients with schizophrenia, with a prevalence of approximately 10%. Anorexia nervosa seems to affect between 1 and 4% of schizophrenia patients. Psychopathological and neurobiological mechanisms, including effects of antipsychotic drugs, should be more extensively explored. *Conclusions.* The comorbidity of EDs in schizophrenia remains relatively unexplored. The clearest message of this review is the importance of screening for and assessment of comorbid EDs in schizophrenia patients. The management of EDs in schizophrenia requires a multidisciplinary approach to attain maximized health outcomes. For clinical practice, we propose some recommendations regarding patient-centered care.

1. Introduction

Schizophrenia is a severe and frequently observed mental illness that affects 1% of the general population. Schizophrenia is characterized by a wide range of symptoms, including positive symptoms (delusions and hallucinations), negative symptoms (social withdrawal, blunted affect), cognitive symptoms (difficulties with memory and attention), and affective dysregulation [1]. Moreover, psychiatric comorbidities are very common among patients with schizophrenia, particularly substance abuse, anxiety, and depressive symptoms [2]. In addition to these psychiatric features, endocrine and cardiometabolic alterations (e.g., type 2 diabetes, obesity, hypertension, and dyslipidemia) are frequently associated with schizophrenia. Indeed, cardiovascular diseases are the leading cause of the high mortality among patients with schizophrenia, which is 2-3 times higher than that of the general population [3, 4].

The etiology of the cardiometabolic disorders in schizophrenia is multifactorial and includes oxidative stress [5], conventional risk factors such as genetic and lifestyle factors, and drug side effects [6]. In addition, as in the general population, eating behaviors and eating disorders (EDs) are crucial in determining the etiology of cardiometabolic disorders in patients with schizophrenia [7]. EDs have been associated with profound physical and psychosocial morbidity and an elevated mortality risk [8, 9].

Although Eugen Bleuler described disturbances in eating behavior as a feature of schizophrenia in the early nineteenth century [10], EDs in schizophrenia remain understudied and poorly understood by health care providers [11, 12]. Indeed, EDs in schizophrenia remain difficult to assess, and schizophrenia patients with EDs usually do not meet all criteria for typical EDs, leading clinicians to consider EDs a secondary problem [13]. Our review focuses on EDs associated with schizophrenia and offers practical methods for their diagnosis and therapeutic management.

For this work, electronic searches were carried out using Medline, ScienceDirect, and Google Scholar for the following terms: "schizophrenia," "eating disorders," "anorexia nervosa," "bulimia nervosa," "binge eating disorder," or "night eating syndrome." The search was limited to articles published in English and French. Youssef Kouidrat and Ali Amad analyzed the studies, including case reports and case series.

2. Eating Disorders Associated with Schizophrenia

2.1. Anorexia Nervosa. With the recent release of the fifth iteration of the Diagnostic and Statistical Manual (DSM-5), diagnostic criteria for anorexia nervosa (AN) have undergone several changes [14]. AN is defined by persistent restriction of energy intake leading to significantly low body weight, intense fear of gaining weight, or persistent behavior that interferes with weight gain and disturbance in the way one's body weight or shape is experienced. The requirement for amenorrhea has been eliminated in DSM-5 [15]. AN is relatively common among young women with a lifetime prevalence up to 4% and a female to male sex ratio of 10 to 1 [16]. The mental illnesses most commonly associated with AN are major depression, anxiety disorders, and obsessive-compulsive disorders [17, 18]. Several evidences from case series have demonstrated the possibility of comorbidity between AN and schizophrenia with different prevalence rates [19–24].

The frequency of AN in schizophrenia has been approximated to be between 1 and 4% [11, 24]; the comorbidity between these disorders seems to vary with sex, at 0.81% for men and 4.01% for women, as found by Gotestam et al. in a large outpatient Norwegian psychiatric population, using a staff-report questionnaire [25]. Interestingly, men with AN are 3.6 times more likely to present with an associated diagnosis of schizophrenia than women [24].

AN can occur as a symptom on the spectrum of manifestations of schizophrenia, and overlapping symptoms in the psychopathology of schizophrenia and AN (such as distortion of body image and fear of being fat) are frequently observed. AN may precede or follow schizophrenia. For example, many male patients who are diagnosed with AN are found to have schizophrenia several years after the initial diagnosis (sometimes even 6 years later) [23, 26, 27].

Additionally, various clinical features of schizophrenia can lead to anorexia. For example, a depressive disorder can be associated with schizophrenia and lead to losses of appetite and weight. Second, due to paranoid delusions, the patient may believe that their food or drink is being poisoned or contaminated and refuse to eat it. Finally, acoustico-verbal hallucinations can be perceived as ordering a complete food refusal.

2.2. Bulimia Nervosa. Bulimia nervosa (BN) is characterized by recurrent episodes of binge eating followed by repeated inappropriate compensatory behaviors to prevent weight gain (such as self-induced vomiting, fasting, or excessive exercise or a misuse of laxatives or other medications) [28]. BN occurs in 1–3% of the population [16]. According to the DSM-5, binge eating and inappropriate compensatory behaviors should both occur, on average, at least once a week for 3 months.

Very little data exist on BN in schizophrenia. Gotestam et al. showed a prevalence of BN with schizophrenia of 0.73% for men and 1.57% for women [25]. In 1997, Deckelman et al. described a case of four young women with BN. In one case, BN clearly preceded the onset of schizophrenia; in the other 3 cases, the bulimic symptoms interacted significantly with the psychotic symptoms at the time of the diagnosis of schizophrenia. These case reports support a model wherein the coexistence of schizophrenia and bulimia may have important clinical implications [29]. Miotto et al. investigated the occurrence of symptoms of psychosis in 112 female patients diagnosed with DSM-IV eating disorders (AN = 61; BN = 51) and in 631 high school girls in the same health district as the patients. Compared with controls, a higher prevalence of symptoms of psychosis has been observed in patients with EDs; however, no cases of comorbid schizophrenia were observed [30]. In conclusion, there are very few studies on BN and schizophrenia, and the hypothesis of an association between these disorders remains to be proven.

2.3. Binge Eating Disorder. Binge eating disorder (BED) has recently been recognized as an ED in the DSM-5. BED is characterized by consuming large amounts of food in a short time period, at once a week for 3 months, and is accompanied by a sensation of losing control over eating. The diagnosis of BED must be associated with at least 3 of the following characteristics: (1) eating much more rapidly than normal, (2) eating until feeling uncomfortably full, (3) eating large amounts of food when not feeling physically hungry, (4) eating alone because being embarrassed of how much one is eating, or (5) feeling disgusted with oneself, depressed, or very guilty after overeating [14]. Moreover, binge eating in BED is not associated with the regular use of inappropriate compensatory behaviors [31].

The prevalence of BED in the general population varies between 0.7% [36] and 4.3% [37], and women are affected approximately 1.5 times more often than men [38]. One study evaluated the symptoms of BED among 31 patients with schizophrenia who were mostly overweight or obese (71% with BMI $\geq 25\,kg/m^2$). In this group, five patients (16%) met the criteria for BED, including three who reported the onset of signs after treatment with atypical antipsychotics [39]. Recently, Lundgren et al. showed a 6% prevalence of BED among 68 obese patients with schizophrenia and bipolar disorder [34]. These prevalence rates are higher than

TABLE 1: Data from descriptive studies evaluating the comorbidity of eating disorders in schizophrenia.

Authors	N	Sex (M/W)	Mean age (SD)	Assessment scale	Type of eating disorder	Prevalence (%)
Gotestam et al. 1995 [25]	10125	3544/6581	19–80	Staff-report questionnaire	AN, BN	**Men:** 0.81% for AN and 0.73% for BN **Women:** 4.01% for AN and 1.57% for BN
Striegel-Moore et al. 1999 [21]	22	22/0	Veterans	ICD	AN, BN	28%
Theisen et al. 2003 [32]	74	47/27	19.8 (±2.2)	QEWP	BED, BN	12.1% for BED 3.7% for BN
Stein et al. 2005 [22]	30	0/30	70 (±6.5)	EAT	AN	13.3%
Kluge et al. 2007 [33]	30	12/18	18–65	DSM-IV	BED	20%
Lundgren et al. 2010 [34]	68*	29/21	43.9 (±10.4)	NEQ, DSM IV, and QEWP	NES, BED	25% for NES 5.9% for BED
Palmese et al. 2011 [35]	100	39/61	46.5 (±10)	NEQ	NES	8%
M. H. Fawzi and M. M. Fawzi 2012 [12]	50	29/21	29.4 (±10.2)	EAT	Not determined	30%

ICD: International Classification of Diseases; QEWP: Questionnaire on Eating and Weight Patterns; EAT: Eating Attitude Test; DSM: Diagnostic and Statistical Manual of Mental Disorders; NEQ: Night Eating Questionnaire.
*Subjects characteristics: schizophrenia: 55.7%; bipolar disorder: 17.1%; major depressive disorder: 25.7%.

those found in the general population (approximately 2%). However, we must be cautious in interpreting this result, given the small sample of patients interviewed.

2.4. Night Eating Syndrome. First described by Stunkard et al. in 1955 [40], various diagnostic criteria for night eating syndrome (NES) have been published in recent years. NES is currently included in the "Other Specified Feeding or Eating Disorder" category of the DSM-5. It is characterized by an abnormally increased food intake in the evening and nighttime, manifested by consumption of at least 25% of intake after the evening meal, and/or nocturnal awakenings with ingestions at least twice per week [41]. Indeed, sleep disorders, which are common in schizophrenia [42], affect the hormonal regulation of food intake and are associated with metabolic disorders, obesity, and cardiovascular disease [43]. NES affects 1.5% of the general population, and between 8.9 and 27% of obese individuals [44].

Out of 175 patients with schizophrenia, Palmese et al. found an 8% prevalence of NES, which was significantly associated with increased rates of insomnia (44%), as assessed by the Pittsburgh Sleep Quality Index (PSQI) [35]. Very recently, out of 100 patients with schizophrenia or schizoaffective disorders and based on the *Night Eating Questionnaire* (NEQ), 8% met the full criteria for NES, with an additional 8% meeting the partial criteria [45]. In 2006, out of 205 psychiatric outpatients (regardless of BMI), Lundgren et al. found that 12% of patients met the criteria for NES [46]. Patients with NES were more likely to take antipsychotic medications than those without NES (38.8% versus 30.8%, resp., $P = 0.04$). In this sample, obese patients were five times more likely to meet the criteria for NES than nonobese patients. In 2010, the same team evaluated the prevalence of NES in a sample of 68 obese patients with schizophrenia and bipolar disorder. Using the NEQ, the prevalence appeared to be approximately 25% [34]. These studies suggest that patients with schizophrenia present an increased risk of NES.

2.5. Other Eating Disorders. The Eating Disorders section of the DSM-5 now includes avoidant/restrictive food intake disorder, pica, and rumination disorder. These 3 disorders were previously listed in the childhood disorders section of the DSM-IV-TR [15]. Small changes were made to the criteria for pica and rumination disorder.

Pica is defined as the repeated ingestion of nonnutritive substances (pebbles, hair, small metal objects, etc.). This disorder is common in children (and is found more rarely in adulthood) with developmental disorders (e.g., autism) or mental retardation [47]. In schizophrenia, it can be defined as an impulsive consumption associated with delusions. Domingo-Claros et al. reported a case of a 29-year-old woman with schizophrenia and severe anemia who was diagnosed with lead poisoning (saturnism) as a result the pica ingestion of small metal jewelry found in her stomach during an endoscopy [48]. Many cases of coprophagia, defined as the ingestion of feces and considered a variant of pica, have been associated with schizophrenia [49]. Finally, many studies suggest a significant association between schizophrenia and potomania, defined as the ingestion of beverages in large quantities, on the order of 8 to 10 liters per day. In cases of water intoxication, severe metabolic imbalances can occur, leading to hyponatremia, convulsions, and coma [50].

In Table 1, descriptive epidemiological studies conducted using widely used scales in the psychiatric population are summarized.

3. Antipsychotics and Eating Behaviors

Antipsychotic drugs remain essential in the therapeutic management of schizophrenia. These treatments have remarkable therapeutic efficacy and result in great improvements in positive symptoms, prevention of deterioration, cognitive function, quality of life, and reduction in the number of (re)hospitalizations [51, 52]. However, they are likely to be associated with varying degrees of metabolic adverse effects, such as weight gain, dyslipidemia, and impaired glucose metabolism. These detrimental metabolic effects are associated with the vast majority of first- and second-generation antipsychotics [53, 54]. Most studies have focused on the importance of weight gain during treatment, and several potential mechanisms have been widely studied. However, the factors related to changes in eating behavior induced by antipsychotics remain surprisingly poorly studied, while changes in food intake and the modification of the signals of satiety have been observed and proposed as mechanisms of weight gain [55].

Very few studies were found concerning food intake modifications associated with antipsychotics. A study evaluating the eating behaviors of 153 patients with schizophrenia using the Three-Factor Eating Questionnaire (TFEQ) and the Dutch Eating Behavior Questionnaire (DEBQ) observed that patients treated with atypical antipsychotics were more responsive to external food cues and had higher scores on the item "loss of control eating behavior" than patients taking first-generation antipsychotics or control subjects [56]. In addition, treatment with clozapine and olanzapine was significantly associated with compulsive overeating and BED [32, 33].

Several mechanisms of weight gain and increased food intake associated with antipsychotics have been proposed and are summarized in the following:

(1) direct effects on antipsychotics receptors,

(2) direct or indirect effects on the neuronal circuits (hypothalamus) controlling food intake and satiety,

(3) disruption of the hypothalamic-pituitary-adrenal axis,

(4) direct effect on insulin sensitivity and insulin secretion,

(5) effects on gastrointestinal hormones involved in food intake,

(6) decreased physical activity and decreased basal metabolism.

Antipsychotic drugs can affect multiple neurotransmitter systems and exert antagonistic actions on dopamine receptors, serotonergics, histamine, muscarinics, and adrenergics [57]. All of these neurotransmitters have been directly or indirectly involved in the pathways associated with the regulation of food intake [58], metabolism [59, 60], and weight balance [61, 62]. Blockades of dopamine (D2 and D3), serotonin (5HT2c), histamine (H1) [63], and muscarinic (M2 and M3) receptors have all been shown to increase appetite [64, 65]. Additionally, by endocrine/metabolic mechanisms, antipsychotics can directly induce the activation of the hypothalamus-pituitary-adrenal axis [66], deficits in insulin secretion [67], and changes in gastrointestinal hormones [68]. Other studies suggested a relationship between the increased food intake induced by an antipsychotic drug and changes in leptin, melatonin, opioid, and endocannabinoid signaling [69]. Moreover, the weight gain liabilities of antipsychotic drugs seem to be partly associated with their ability to increase appetite [70].

Despite the relevance of these studies, it is clear that the mechanisms underlying the effects of antipsychotics on eating behavior are insufficiently understood. A better understanding of the role of changes in eating behaviors during antipsychotic treatment is necessary for both clinicians and patients. Indeed, any change in appetite could be a harbinger of weight gain, and, thus, preventive measures (choice of antipsychotic treatment, patient education and/or counseling on lifestyle and dietary rules) with a demonstrated efficacy should be taken [71]. In addition, patients and their families should be informed in advance of these side effects so that they are better able to manage them.

4. Discussion and Recommendations

In clinical practice, many combinations of EDs and schizophrenia are possible, as these diagnoses are certainly not mutually exclusive. The EDs may occur together with or independent of the psychotic symptoms of patients [13]. In some clinical situations, ED coexists as a separate clinical entity of schizophrenia. Sometimes, the ED represents a symptom that may be the first manifestation of a psychotic disorder, such as schizophrenia.

However, despite a high prevalence of comorbidity between schizophrenia and EDs, this topic remains relatively unexplored. According to our literature review, the prevalence of EDs differed according to the methodology, sample sizes, and scales of the studies. Thus, AN affects between 1 and 4% of patients with schizophrenia. In addition, BED and NES have an average prevalence of 5–20% in the schizophrenia population (approximately 5 times higher than in the general population) [34, 45].

The origin of the development of EDs in these patients remains unclear, and related psychopathological and neurobiological mechanisms need to be further explored. Otherwise, a number of limitations of the existing descriptive studies should be highlighted. These mainly pertain to differences in methodological approach (cross-sectional studies, small samples, outpatient/inpatient, and self-administered questionnaires versus semistructured interviews). Many confounding factors are insufficiently taken into account, such as age, sex, disease duration, and treatment with other psychoactive drugs. Indeed, in addition to antipsychotics, patients often consume anxiolytics, antidepressants, and other mood stabilizers with well-documented side effects of increased appetite and weight gain [72]. Finally, the impact of a bad socioeconomic environment, which frequently affects this vulnerable population, is rarely analyzed in studies. This socioeconomic insecurity is directly responsible for their limited access to medical care and healthy food and represents a major obstacle to the implementation of lifestyle and dietary rules, instead contributing to an unbalanced diet and insufficient physical exercise [6]. Moreover, the pharmacological treatment of EDs remains an underdeveloped field [73].

From a clinical point of view, we want to emphasize the importance of screening and assessment for comorbid EDs in patients presenting with schizophrenia. For example, antipsychotics have been implicated in binge eating symptomatology and other compulsive disorders [32, 33]. These compulsive symptoms may improve or cease when the antipsychotic is withdrawn or replaced. The clinician should distinguish this situation from a preexisting eating disorder. Interestingly, many screening tools for EDs exist, such as questionnaires or semistructured interviews, and should be included in these research protocols. Revised versions with a reduced number of items are now available. Their use within a multidisciplinary framework (physician, psychologist, and dietician) can allow a better approach to the EDs, leading to more accurate and reproducible assessment in monitoring. In addition, some of these self-rating scales have been translated and validated in several languages.

In conclusion, we should keep in mind that somatic and/or behavior comorbidities are often associated with schizophrenia. Given their frequency and negative impact on quality of life, the assessment of these specific EDs in schizophrenia needs to be improved. The screening and management of patients suffering from schizophrenia with EDs must be multidisciplinary. Coordinated actions among psychiatrists, general practitioners, psychotherapists, endocrinologists, nurses, dieticians and patients' families might be a valuable assistance to optimal care [74, 75]. Further studies should be performed in this domain because the available literature on the subject is very poor. The recommendations proposed for clinical practice are summarized in the following.

(i) Assess eating behaviors and screen for EDs, using validated tools if necessary.

(ii) Recognize the somatic risks associated with EDs and assessing the patient's nutritional status (e.g., malnutrition, weight gain, and cardiometabolic disorders).

(iii) Interview the patient about his or her quality and duration of sleep.

(iv) Educate patients and family members on the side effects of antipsychotics (change in appetite, weight gain, risk of glucose intolerance, and lipid abnormalities).

(v) Adjust, if possible, the patient's antipsychotic treatment in accordance with his or her metabolic profile.

(vi) Organize multidisciplinary and early management of EDs.

(vii) Develop a personalized and comprehensive treatment strategy, including lifestyle measures (diet, adapted physical activity, and sleep hygiene).

(viii) Use cognitive behavioral therapies that have proven effective in the field of EDs.

Conflict of Interests

The authors declare that there is no conflict of interests regarding the publication of this paper.

References

[1] J. van Os and S. Kapur, "Schizophrenia," *The Lancet*, vol. 374, no. 9690, pp. 635–645, 2009.

[2] P. F. Buckley, B. J. Miller, D. S. Lehrer, and D. J. Castle, "Psychiatric comorbidities and schizophrenia," *Schizophrenia Bulletin*, vol. 35, no. 2, pp. 383–402, 2009.

[3] S. Saha, D. Chant, and J. McGrath, "A systematic review of mortality in schizophrenia: is the differential mortality gap worsening over time?" *Archives of General Psychiatry*, vol. 64, no. 10, pp. 1123–1131, 2007.

[4] C. H. Hennekens, A. R. Hennekens, D. Hollar, and D. E. Casey, "Schizophrenia and increased risks of cardiovascular disease," *American Heart Journal*, vol. 150, no. 6, pp. 1115–1121, 2005.

[5] Y. Kouidrat, A. Amad, R. Desailloud et al., "Increased advanced glycation end-products (AGEs) assessed by skin autofluorescence in schizophrenia," *Journal of Psychiatric Research*, vol. 47, no. 8, pp. 1044–1048, 2013.

[6] M. de Hert, C. U. Correll, J. Bobes et al., "Physical illness in patients with severe mental disorders. I. Prevalence, impact of medications and disparities in health care," *World Psychiatry*, vol. 10, no. 1, pp. 52–77, 2011.

[7] A. Golay, E. Brock, R. Gabriel et al., "Taking small steps towards targets—perspectives for clinical practice in diabetes, cardiometabolic disorders and beyond," *International Journal of Clinical Practice*, vol. 67, no. 4, pp. 322–332, 2013.

[8] K. L. Klump, C. M. Bulik, W. H. Kaye, J. Treasure, and E. Tyson, "Academy for eating disorders position paper: eating disorders are serious mental illnesses," *International Journal of Eating Disorders*, vol. 42, no. 2, pp. 97–103, 2009.

[9] J. Treasure, A. M. Claudino, and N. Zucker, "Eating disorders," *The Lancet*, vol. 375, no. 9714, pp. 583–593, 2010.

[10] P. Hoff, "Eugen Bleuler's concept of schizophrenia and its relevance to present-day psychiatry," *Neuropsychobiology*, vol. 66, no. 1, pp. 6–13, 2012.

[11] C. Foulon, "Schizophrenia and eating disorders," *Encephale*, vol. 29, no. 5, pp. 463–466, 2003.

[12] M. H. Fawzi and M. M. Fawzi, "Disordered eating attitudes in Egyptian antipsychotic naive patients with schizophrenia," *Comprehensive Psychiatry*, vol. 53, no. 3, pp. 259–268, 2012.

[13] S. Y. Yum, G. Caracci, and M. Y. Hwang, "Schizophrenia and eating disorders," *Psychiatric Clinics of North America*, vol. 32, no. 4, pp. 809–819, 2009.

[14] American Psychiatric Association, *Diagnostic and Statistical Manual of Mental Disorders: DSM-5*, American Psychiatric Association, Arlington, Va, USA, 2013.

[15] C. Call, B. T. Walsh, and E. Attia, "From DSM-IV to DSM-5: changes to eating disorder diagnoses," *Current Opinion in Psychiatry*, vol. 26, no. 6, pp. 532–536, 2013.

[16] F. R. E. Smink, D. Van Hoeken, and H. W. Hoek, "Epidemiology, course, and outcome of eating disorders," *Current Opinion in Psychiatry*, vol. 26, no. 6, pp. 543–548, 2013.

[17] M. K. Heaner and B. T. Walsh, "A history of the identification of the characteristic eating disturbances of Bulimia Nervosa, Binge Eating Disorder and Anorexia Nervosa," *Appetite*, vol. 65, pp. 185–188, 2013.

[18] H. Roux, E. Chapelon, and N. Godart, "Épidémiologie de l'anorexie mentale: revue de la littérature," *L'Encéphale*, vol. 39, no. 2, pp. 85–93, 2013.

[19] L. K. G. Hsu, E. S. Meltzer, and A. H. Crisp, "Schizophrenia and anorexia nervosa," *Journal of Nervous and Mental Disease*, vol. 169, no. 5, pp. 273–276, 1981.

[20] J. M. Ferguson and N. F. Damluji, "Anorexia nervosa and schizophrenia," *International Journal of Eating Disorders*, vol. 7, no. 3, pp. 343–352, 1988.

[21] R. H. Striegel-Moore, V. Garvin, F. A. Dohm, and R. A. Rosenheck, "Psychiatric comorbidity of eating disorders in men: a national study of hospitalized veterans," *International Journal of Eating Disorders*, vol. 25, no. 4, pp. 399–404, 1999.

[22] D. Stein, C. Zemishlani, B. Shahal, and Y. Barak, "Disordered eating in elderly female patients diagnosed with chronic schizophrenia," *The Israel Journal of Psychiatry and Related Sciences*, vol. 42, no. 3, pp. 191–197, 2005.

[23] B. Cinemre and B. Kulaksizoğlu, "Case report: comorbid anorexia nervosa and schizophrenia in a male patient," *Turk Psikiyatri Dergisi*, vol. 18, no. 1, pp. 87–91, 2007.

[24] R. B. Khalil, D. Hachem, and S. Richa, "Eating disorders and schizophrenia in male patients: a review," *Eating and Weight Disorders*, vol. 16, no. 3, pp. e150–e156, 2011.

[25] K. G. Gotestam, L. Eriksen, and H. Hagen, "An epidemiological study of eating disorders in Norwegian psychiatric institutions," *International Journal of Eating Disorders*, vol. 18, no. 3, pp. 263–268, 1995.

[26] P. Cheung and E. Wilder-Smith, "Anorexia nervosa and schizophrenia in a male Chinese," *International Journal of Eating Disorders*, vol. 18, no. 1, pp. 103–106, 1995.

[27] B. Kiraly and E. A. Joy, "Case report. Anorexia nervosa and psychosis in a male triathlete," *Current Sports Medicine Reports*, vol. 2, no. 6, pp. 317–319, 2003.

[28] G. T. Wilson and R. Sysko, "Frequency of binge eating episodes in bulimia nervosa and binge eating disorder: diagnostic considerations," *International Journal of Eating Disorders*, vol. 42, no. 7, pp. 603–610, 2009.

[29] M. C. Deckelman, L. B. Dixon, and R. R. Conley, "Comorbid bulimia nervosa and schizophrenia," *International Journal of Eating Disorders*, vol. 22, no. 1, pp. 101–105, 1997.

[30] P. Miotto, B. Pollini, A. Restaneo et al., "Symptoms of psychosis in anorexia and bulimia nervosa," *Psychiatry Research*, vol. 175, no. 3, pp. 237–243, 2010.

[31] Z. Cooper and C. G. Fairburn, "Refining the definition of binge eating disorder and nonpurging bulimia nervosa," *International Journal of Eating Disorders*, vol. 34, no. S1, pp. S89–S95, 2003.

[32] F. M. Theisen, A. Linden, I. R. König, M. Martin, H. Remschmidt, and J. Hebebrand, "Spectrum of binge eating symptomatology in patients treated with clozapine and olanzapine," *Journal of Neural Transmission*, vol. 110, no. 1, pp. 111–121, 2003.

[33] M. Kluge, A. Schuld, H. Himmerich et al., "Clozapine and olanzapine are associated with food craving and binge eating: results from a randomized double-blind study," *Journal of Clinical Psychopharmacology*, vol. 27, no. 6, pp. 662–666, 2007.

[34] J. D. Lundgren, M. V. Rempfer, C. E. Brown, J. Goetz, and E. Hamera, "The prevalence of night eating syndrome and binge eating disorder among overweight and obese individuals with serious mental illness," *Psychiatry Research*, vol. 175, no. 3, pp. 233–236, 2010.

[35] L. B. Palmese, P. C. DeGeorge, J. C. Ratliff et al., "Insomnia is frequent in schizophrenia and associated with night eating and obesity," *Schizophrenia Research*, vol. 133, no. 1–3, pp. 238–243, 2011.

[36] A. Basdevant, M. Pouillon, N. Lahlou, M. Le Barzic, M. Brillant, and B. Guy-Grand, "Prevalence of binge eating disorder in different populations of French women," *International Journal of Eating Disorders*, vol. 18, no. 4, pp. 309–315, 1995.

[37] R. L. Spitzer, S. Yanovski, T. Wadden et al., "Binge eating disorder: its further validation in a multisite study," *International Journal of Eating Disorders*, vol. 13, no. 2, pp. 137–153, 1993.

[38] M. de Zwaan, "Binge eating disorder and obesity," *International Journal of Obesity*, vol. 25, supplement 1, pp. S51–S55, 2001.

[39] C. E. Ramacciotti, R. A. Paoli, M. Catena et al., "Schizophrenia and binge-eating disorders," *Journal of Clinical Psychiatry*, vol. 65, no. 7, pp. 1016–1017, 2004.

[40] A. J. Stunkard, W. J. Grace, and H. G. Wolff, "The night-eating syndrome; a pattern of food intake among certain obese patients," *The American Journal of Medicine*, vol. 19, no. 1, pp. 78–86, 1955.

[41] K. C. Allison, J. D. Lundgren, J. P. O'Reardon et al., "Proposed diagnostic criteria for night eating syndrome," *International Journal of Eating Disorders*, vol. 43, no. 3, pp. 241–247, 2010.

[42] S. Cohrs, "Sleep disturbances in patients with schizophrenia: impact and effect of antipsychotics," *CNS Drugs*, vol. 22, no. 11, pp. 939–962, 2008.

[43] K. Spiegel, E. Tasali, R. Leproult, and E. van Cauter, "Effects of poor and short sleep on glucose metabolism and obesity risk," *Nature Reviews Endocrinology*, vol. 5, no. 5, pp. 253–261, 2009.

[44] C. S. Rand, A. M. Macgregor, and A. J. Stunkard, "The night eating syndrome in the general population and among postoperative obesity surgery patients," *International Journal of Eating Disorders*, vol. 22, no. 1, pp. 65–69, 1997.

[45] L. B. Palmese, J. C. Ratliff, E. L. Reutenauer, K. M. Tonizzo, C. M. Grilo, and C. Tek, "Prevalence of night eating in obese individuals with schizophrenia and schizoaffective disorder," *Comprehensive Psychiatry*, vol. 54, no. 3, pp. 276–281, 2013.

[46] J. D. Lundgren, K. C. Allison, S. Crow et al., "Prevalence of the night eating syndrome in a psychiatric population," *American Journal of Psychiatry*, vol. 163, no. 1, pp. 156–158, 2006.

[47] C. B. Delaney, K. T. Eddy, A. S. Hartmann, A. E. Becker, H. B. Murray, and J. J. Thomas, "Pica and rumination behavior among individuals seeking treatment for eating disorders or obesity," *International Journal of Eating Disorders*, 2014.

[48] A. Domingo-Claros, E. Alonso, and E. de La Banda, "Schizophrenia and refractory anaemia with ring sideroblasts," *British Journal of Haematology*, vol. 125, no. 5, p. 543, 2004.

[49] D. A. Beck and N. R. Frohberg, "Coprophagia in an elderly man: a case report and review of the literature," *International Journal of Psychiatry in Medicine*, vol. 35, no. 4, pp. 417–427, 2005.

[50] E. Mercier-Guidez and G. Loas, "Polydipsia and water intoxication in 353 psychiatric inpatients: an epidemiological and psychopathological study," *European Psychiatry*, vol. 15, no. 5, pp. 306–311, 2000.

[51] A. G. Awad and L. N. P. Voruganti, "The impact of newer atypical antipsychotics on patient-reported outcomes in schizophrenia," *CNS Drugs*, vol. 27, no. 8, pp. 625–636, 2013.

[52] S. Leucht, A. Cipriani, L. Spineli et al., "Comparative efficacy and tolerability of 15 antipsychotic drugs in schizophrenia: a multiple-treatments meta-analysis," *The Lancet*, vol. 382, no. 9896, pp. 951–962, 2013.

[53] D. B. Allison, J. L. Mentore, M. Heo et al., "Antipsychotic-induced weight gain: a comprehensive research synthesis,"

American Journal of Psychiatry, vol. 156, no. 11, pp. 1686–1696, 1999.

[54] J. W. Newcomer, "Second-generation (atypical) antipsychotics and metabolic effects: a comprehensive literature review," *CNS Drugs*, vol. 19, supplement 1, pp. 1–93, 2005.

[55] T. Lencz, D. G. Robinson, B. Napolitano et al., "DRD2 promoter region variation predicts antipsychotic-induced weight gain in first episode schizophrenia," *Pharmacogenetics and Genomics*, vol. 20, no. 9, pp. 569–572, 2010.

[56] O. Sentissi, A. Viala, M. C. Bourdel et al., "Impact of antipsychotic treatments on the motivation to eat: preliminary results in 153 schizophrenic patients," *International Clinical Psychopharmacology*, vol. 24, no. 5, pp. 257–264, 2009.

[57] F. C. J. Starrenburg and J. P. A. M. Bogers, "How can antipsychotics cause diabetes mellitus? Insights based on receptor-binding profiles, humoral factors and transporter proteins," *European Psychiatry*, vol. 24, no. 3, pp. 164–170, 2009.

[58] K. Weston-Green, X.-F. Huang, M. Han, and C. Deng, "The effects of antipsychotics on the density of cannabinoid receptors in the dorsal vagal complex of rats: implications for olanzapine-induced weight gain," *International Journal of Neuropsychopharmacology*, vol. 11, no. 6, pp. 827–835, 2008.

[59] J.-K. Sharpe, N. M. Byrne, T. J. Stedman, and A. P. Hills, "Resting energy expenditure is lower than predicted in people taking atypical antipsychotic medication," *Journal of the American Dietetic Association*, vol. 105, no. 4, pp. 612–615, 2005.

[60] J.-K. Sharpe, T. J. Stedman, N. M. Byrne, C. Wishart, and A. P. Hills, "Energy expenditure and physical activity in clozapine use: implications for weight management," *Australian & New Zealand Journal of Psychiatry*, vol. 40, no. 9, pp. 810–814, 2006.

[61] G. P. Reynolds and S. L. Kirk, "Metabolic side effects of antipsychotic drug treatment—pharmacological mechanisms," *Pharmacology and Therapeutics*, vol. 125, no. 1, pp. 169–179, 2010.

[62] T. A. P. Lett, T. J. M. Wallace, N. I. Chowdhury, A. K. Tiwari, J. L. Kennedy, and D. J. Müller, "Pharmacogenetics of antipsychotic-induced weight gain: review and clinical implications," *Molecular Psychiatry*, vol. 17, no. 3, pp. 242–266, 2012.

[63] S. F. Kim, A. S. Huang, A. M. Snowman, C. Teuscher, and S. H. Snyder, "Antipsychotic drug-induced weight gain mediated by histamine H1 receptor-linked activation of hypothalamic AMP-kinase," *Proceedings of the National Academy of Sciences of the United States of America*, vol. 104, no. 9, pp. 3456–3459, 2007.

[64] C. U. Correll, T. Lencz, and A. K. Malhotra, "Antipsychotic drugs and obesity," *Trends in Molecular Medicine*, vol. 17, no. 2, pp. 97–107, 2011.

[65] R. Coccurello and A. Moles, "Potential mechanisms of atypical antipsychotic-induced metabolic derangement: clues for understanding obesity and novel drug design," *Pharmacology and Therapeutics*, vol. 127, no. 3, pp. 210–251, 2010.

[66] T. Baptista, J. Zárate, R. Joober et al., "Drug induced weight gain, an impediment to successful pharmacotherapy: focus on antipsychotics," *Current Drug Targets*, vol. 5, no. 3, pp. 279–299, 2004.

[67] A. F. Chintoh, S. W. Mann, L. Lam et al., "Insulin resistance and decreased glucose-stimulated insulin secretion after acute olanzapine administration," *Journal of Clinical Psychopharmacology*, vol. 28, no. 5, pp. 494–499, 2008.

[68] E. Palik, K. D. Birkás, G. Faludi, I. Karádi, and K. Cseh, "Correlation of serum ghrelin levels with body mass index and carbohydrate metabolism in patients treated with atypical antipsychotics," *Diabetes Research and Clinical Practice*, vol. 68, supplement 1, pp. S60–S64, 2005.

[69] H. A. Nasrallah, "Atypical antipsychotic-induced metabolic side effects: insights from receptor-binding profiles," *Molecular Psychiatry*, vol. 13, no. 1, pp. 27–35, 2008.

[70] U. Werneke, D. Taylor, and T. A. B. Sanders, "Behavioral interventions for antipsychotic induced appetite changes," *Current Psychiatry Reports*, vol. 15, no. 3, article 347, 2013.

[71] V. L. Stauffer, I. Lipkovich, V. P. Hoffmann, A. N. Heinloth, H. S. Scott, and B. J. Kinon, "Predictors and correlates for weight changes in patients co-treated with olanzapine and weight mitigating agents; a post-hoc analysis," *BMC Psychiatry*, vol. 9, article 12, 2009.

[72] A. Serretti and L. Mandelli, "Antidepressants and body weight: a comprehensive review and meta-analysis," *Journal of Clinical Psychiatry*, vol. 71, no. 10, pp. 1259–1272, 2010.

[73] J. E. Mitchell, J. Roerig, and K. Steffen, "Biological therapies for eating disorders," *International Journal of Eating Disorders*, vol. 46, no. 5, pp. 470–477, 2013.

[74] D. Le Grange, J. Lock, K. Loeb, and D. Nicholls, "Academy for eating disorders position paper: the role of the family in eating disorders," *International Journal of Eating Disorders*, vol. 43, no. 1, pp. 1–5, 2010.

[75] W. S. Agras and A. H. Robinson, "Forty years of progress in the treatment of the eating disorders," *Nordic Journal of Psychiatry*, vol. 62, supplement 47, pp. 19–24, 2008.

22

Effect of a System-Oriented Intervention on Compliance Problems in Schizophrenia: A Pragmatic Controlled Trial

Hanne Skarsholm,[1] Henrik Stoevring,[2] and Bent Nielsen[3]

[1] *The Psychiatry in the Region of Southern Denmark, Søndre, Sdr. Boulevard 29, 5000 Odense C, Denmark*
[2] *Department of Public Health, Aarhus University, 8000 Aarhus C, Denmark*
[3] *Department of Psychiatry, The Psychiatry in the Region of Southern Denmark, 5000 Odense, Denmark*

Correspondence should be addressed to Hanne Skarsholm; hskarsholm@health.sdu.dk

Academic Editor: Robin Emsley

Background. Numerous studies have been conducted with a view to developing strategies for improvement of medical compliance in patients with schizophrenia. All of the studies conducted so far have had an individual approach to compliance based on the assumption that noncompliance is determined individually due to inappropriate behavior in the patient. We conducted a pragmatic controlled trial with a system-oriented approach, to provide a new perspective on compliance and test the efficacy of a multifactorial intervention at the system level in a routine clinical setting, an approach that has not previously been used for the improvement of compliance. *Methods.* 30 patients were allocated to the system-oriented therapy and 40 patients were allocated to the reference intervention, which consisted of individually based compliance therapy. The follow-up period was six months. Primary endpoint was improvement in compliance, measured by improvement in a compliance scale specifically developed for the project. *Results.* When accounting for missing values with a multiple imputation approach, we found a tendency toward a difference in both the compliance scale and PANSS favoring the system-oriented therapy, although it did not reach statistical significance. A significant difference in incidence of adverse events and time to first readmission was found. Attrition rates were significantly higher in the reference group and nonsignificant among individuals with lower compliance, which may have diluted effect estimates. This was reflected by significant differences found in an analysis based on a last observation carried forward approach. *Conclusion.* This study suggests that compliance problems are better solved by a multifactorial intervention at the system level than at the individual level.

1. Background

Schizophrenia is a severe mental illness [1], for which the cornerstone of treatment is antipsychotic medication [2]. Compliance with the medications is poor, as only approximately 50% of the prescribed medication is consumed [3], even though a compromised compliance has extensive clinical and economic consequences [4, 5]. Consequently, numerous studies have been conducted to develop strategies for the improvement of compliance in schizophrenia [6–18]. These studies have all had an individual approach to compliance based on the assumption that noncompliance is individually determined and due to inappropriate behavior of the patient. Alternatively noncompliance could be regarded as an "incident" caused by a "system failure" [19], that is, a product of failed processes within the organization. From this perspective, key elements in improving compliance would be to establish monitoring to minimize errors, build barriers that prevent errors, and perform careful analysis when errors are made in order to identify causes and prevent recurrence. This approach uses principles of clinical risk management and quality assurance principles [20].

Based on a system-oriented approach, we will in this study bring a new perspective on compliance and test the efficacy of a multifactorial intervention at the system level in comparison with a more traditional individual based intervention with respect to improving compliance in patients with schizophrenia, which as far as we know has not previously been done.

The study is a pragmatic controlled trial in the sense that interventions were delivered in a routine general adult

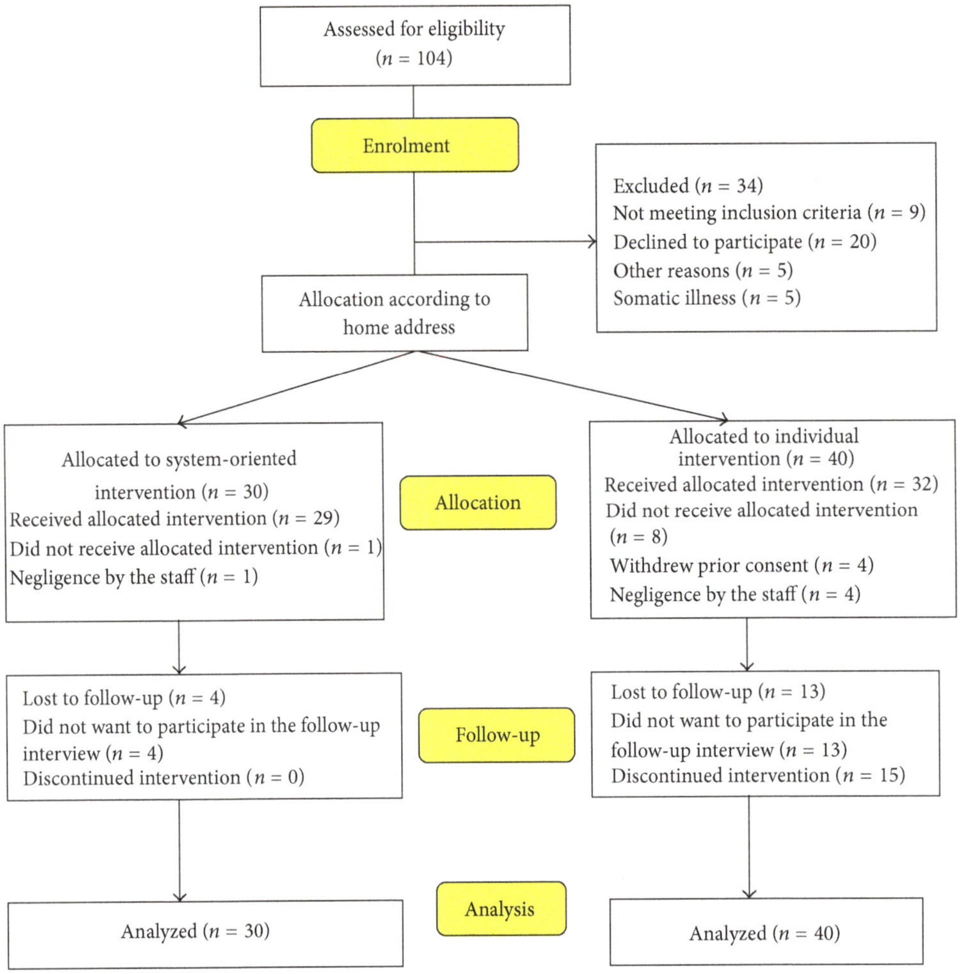

FIGURE 1: Flow chart.

psychiatric setting so as to maximize generalisability of its results.

2. Methods

2.1. Study Setting and Design. Two open psychiatric sections at the Department of Psychiatry, Odense, Denmark, participated in the study with their community mental health teams assigned to the respective sections. Each section and assigned team received patients from geographically well-defined areas in Odense and there was no significant difference in the patient population or staff composition in observed characteristics. The patients were allocated to one of the two participating psychiatric sections according to their home address. In one section, the system-oriented intervention was implemented, and the individual-oriented approach was in the other section.

The flow diagram shows the study design schematically (Figure 1).

Patients, who fulfilled the inclusion criteria, were invited to participate in the study within a few days after admission. If they accepted, informed written consent was obtained and an index interview conducted before the intervention was started. The follow-up period ended with an interview after six months.

Medical records were collected to obtain information on readmissions and bed days from baseline and in the subsequent 12 months.

The two intervention groups were considered to represent a reference intervention and an experimental intervention, respectively. We chose to use a reference group rather than a control group with treatment as usual, since compliance problems tend to disappear when focusing on them, regardless of the nature of the intervention [21].

2.2. Study Population. Criteria for including patients admitted in the study period were ICD-10 diagnosis of schizophrenia or schizoaffective disorder; age of 23–70 years; Danish ethnicity; being supposed to be followed up by the community mental health teams; and not being subject to legal action.

104 patients were assessed to be included of which 34 were excluded; see Figure 1. The intervention groups thus consisted of 30 patients in the system-oriented intervention group and 40 patients in the individual group.

The study was conducted in accordance with the Declaration of Helsinki and approved by The Ethics Committee, Region of Southern Denmark, Denmark.

2.3. Interventions

2.3.1. The System-Oriented Intervention. The system-oriented intervention will be briefly introduced here—for further details please see Skarsholm and Nielsen [22].

The system-oriented intervention was based on five standards (qualitative), which intended to improve medical compliance. The five standards dealt with the following topics: information, compliance, reminders, medication reconciliation, and clinical guidelines for treatment with antipsychotic medications.

(1) Information. Standard concerning information on antipsychotic drug treatment.

The standard contained a brochure on antipsychotic drug treatment and a questionnaire as a basis for conversation between the patient and his or her primary care provider about the patient's experience of information.

(2) Compliance. Standard concerning focus on identifying and solving compliance problems.

The standard was designed to ensure a regular focus on compliance issues in conversations between patient and nurse by using a screening form for identification of compliance problems. Identified obstacles should be sought removed.

(3) Reminders. Standard concerning reminder systems.

The content of this standard was a "reminder box." It contained among f x medicine cards, medicine dosage boxes, electronic alarm systems for reminding of medication intake, and reminder of prescription renewal. There were no restrictions on the content of the box, and it was allowed to add relevant reminders during the project period.

(4) Medication Reconciliation. Standard concerning medication reconciliation at transfer.

This standard focused on avoidance of potential medication errors when transferring between different sectors. The concept of medication reconciliation involves control of medication in any relocation including discharge.

(5) Clinical Guidelines for Treatment with Antipsychotic Medications. The guidelines were developed by psychiatrists and clinical pharmacologists affiliated to Odense University Hospital after the extensive literature studies. The clinical guidelines should provide the standard for good clinical practice in antipsychotic drug therapy.

The performance of the standards was recorded in monitoring schemes and evaluated at audits twice a year with subsequent feedback to the clinical team.

For patients readmitted with compliance problems a special in-depth audit, so-called "aggregate root cause analysis" (http://www.patientsafety.gov/), was performed, which means that multiple occurrences of the same character accrued over a given time were analyzed simultaneously in order to identify causes for noncompliance and give feedback to the care providers. This method is ideal where there are likely frequent occurrences within a given period, especially when these occurrences look like each other, meaning that you can identify common trends in the causes you find for non-compliance in the analyses.

Prior to the inclusion of patients the involved staff participated in a four-day course consisting of training in psychopharmacology, psychopathology, quality and risk management, root cause analysis, and compliance promotion.

2.3.2. The Individual Intervention. The individual intervention consisted of compliance therapy, which was a manual based short-term therapy, based on an individual, cognitive-behavioral therapeutic approach to improvement of compliance in people with schizophrenia. It was built on the principles of "motivational interviewing" [23] and "concordance skills" [24]. It consisted of 6 sessions and 3 booster sessions each of 30–45 minutes' length.

The therapy consisted of 6 areas: (1) assessments of current medication, attitudes towards medication, and adverse events, (2) solving problems related to medication, (3) reviewing former positive and negative experiences with different treatment strategies, (4) study of ambivalence, (5) concerns and expectations in relation to medicine, and (6) the future, including relapse prevention and warning signals.

In all phases the motivational interviewing style was used, which included clarifying the discrepancy between the patient's desires and behavior in relation to medicine. The aim of the therapy was to achieve joint decision making about medicines, since a central tenet of the therapy was that a joint decision will increase compliance.

Prior to the inclusion of patients a four-day course was held for the staff involved in the individual intervention group, consisting of education in psychopharmacology and psychopathology and training in "motivational interviewing." The teacher in "motivational interviewing" was trained by the founder of the therapy and was responsible for the ongoing supervision during the project.

Both interventions were intended to be initiated in the ward and continued in the community mental health teams.

2.4. Objectives and Outcomes. The primary endpoint was improvement on a compliance scale specifically developed for the project and consisting of 4 items: (1) compliance self-assessment by the patient, (2) Drug Attitude Inventory (DAI-10) [24], (3) appointment keeping with the common mental health system, and (4) PANSS-item G12 concerning judgment about illness and need for treatment [25]. All items are proven methods to assess compliance [26–32], but no method is considered to be the gold standard. A combination of measures maximizes accuracy [3].

Validation of the scale resulted in Crohnbach's alpha coefficient of 0.81. Loevinger's coefficient, H, was 0.61, 0.64, 0.52, and 0.62 of items 1, 2, 3, and 4, respectively. Possible scores on the compliance scale ranged from 0 to 8 points.

The secondary endpoints were improvement in a number of recognized clinical scales, as an indirect measure of improved compliance: Positive and Negative Syndrome Scale's (PANSS) remission criteria [25], Global Assessment of Functioning Scale (GAF) [33], and Subjective Well-Being on Neuroleptic Treatment Scale (SWN) [34].

The UKU side effects rating scale (UKU) [35] was also used as the presence of side effects indicates actual consumption of the medication.

The tertiary endpoints were time from discharge to first rehospitalization and bed day consumption within 12 months.

2.5. Statistical Analysis. Prior to enrolment of patients a power calculation was undertaken. We assumed an improvement in compliance score of at least 1.00 points on average. We also assumed that there would be a baseline standard deviation of compliance points of maximum 1.00. Under these conditions a minimum of 40 participants in the project was needed in order to achieve a power of 80% at a significance level of 5%.

For comparison of unpaired, numeric, nonnormally distributed data, the Mann-Whitney test was applied. For comparison of unpaired, numeric, normally distributed data, the *t*-test was used. To provide confidence intervals for estimated differences of nonnormally distributed data, robust variance estimates were used. For comparison of categorical data, Fisher's exact test was applied. The two-sided significance level was set to 5%.

All participants were primarily analyzed by the intention-to-treat principle with the method of multiple imputation (MI) and alternatively with the last-observation-carried-forward (LOCF) method.

To account for missing data by MI, we identified the baseline variables that were best predictors of whether a subject completed follow-up and used these in a multiple imputation to predict missing values of the outcomes. Based on the literature we assumed that low GAF score, age, duration of illness, compliance at baseline, and abuse status were both related to whether a patient would fail to complete follow-up and what the missing values would have been had they not been missing. 10 sets of multiply imputed data were generated and analyzed.

All analyses were conducted in Stata 10.

3. Results

3.1. Characteristics and Disposition of Patients. Table 1 shows the baseline comparison of patients for a variety of demographic and clinical conditions. There were no significant differences between the two groups at baseline.

3.2. Discontinuation and the Intervention Process. There was a significantly greater proportion of the individual compared to the system-oriented group that did not complete follow-up (15/40 versus 4/30, *P* value 0.017). In the individual intervention group, each participant received on average 3 sessions (SD 2.1) and 0 booster sessions (SD 0.7).

The system-oriented intervention had a fulfillment of the standards of 43% in the hospital. In the common mental health teams, the standards were met by 57%. The compliance with the standards was highest at the beginning of the study (attention bias).

Four aggregate root cause analyses were performed during the intervention period. They concurrently revealed instances of nonuse of standards and failure to use information and knowledge about the patient's condition.

3.3. Effect of the Intervention on the Compliance Scale (Primary Endpoint). Analysis of data with MI yielded a coefficient of 0.476 (SE 0.362 and CI −0.247–1.120); that is, there was a positive effect on compliance associated with being in the system-oriented group rather than the individual group after adjustment for compliance at baseline, abuse status, and GAF. Abuse status and GAF are known from the literature to affect compliance and were hence controlled for to improve precision. The result was not significant, *P* value 0.193 (Table 2).

3.4. Effect of the Intervention on the Rating Scales (Secondary Endpoints)

Remission. There was no significant difference at follow-up.

PANSS. Regression using MI leads to a regression coefficient of PANSS at follow-up in the intervention group when adjusted for PANSS at baseline of −4.478 (CI −9.259–0.403), *P* value 0.072.

LOCF revealed a significantly lower PANSS score on the remission items in the system-oriented group at follow-up, on average a score of 22 compared to 26 in the individual group, *P* value 0.036. When the individual's baseline value was included, *P* value of the differences was 0.001 by *t*-tests in favor of the system-oriented group. Estimate of the difference between the two groups by regression was 4.93 (CI −7.835 to −2.015).

GAF and SWN. No significant difference could be identified (MI and LOCF).

UKU. Analysis based on MI leads to an OR of 4.218 (CI 1.427 to 12.470) comparing the system- to the individual-oriented intervention. Based on LOCF 17 (43%) in the individual group and 21 (70%) in the system-oriented group were assessed as having adverse events, *P* value 0.030.

3.5. Data on Bed Days (Tertiary Endpoints). These data were collected from medical records of all the 70 patients. Figure 2 shows the proportion of project participants divided by intervention group, who have not been readmitted at a given point of time.

The system-oriented group had significantly longer time to readmission, *P* value 0.049.

There was no significant difference in the duration of the index hospitalization in the two groups or the average bed day consumption throughout the 12 months.

3.6. Nonparticipants. There were 16 patients who met the criteria for enrolment but who did not want to participate

Table 1: Baseline demographic and clinical characteristics.

	Individual intervention, N (%) Mean (SD) Median [10; 90% percentile]	Systemic intervention, N (%) Mean (SD) Median [10; 90% percentile]	P
Number	40	30	
Sex (%)			
Male	17 (42.5)	14 (46.7)	
Female	23 (57.5)	16 (53.3)	0.810
Age, yr (SD)	43.4 (10.6)	40.1 (10.0)	0.195
High school (%)	19 (47.5)	12 (40.0)	0.190
Education (%)	18 (45)	15 (50)	0.810
Livelihood (%)			
Employed	2 (5.0)	1 (3.3)	
Student	1 (2.5)	0 (0.0)	
Early retirement (financed by the state)	35 (87.5)	26 (86.7)	
Cash benefits	1 (2.5)	2 (6.7)	
Others	1 (2.5)	1 (3.3)	0.949
Crime (%)			
Arrested	10 (25.0)	9 (31.0)	0.597
New diagnosed (%)	2 (5.0)	2 (6.7)	1.000
Number of admissions	8.5 [2; 31.5]	10 [1; 50]	0.384
Duration of illness, yr	19 [4; 30]	11 [5; 32]	0.301
Abuse			
Alcohol and/or drugs	10 (25.6)	14 (46.7)	0.080
Alcohol (+ drugs)	8 (20.5)	13 (43.3)	0.064
Community mental health team	26 (65.0)	21 (0.7)	0.798
Psychosocial functioning (GAF)	33 [25; 40]	33 [25; 45]	0.727
Taking medication	34 (85.0)	28 (93.3)	0.425
Medications			
First-generation drug	9 (22.5)	8 (26.7)	0.781
Second-generation drug	31 (77.5)	26 (86.7)	0.371
Clozapine	10 (25.0)	10 (33.3)	0.594
Depot antipsychotics	10 (25.0)	11 (36.7)	0.307
Polypharmacy	10 (25.0)	10 (33.3)	0.594
Side effects			
Physician assessment	25 (62.5)	20 (66.7)	0.804

Missing values: crime 1, number of admissions 1, duration of illness 30, abuse 1, SWN 4, PANSS, all scores 1, remission 1, GAF 2, and side effects 7.
SWN: Subjective Well-Being under Neuroleptic Treatment. PANSS: Positive and Negative Symptom Scale. GAF: Global Assessment of Functioning Scale. Remission: score max 3 on all of the PANSS remission items.

in the project (Figure 1). These were significantly older than participants.

4. Discussion

When accounting for missing values with a multiple imputation approach, we found a tendency toward a difference in both the compliance scale and PANSS favoring the system-oriented therapy, although it did not reach statistical significance. A significant difference in incidence of adverse events and time to first readmission was found. Attrition rates were significantly higher in the reference group and nonsignificantly among individuals with lower compliance, which may have diluted effect estimates. This was reflected by significant differences found in an analysis based on a last observation carried forward approach.

More results were not significant using MI because MI takes into account the uncertainty of the missing data. MI thus best reflects the actual uncertainty of results.

The patients were allocated to one of the two participating psychiatric sections according to their home address in order to avoid confounding by indication. Still the combination of an unblinded treatment in a pragmatic trial with patient self-assessment holds potential for bias. To protect against this, pragmatic trials may benefit from including objective outcome measures in addition to subjective measures [36].

Table 2: Effect on the compliance scale.

(a) Difference in compliance score from baseline to follow-up, LOCF

	Difference, compliance score mean (CI)	P value
The individual therapy, $N = 40$	0.400 (−0.174–0.974)	>0.05
The system-oriented therapy, $N = 30$	1.103 (0.434–1.733)	<0.05

(b) Test on difference between intervention groups

	Coefficient	SE	CI	P value
Regression, MI	0.476	0.362	−0.247–1.120	0.193
Regression, LOCF	0.724	0.338	0.050–1.398	0.036

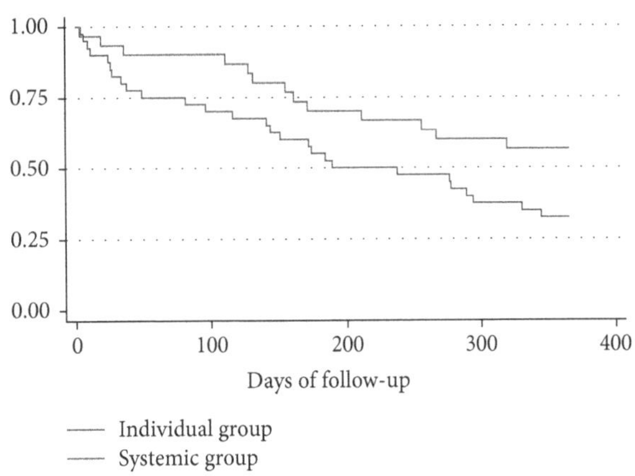

Figure 2: Kaplan-Meier survival proportion.

This was the case in our study, where time to readmission was an objective outcome, which furthermore was available for all at end of follow-up and showed results in the same direction as when analyzing subjective outcome measures.

The systemic intervention had an effect on the compliance level and was better tolerated than the individual-oriented intervention since no patients in the systemic intervention group withdrew from the project during the intervention period.

It was expected that during the project period there would be an increasing degree of compliance with the standards, but this was not achieved. The fulfillment was highest in the first period, which may be regarded as an attention bias (Hawthorne effect).

It was difficult to optimize the quality of daily routines as indicated by the four root cause analyses largely having similar conclusions. More focus on "knowledge sharing" was needed—focus on the factors influencing uptake and retention of new knowledge among health care staff [37].

No significant effect of the individual intervention was obtained. The individual intervention was poorly carried out. It was supposed to consist of 6 sessions and 3 booster sessions; yet the patients received on average 3 sessions and 0 booster sessions. Furthermore evaluation by the supervisor gave the impression of inadequate acquisition of the method (motivational interviewing) of those who were supposed to carry out the therapy. The supervisor estimated that training would have to be doubled for it to become adequate. After completion of the investigation, contact with W. Miller, who founded the therapy, clarified that experience has shown large variations in the amount of training needed to achieve sufficient skills to perform adequately (private communications). In the literature, divergent effects of compliance therapy and adherence therapy have been reported [8, 10, 12, 38, 39].

A study from 2010 [18] found no effect of adherence therapy on either clinical symptoms as measured by PANSS or medical adherence. The study was probably affected by selection bias, since only 26 of the 130 possible individuals accepted participation.

Consequently, the effect of compliance therapy and adherence therapy must still be regarded as uncertain, especially after the recent studies [40].

With 70 participants, we achieved more than the 40 participants assumed to be sufficient according to the power calculation. However, the actual size of the observed effect and standard deviations demanded a bigger amount of participants to achieve significant results. Usually pragmatic trials require large sample sizes to detect small treatment effects in a heterogeneous population [36].

The project was designed as a pragmatic controlled study, which gives a realistic impression of the effect of intervention, as it would be when carried out in a routine clinical setting, because such trials are performed in the context of usual care and use broad eligibility criteria [41]. It seeks to address the overall effectiveness of a given therapy [36, 42] and is therefore useful when considering the benefits of implementing a new treatment, even if this way of conducting a study may sacrifice intern validity to achieve generalisability [36, 43].

The patients were allocated to hospital section, and thus intervention type, from their residential address in order to avoid selection bias, specifically "confounding by indication."

The literature recommends cluster randomization for testing system-level interventions since patient randomization may be vulnerable to contamination. Patients in the reference group may be influenced by the system-level changes [44]. Therefore, the two interventions were applied at two different sections.

This design allowed us to implement and test a system-based intervention, which has not been previously done in this vulnerable group of patients.

5. Conclusion

This study suggests that compliance problems are best solved by a multifactorial intervention on the system level. Yet the point that the system-oriented intervention was superior to the individual intervention can be questioned; since the patients only received small amounts of this intervention, it still can serve as a reference intervention recording to the fact that compliance problems tend to disappear when focusing on them (attention bias).

The system-oriented intervention is likely suitable to be applied to compliance problems in other groups of vulnerable patients with chronic diseases.

This study may be considered a first step in investigating the potential effect of system-based interventions on improving patient compliance—a perspective which in our view has not received sufficient attention in the past. Although not all the estimated effects reached significance, they all favored the systemic intervention and they should therefore serve as the basis of larger and more definitive studies of this kind.

Conflict of Interests

The authors declare that there is no conflict of interests regarding the publication of this paper.

References

[1] H. Lublin, J. Eberhard, and S. Levander, "Current therapy issues and unmet clinical needs in the treatment of schizophrenia: a review of the new generation antipsychotics," *International Clinical Psychopharmacology*, vol. 20, no. 4, pp. 183–198, 2005.

[2] J. M. Kane and C. U. Correll, "Pharmacologic treatment of schizophrenia," *Dialogues in Clinical Neuroscience*, vol. 12, no. 3, pp. 345–357, 2010.

[3] L. Osterberg and T. Blaschke, "Adherence to medication," *New England Journal of Medicine*, vol. 353, no. 5, pp. 487–497, 2005.

[4] D. C. Goff, M. Hill, and O. Freudenreich, "Strategies for improving treatment adherence in schizophrenia and schizoaffective disorder," *Journal of Clinical Psychiatry*, vol. 71, supplement 2, pp. 20–26, 2010.

[5] P. S. Masand, M. Roca, M. S. Turner, and J. M. Kane, "Partial adherence to antipsychotic medication impacts the course of illness in patients with schizophrenia: a review," *Primary Care Companion to the Journal of Clinical Psychiatry*, vol. 11, no. 4, pp. 147–154, 2009.

[6] M. S. Razali and H. Yahya, "Compliance with treatment in schizophrenia: a drug intervention program in a developing country," *Acta Psychiatrica Scandinavica*, vol. 91, no. 5, pp. 331–335, 1995.

[7] R. Gray, "Does patient education enhance compliance with clozapine? A preliminary investigation," *Journal of Psychiatric and Mental Health Nursing*, vol. 7, no. 3, pp. 285–286, 2000.

[8] C. O'Donnell, G. Donohoe, L. Sharkey et al., "Compliance therapy: a randomised controlled trial in schizophrenia," *The British Medical Journal*, vol. 327, no. 7419, pp. 834–836, 2003.

[9] R. Gray, T. Wykes, M. Edmonds, M. Leese, and K. Gournay, "Effect of a medication management training package for nurses on clinical outcomes for patients with schizophrenia: cluster randomised controlled trial," *The British Journal of Psychiatry*, vol. 185, pp. 157–162, 2004.

[10] R. Gray, M. Leese, J. Bindman et al., "Adherence therapy for people with schizophrenia: European multicentre randomised controlled trial," *The British Journal of Psychiatry*, vol. 189, pp. 508–514, 2006.

[11] G. Pitschel-Walz, J. Bäuml, W. Bender, R. R. Engel, M. Wagner, and W. Kissling, "Psychoeducation and compliance in the treatment of Schizophrenia: results of the Munich psychosis information project study," *Journal of Clinical Psychiatry*, vol. 67, no. 3, pp. 443–452, 2006.

[12] S. Maneesakorn, D. Robson, K. Gournay, and R. Gray, "An RCT of adherence therapy for people with schizophrenia in Chiang Mai, Thailand," *Journal of Clinical Nursing*, vol. 16, no. 7, pp. 1302–1312, 2007.

[13] L. H. Beebe, K. Smith, C. Crye et al., "Telenursing intervention increases psychiatric medication adherence in schizophrenia outpatients," *Journal of the American Psychiatric Nurses Association*, vol. 14, no. 3, pp. 217–224, 2008.

[14] T. J. Hudson, R. R. Owen, C. R. Thrush, T. L. Armitage, and P. Thapa, "Guideline implementation and patient-tailoring strategies to improve medication adherence for schizophrenia," *Journal of Clinical Psychiatry*, vol. 69, no. 1, pp. 74–80, 2008.

[15] D. I. Velligan, P. M. Diamond, J. Mintz et al., "The use of individually tailored environmental supports to improve medication adherence and outcomes in schizophrenia," *Schizophrenia Bulletin*, vol. 34, no. 3, pp. 483–493, 2008.

[16] P. J. Weiden, N. R. Schooler, J. C. Weedon, A. Elmouchtari, A. Sunakawa, and S. M. Goldfinger, "A randomized controlled trial of long-acting injectable risperidone vs continuation on oral atypical antipsychotics for first-episode schizophrenia patients: initial adherence outcome," *Journal of Clinical Psychiatry*, vol. 70, no. 10, pp. 1397–1406, 2009.

[17] S. W. C. Chan, B. Yip, S. Tso, B. S. Cheng, and W. Tam, "Evaluation of a psychoeducation program for Chinese clients with schizophrenia and their family caregivers," *Patient Education and Counseling*, vol. 75, no. 1, pp. 67–76, 2009.

[18] K. H. Anderson, S. Ford, D. Robson, J. Cassis, C. Rodrigues, and R. Gray, "An exploratory, randomized controlled trial of adherence therapy for people with schizophrenia," *International Journal of Mental Health Nursing*, vol. 19, no. 5, pp. 340–349, 2010.

[19] N. Barber, "Should we consider non-compliance a medical error?" *Quality and Safety in Health Care*, vol. 11, no. 1, pp. 81–84, 2002.

[20] P. Knudsen, H. Herborg, A. R. Mortensen, M. Knudsen, and A. Hellebek, "Preventing medication errors in community pharmacy: root-cause analysis of transcription errors," *Quality and Safety in Health Care*, vol. 16, no. 4, pp. 285–290, 2007.

[21] R. Gray, T. Wykes, and K. Gournay, "From compliance to concordance: a review of the literature on interventions to enhance compliance with antipsychotic medication," *Journal of Psychiatric and Mental Health Nursing*, vol. 9, no. 3, pp. 277–284, 2002.

[22] H. Skarsholm and B. Nielsen, "Development and implementation of an integrated care pathway for managing compliance problems in patients with schizophrenia," *International Journal of Care Pathways*, vol. 16, no. 4, pp. 139–145, 2012.

[23] W. Miller and S. Rollnick, *Motivational Interviewing*, Guilford Press, 1st edition, 2002.

[24] R. Gray and D. Robson, *Concordance Skills—A Manual for Health Workers*, Institute of Psychiatry at Maudsley, King's College London, University of London, London, UK, 2004.

[25] N. C. Andreasen, W. T. Carpenter Jr., J. M. Kane, R. A. Lasser, S. R. Marder, and D. R. Weinberger, "Remission in schizophrenia: proposed criteria and rationale for consensus," *The American Journal of Psychiatry*, vol. 162, no. 3, pp. 441–449, 2005.

[26] T. P. Hogan, A. G. Awad, and R. Eastwood, "A self-report scale predictive of drug compliance in schizophrenics: reliability and discriminative validity," *Psychological Medicine*, vol. 13, no. 1, pp. 177–183, 1983.

[27] D. I. Velligan, Y. W. F. Lam, D. C. Glahn et al., "Defining and assessing adherence to oral antipsychotics: a review of the

literature," *Schizophrenia Bulletin*, vol. 32, no. 4, pp. 724–742, 2006.

[28] D. I. Velligan, M. Wang, P. Diamond et al., "Relationships among subjective and objective measures of adherence to oral antipsychotic medications," *Psychiatric Services*, vol. 58, no. 9, pp. 1187–1192, 2007.

[29] W. M. Macharia, G. Leon, B. H. Rowe, B. J. Stephenson, and R. B. Haynes, "An overview of interventions to improve compliance with appointment keeping for medical services," *Journal of the American Medical Association*, vol. 267, no. 13, pp. 1813–1817, 1992.

[30] J. P. Lacro, L. B. Dunn, C. R. Dolder, S. G. Leckband, and D. V. Jeste, "Prevalence of and risk factors for medication nonadherence in patients with schizophrenia: a comprehensive review of recent literature," *Journal of Clinical Psychiatry*, vol. 63, no. 10, pp. 892–909, 2002.

[31] M. Nosé, C. Barbui, and M. Tansella, "How often do patients with psychosis fail to adhere to treatment programmes? A systematic review," *Psychological Medicine*, vol. 33, no. 7, pp. 1149–1160, 2003.

[32] J. M. Kane, "Treatment adherence and long-term outcomes," *CNS Spectrums*, vol. 12, no. 10, pp. 21–26, 2007.

[33] H. H. Goldman, A. E. Skodol, and T. R. Lave, "Revising axis V for DSM-IV: a review of measures of social functioning," *The American Journal of Psychiatry*, vol. 149, no. 9, pp. 1148–1156, 1992.

[34] D. Naber, S. Moritz, M. Lambert et al., "Improvement of schizophrenic patients' subjective well-being under atypical antipsychotic drugs," *Schizophrenia Research*, vol. 50, no. 1, pp. 79–88, 2001.

[35] O. Lingjaerde, U. G. Ahlfors, P. Bech, S. J. Dencker, and K. Elgen, "The UKU side effect rating scale. A new comprehensive rating scale for psychotropic drugs and a cross-sectional study of side effects in neuroleptic-treated patients," *Acta Psychiatrica Scandinavica*, vol. 334, pp. 1–100, 1987.

[36] J. H. Ware and M. B. Hamel, "Statistics in medicine: pragmatic trials—guides to better patient care?" *New England Journal of Medicine*, vol. 364, no. 18, pp. 1685–1687, 2011.

[37] W. B. Berta and R. Baker, "Factors that impact the transfer and retention of best practices for reducing error in hospitals," *Health Care Management Review*, vol. 29, no. 2, pp. 90–97, 2004.

[38] R. Ilott, "Does compliance therapy improve use of antipsychotic medication?" *The British Journal of Community Nursing*, vol. 10, no. 11, pp. 514–519, 2005.

[39] A. M. McIntosh, L. Conlon, S. M. Lawrie, and A. C. Stanfield, "Compliance therapy for schizophrenia," *Cochrane Database of Systematic Reviews*, vol. 3, Article ID CD003442, 2006.

[40] R. Gray, J. White, M. Schulz, and C. Abderhalden, "Enhancing medication adherence in people with schizophrenia: an international programme of research," *International Journal of Mental Health Nursing*, vol. 19, no. 1, pp. 36–44, 2010.

[41] P. Maningat and J. L. Breslow, "Needed: pragmatic clinical trials for statin-intolerant patients," *New England Journal of Medicine*, vol. 365, no. 24, pp. 2250–2251, 2011.

[42] P. J. Helms, ""Real world" pragmatic clinical trials: what are they and what do they tell us?" *Pediatric Allergy and Immunology*, vol. 13, no. 1, pp. 4–9, 2002.

[43] D. Price, S. D. Musgrave, L. Shepstone et al., "Leukotriene antagonists as first-line or add-on asthma-controller therapy," *New England Journal of Medicine*, vol. 364, no. 18, pp. 1695–1707, 2011.

[44] D. A. Richards, K. Lovell, S. Gilbody et al., "Collaborative care for depression in UK primary care: a randomized controlled trial," *Psychological Medicine*, vol. 38, no. 2, pp. 279–287, 2008.

23

Traditional Knowledge and Formulations of Medicinal Plants Used by the Traditional Medical Practitioners of Bangladesh to Treat Schizophrenia Like Psychosis

Md. Nasir Ahmed and Md. Nur Kabidul Azam

Ethnobotany & Ethnomedicine Division, TechB Herbal Solution, Bheramara, Kushtia 7040, Bangladesh

Correspondence should be addressed to Md. Nasir Ahmed; nasir.ahmedbd@hotmail.com

Academic Editor: Jouko Miettunen

Schizophrenia is a subtle disorder of brain development and plasticity; it affects the most basic human processes of perception, emotion, and judgment. In Bangladesh the traditional medical practitioners of rural and remote areas characterized the schizophrenia as an insanity or a mental problem due to possession by ghosts or evil spirits and they have used various plant species' to treat such symptoms. The aim of the present study was to conduct an ethnomedicinal plant survey and documentation of the formulations of different plant parts used by the traditional medical practitioners of Rangamati district of Bangladesh for the treatment of schizophrenia like psychosis. It was observed that the traditional medical practitioners used a total of 15 plant species to make 14 formulations. The plants were divided into 13 families, used for treatment of schizophrenia and accompanying symptoms like hallucination, depression, oversleeping or insomnia, deterioration of personal hygiene, forgetfulness, and fear due to evil spirits like genies or ghost. A search of the relevant scientific literatures showed that a number of plants used by the medicinal practitioners have been scientifically validated in their uses and traditional medicinal knowledge has been a means towards the discovery of many modern medicines. Moreover, the antipsychotic drug reserpine, isolated from the dried root of *Rauvolfia serpentina* species, revolutionized the treatment of schizophrenia. So it is very much possible that formulations of the practitioner, when examined scientifically in their entireties, can form discovery of lead compounds which can be used as safe and effective antipsychotic drug to treat schizophrenia.

1. Introduction

Schizophrenia is a psychological disorder characterized by psychotic symptoms: hallucinations and delusions that significantly affect emotions, behavior, and, most notably, mental processes and mental contents. Psychosis is a condition of mental illness that causes a person to lose his or her sense of reality. Schizophrenia is a type of psychosis meaning spilt mind which often describes as a mental disorder characterized by impairments in the perception or expression of reality and by significant social or occupational dysfunction. People with this disease have delusions, hallucinations, disorganized speech, grossly disorganized behavior, or catatonic behavior [1, 2]. The world over, from China or Finland to the United States or New Guinea, approximately 1% of the population will develop schizophrenia at some point in their lives [3, 4]. Schizophrenia is one of the top five causes of disability among adults in developed nations, ranking with heart disease, arthritis, drug use, and HIV [5]. In the United States, about 5% of people with schizophrenia (about 100,000 individuals) are homeless, 5% are in hospitals, and 6% are in jail or prison [6]. Together, these three groups of people represent about 16% of Americans with schizophrenia; in contrast, 34% of people with this disorder live independently. According to World Health Organization (WHO) at least 40 million people in the world suffer from mental disorders such as schizophrenia and dementia [7]. Over 10% of schizophrenia patients ultimately commit suicide [8, 9]; this makes the disease a serious psychiatric illness among the various nationalities of the world.

Bangladesh is a densely populated area where prevalence of psychiatric illness is not less than that of any other country in the world. A study showed that 29% of patients attending general practice were suffering from functional disorder and 6% from both functional and organic disorders. The same study demonstrated that 47% of patients were suffering from neurotic disorder, 37% from psychosomatic disorder, 10% from affective disorder, 1.44% from schizophrenia, 2.88% from substance use disorder, and 2% from organic psychiatric syndrome [10]. Another study conducted in Outpatient Department of National Institute of Mental Health (NIMH), Dhaka, Bangladesh, revealed that 37.4% of patients were suffering from schizophrenia and schizophrenia like psychotic disorders, 16.14% from anxiety disorders, 11.19% from major depressive disorder, and 8.95% from bipolar mood disorder [11]. In the Dhaka city, most of the patients (70.4%) were from urban background and from rural area 29.6% patients [12]. According to other studies it was seen that across various countries, schizophrenia is more common among people in urban areas and lower socioeconomic classes than among people in rural areas and higher socioeconomic classes [13, 14].

Antipsychotic agents are the cornerstone of acute and maintenance treatment of schizophrenia and are effective in the treatment of hallucinations, delusions, and thought disorders, regardless of etiology. In recent decades, the modern psychiatry has introduced herbal medicine in the treatment of psychiatric disorders including schizophrenia. After the rise of a pharmaceutical industry in the last century and significant progress in the treatment, a period of disappointment comes in accepting the fact that synthetic drugs are not almighty. Due to this fact, there has been a growing interest in the last decades for the treatment of psychiatric disorders including schizophrenia by using alternative and complementary methods [15] and a study revealed that 44% of psychiatric patients with schizophrenia (9%) had used herbal medicine (mainly for psychiatric purposes) during the previous 12 months [16].

Plants contain various phytochemicals and these phytochemicals can play an important role in reducing occurrences of many diseases by boosting up various organ functions of the human body. Many traditional healing herbs and their parts have been shown to have medicinal value and can be used to prevent, alleviate, or cure several human diseases [17]. It has also been observed that number of modern drugs has been derived from plants used by the indigenous people [18]. Modern drugs like aspirin, atropine, ephedrine, digoxin, morphine, quinine, reserpine, and tubocurarine are examples, which were originally discovered through observations of traditional cure methods of indigenous peoples [19]. Presently, there is a resurgence of herbal medicine as people want more control in their personal healthcare. The U.S. herbal market is growing tremendously with consumer demand way ahead of regulatory agencies. It is interesting to note that four (Ginkgo, St. John's Wort, Valerian, and Kava) of the top ten herbs purchased in the U.S. (according to 1999 Whole Foods Survey) have psychotropic activity. Recent trends in research into African plant uses show that traditional medicine is commonly used to treat neurological disorders in the West African region, and some recent publications are available [20].

In Bangladesh, traditional medical practice is still ongoing. The traditional medical practitioners (generally known as *Kabirajes* by the mainstream community) perform a central role in providing primary healthcare to the rural inhabitants of Bangladesh. There are 86,000 villages in the country and almost every village has one or two traditional *Kabirajes*. They are the providers of primary healthcare to village populations of Bangladesh and moreover they are the important sources of ethnomedicinal knowledge. The practices of the *Kabirajes* extend throughout both urban and rural areas of the country, although rural practice is more extensive than urban practice.

The advantage of the *Kabirajes* is that they rely chiefly on medicinal plants for treatment. The formulations are rarely complex and usually consist of simple extraction of juice of whole plant or plant part through squeezing plant part. The juice is then administered orally or typically applied depending on the nature of diseases. The previous ethnomedicobotanical studies conducted among folk and tribal medicinal practitioners of the country have noticed considerable variation between the medicinal plants selected by different *Kabirajes* for treatment of a given ailment [21–25]. The aim of the present study was to document the traditional medicine knowledge as well formulations of medicinal plants used by the traditional medical practitioners of Rangamati district in the Chittagong Hill Tracts (CHT) region of Bangladesh for the treatment of schizophrenia like psychosis.

2. Materials and Methods

2.1. Study Area. For the present study, survey was done between March to Mid-April' 2013, in the largest district of the country called Rangamati which is located in the CHT region. It is consists of 10 upazilas and bordered by the Tripura state of India to the north and Bandarban district to the south. The area of the district is 6116 km^2 of which 1292 km^2 is riverine and 4825 km^2 is under forest vegetation. The main survey was conducted in the Rangamati Sadar Upazila (located at 22.6500°N 92.1833°E), which consists of 6 unions, on the information about medicinal plants commonly used for treatment of psychotic disorders with particular attention to schizophrenia. The study area for this specific ethnomedicinal survey was selected by the authors themselves regarding information on the noted traditional medical practices. Moreover, the study area as well as the total CHT region is very rich in species diversity. We are conducting systematic ethnomedicinal survey of Bangladesh since 2011 as to explore how do the *Kabirajes* of Bangladesh select medicinal plants for treatment of any ailment. In order to address such question we conducted this specific survey among *Kabirajes* of Rangamati Sadar Upazila of Bangladesh (Figure 1). The above question is more important from the viewpoint that how and why medicinal plants are selected by the TMPs can lead the way towards a better linking between traditional knowledge with biomedical science [26, 27].

2.2. Mode of Interview and Plant Data Collection. The collection of data through interviews of 3 traditional medical

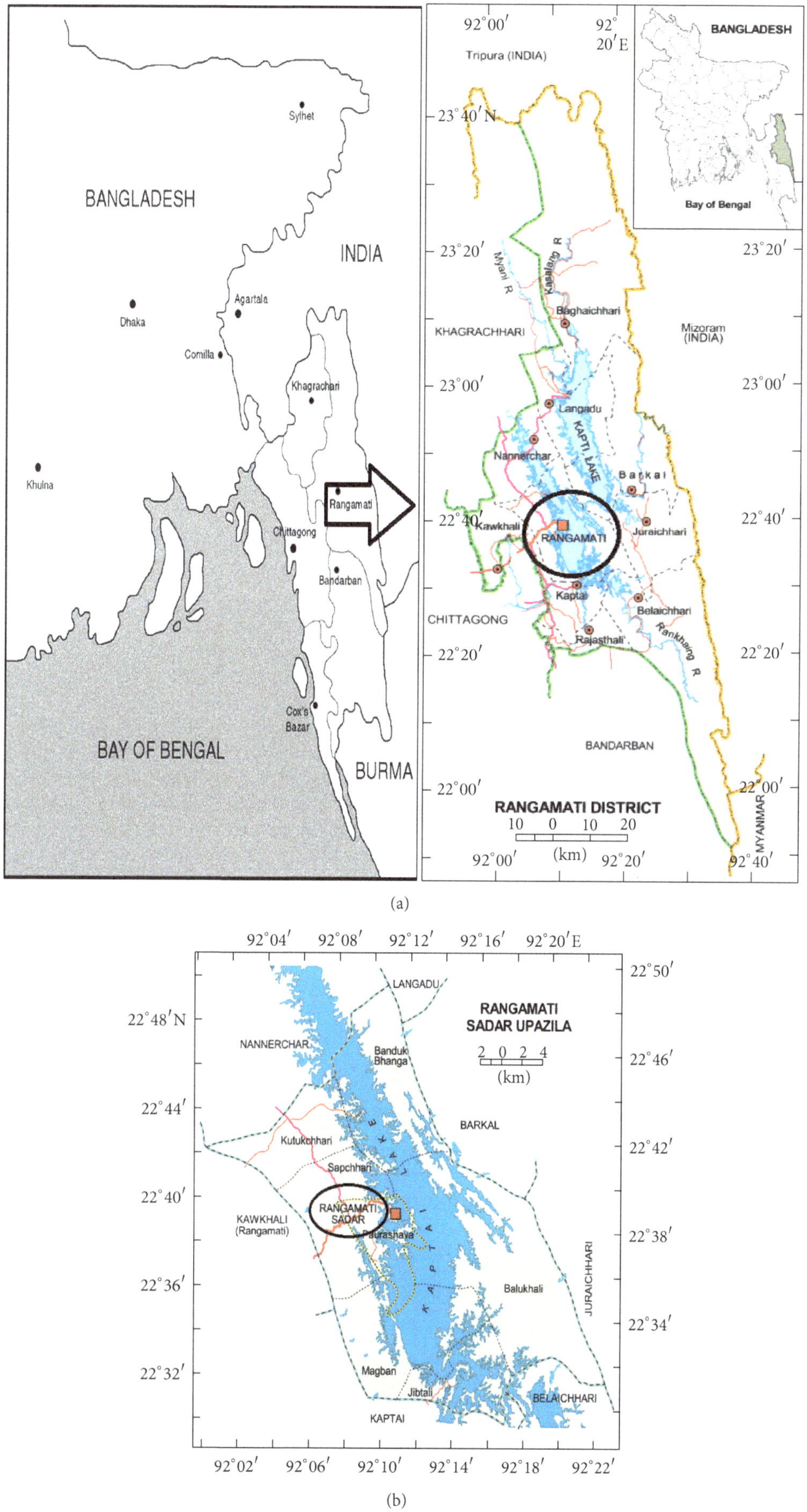

FIGURE 1: Map of Bangladesh showing the Rangamati district. Study site is marked on the map with black round shade.

practitioners (TMP; aged between 61–67) was conducted by the researchers themselves with the help of a semistructured questionnaire. The number of 3 TMPs was chosen on the basis of recommendation of the local inhabitants as to being more proficient and reputed to their practices. In the preliminary survey, the TMPs were specifically asked as to whether they know and treat schizophrenia, the basis for their diagnosis, and their mode of treatment when the disease has been diagnosed as schizophrenia. According to folk medical practitioners, the symptoms were hallucinations, over sleeping in the day, insomnia, staying alone in the dark room, anxiety, being silent or not so much interested to keep attached with family members, and most commonly getting fear due to invisible person (as per patient's thoughts). The traditional medical practitioners defined this fear to be due to evil spirits, genies, or ghosts. The basic method followed was one of guided fieldwork [28–30]. Information collected from the *Kabirajes* consisted of medicinal plants or plant parts used, formulations, and dosage. The information was noted down during the daytime interviews. At the end of each interview plant specimens shown by the traditional medical practitioners were collected, dried, and later brought back to the Dhaka for identification at the Bangladesh National Herbarium and all the voucher specimens were deposited there. Nomenclature of plants was compiled from the plant list database [31]. For this specific ethnomedicinal survey, the number of visits was made to the traditional medical practitioners to gain their confidence.

3. Results

It was observed that the 3 traditional medical practitioners (TMP) of the Rangamati district used a total of 14 formulations from the 15 plant species, distributed into 13 families for treatment of schizophrenia like psychotic episodes. The Rubiaceae and Lamiaceae families were contributing 2 plants, the rest of the plant families contributed one plant each. The various plant parts were used including leaf, roots, bark, stem, flower, seed, and fruit. This study recorded that several parts or individual plant species are used as medicine. Leaves constituted the major plant part used, forming 47.62% of total uses. Barks and seeds each constituted 14.28% of total uses. The other plant parts mentioned constituted, respectively, 9.52, 4.76, 4.76, and 4.76% of total uses (Figure 2).

The medicinal knowledge of TMPs was derived from the earlier generation practitioners, with whom every TMP had to serve a period of apprenticeship and training before they could practice independently. This medicinal knowledge has come out of practice through the centuries and every practitioner had their own lists of plants for treatment of any particular disease or disorder. As mentioned earlier all 3 TMPs were interviewed separately, so the plants advised by the TMPs did not reflect any individual opinion. It can be concluded by the interviewers that schizophrenia and other related psychotic problems have existed for centuries among the people surveyed and various TMPs have developed their own medicinal plant formulations for treatment of schizophrenia like psychosis, possibly through trial and error methods over centuries long practices.

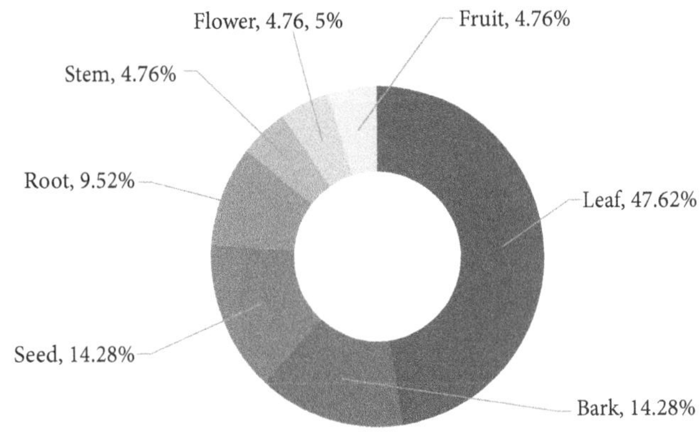

FIGURE 2: Parts of medicinal plants used by the traditional medical practitioners of Rangamati Sadar Upazila to treat schizophrenia like psychosis.

Any sort of complex formulations was avoided by the TMPs for the treatment of schizophrenia like psychosis. Generally fruits and seeds were consumed directly or with water. In most cases, juice obtained from squeezed plant part was advised to be taken or pills made from paste of plant part taken orally. It was noted that mashed leaves of *Piper retrofractum* are taken with rice. A combination of bark and seed of *Thevetia peruviana* paste is taken orally. Another formulation suggested by a TMP was that juice from macerated *Euphorbia neriifolia* leaves is taken orally; the formulation was also used to keep head cool and to increase memory of a patient as per the TMP. There were also mentioned some more easy formulations: smell of flower of *Abroma augusta* is taken with the nose and leaves of *Vitex negundo* were carried alongside the body. If a patient is in severe condition then the leaves of *Cannabis sativa* were used to make vapor and the vapor is taken by the nose, as advised by a TMP. Leaf juice of *Ocimum americanum* is mixed with seeds of *Brassica juncea* and taken orally till cure. Most of the formulations were usually administrated orally with three exceptions. The rest of the formulations were given in Table 1.

In our present study, TMPs recommended different forms of medication including juice (3 species), pill, vegetable and paste (2 each), tablet, vapor, oil message, decoction (1 species each), and others (3). Most often standard medicines are prescribed in mixed ingredient form by mixing several valuable medicinal plants or several plant parts of one plant species. TMPs believe that using plant or plant part mixtures in the preparation of medicine is important as a single plant alone may not be sufficient to cure any disease completely and the combination of several medicinal plants increases the quality and efficacy of medicine. Similar observations have also been found in Nepal and India [32, 33].

4. Discussions

Investigation into the mechanism of action of the drugs used to treat schizophrenia has not provided clear understanding of the pathogenesis of the disease. While schizophrenia

TABLE 1: Medicinal plants used by the traditional medical practitioners of Rangamati district for treatment of schizophrenia like psychotic episodes.

Serial number	Formulations and dosage	Parts used	Botanical name/vernacular name
1	Leaves of *Piper retrofractum* (Piperaceae) are taken orally in mashed form as vegetable with rice till cure.	Leaf	*Piper retrofractum* Vahl/Choi
2	Juice obtained from macerated leaves or roots of *Ficus hirta* (Moraceae) is taken orally till cure.	Leaf, root	*Ficus hirta* Vahl./Pakur
3	A combination of bark and seed of *Thevetia peruviana* (Apocynaceae) paste is taken orally till cure.	Bark, seed	*Thevetia peruviana* (Pers.) K. Schum./Holde Korobi
4	A combination of leaf and seed paste from *Datura metel* L. (Solanaceae) is taken orally or macerated leaves are pressed to the nose.	Leaf, seed	*Datura metel* L./Dhutura
5	Juice from macerated *Euphorbia neriifolia* (Euphorbiaceae) leaves is taken orally.	Leaf	*Euphorbia neriifolia* L./Monshaseez
6	Juice is collected from macerated bark of *Randia dumetorum* (Rubiaceae). It is then dried and turned into powder, which is mixed with sugar. Tablets weighing 5 g each are made from the mixture and taken till cure	Bark	*Randia dumetorum* (Retz.) Lam/Monkata
7	*Aegle marmelos* (Rutaceae) leaves and roots crushed and made into 1/2 tola amount pills. Pills are taken twice daily for three days. (1 tola = 11.66 g)	Leaf, root	*Aegle marmelos* (L.) Corr./Bel
8	*Litsea polyantha* (Lauraceae) bark is macerated with 1 g sugar to obtain juice, which is then taken orally.	Bark	*Litsea polyantha* Juss./Uruijja, Menda
9	Leaves of *Coccinia grandis* (Cucurbitaceae) are boiled and the decoction is taken orally.	Leaf	*Coccinia grandis* (L.) J. Voigt/Telakuchi
10	Leaf juice of *Ocimum americanum* (Lamiaceae) are mixed with mashed seeds of *Brassica juncea* (Cruciferae) and taken orally till cure.	Leaf, seed	*Ocimum americanum* L./Radha tulshi *Brassica juncea* (L.) Czern./Shorisha
11	Smell of flower of *Abroma augusta* (Malvaceae) is taken with the nose or crushed stems are taken with *Aloe vera* and sugar twice daily for seven days till cure.	Flower, steam	*Abroma augusta* L.f./Ulot Kombol
12	Leaves of *Vitex negundo* (Lamiaceae) are kept or carried alongside the body. Another formulation is to take pills in the morning made from the leaves.	Leaf	*Vitex negundo* L./Nishinda
13	Leaves from *Cannabis Sativa* (Cannabaceae) are used to make oil then message on the scalp till cure. If a patient is in severe condition then the leaves were used to make vapor and the vapor is taken by the nose.	Leaf	*Cannabis Sativa* L./Bhang, Siddhi
14	Ripe fruit of *Morinda citrifolia* (Rubiaceae) is eaten as raw and mashed leaves were eaten as vegetable.	Fruit, leaf	*Morinda citrifolia* Linn./Holdi Kachu, Noni

is highly heritable, the genetics are complex and the interpretation of genetic data has proven difficult. Now advances in phenotypic analysis, neuroimaging, genetics, and molecular pathology provide the basis for optimism [34]. Schizophrenia can be understood as a subtle disorder of brain development [35–37].

4.1. Neural Communication in Schizophrenia. Recent findings have shown changes in markers in a number of neurotransmitter systems in the brains of subjects with schizophrenia which include the dopaminergic, serotonergic, glutamatergic, and GABAergic systems of the CNS. Many of these changes also appear to be regionally specific, and abnormalities in nonneurotransmitter specific pathways have been found in schizophrenia [38]. A major component of the studies used postmortem CNS tissue because these sites are amenable to manipulation by therapeutic agents, in many cases they are the sites of action of drugs which provide antipsychotic activity [39]. Ultimately neurobiology of schizophrenia may help illuminate the nature of normal thought, perception and emotion.

The findings that antipsychotic drugs are dopamine D2 receptor antagonists and the *dopamine hypothesis* propose that an overproduction of dopamine or an increase in the number or sensitivity of dopamine receptors is responsible for schizophrenia. According to this hypothesis, the excess dopamine or extra sensitivity to this neurotransmitter triggers a flood of unrelated thoughts, feelings, and perceptions. Delusions are then attempt to organize these disconnected events into a coherent, understandable experience [40, 41].

There has been an increasing acceptance that antipsychotic drugs that bind to both the dopamine D_2-like receptor family and the *serotonin* $(5HT)_{2A}$ receptor have been improved clinical outcomes [42]. Using DNA from peripheral tissue, a number of studies have suggested that mutations in the gene for the $5HT_{2A}$ receptor are associated with schizophrenia [43].

The hypothesis that changed *glutamatergic* function is involved in the pathology of schizophrenia and a glutamate receptor ion channel blocker reduce or exacerbate a schizophrenia like psychosis [44]. The N-methyl-D-aspartate (NMDA) glutamate receptor has been shown to play a crucial role in learning and memory, and hence abnormalities in its functioning may explain some of the deficits associated with schizophrenia, such as deficits in working memory. Studies have found unusually high levels of glutamate in people with schizophrenia, particularly in the frontal lobe [45, 46]; such an excess of glutamate may disrupt the timing of neural activation in the frontal lobe, which in turn may impair cognitive activities that depend on the smooth coordination of different operations, such as working memory, where information must be actively retained in short-term memory as it is operated upon [47].

Research findings suggest that stress can contribute to schizophrenia because stress affects *cortisol* production, which in turn affects the brain. The relationship with cortisol appears even in childhood. Children who are at risk for schizophrenia react more strongly to stress, and their baseline levels of cortisol are higher than those of other children [48]. The relationship between stress, cortisol, and symptoms of schizophrenia has also been noted during adolescence [49]. Even after adolescence, people with schizophrenia have higher levels of stress-related hormones, including cortisol [50].

Several lines of evidence implicated the *GABAergic* system in the pathology of schizophrenia. The study of mRNA encoding the different subunits has now extended original findings on radioligand binding to show an increase in levels of mRNA encoding the α-1 subunit of the $GABA_A$ receptor in Brodmann's areas 9 and 10 from subjects with schizophrenia [51]. There are changes in expression of $GABA_A$ receptor subunit in schizophrenia which are the finding that there is a marked decrease in levels of mRNA encoding for the short form of the $\gamma 2$ subunit of the $GABA_A$ receptor in the prefrontal cortex from schizophrenia [52].

4.2. Herbal Medications in the Enhancement of Brain Function. Humans consume a wide range of foods, drugs, and dietary supplements that are derived from plants and which modify the functioning of the central nervous system (CNS). The psychoactive properties of these substances are attributable to the presence of plant secondary metabolites; in many cases, the effects of these phytochemicals on the human CNS might be linked either to their ecological roles in the life of the plant or to molecular and biochemical similarities in the biology of plants and higher animals [53]. Schizophrenia as well as other psychotic disorders is likely to involve a complex interplay of many brain systems and neurotransmitters including dopamine, serotonin, and glutamate, and there is extensive evidence that schizophrenia is a biological disease of the brain. The primary mechanism of action involves modulation of neuronal communication, via specific plant metabolites binding to neurotransmitter/neuromodulator receptors [54] and via alteration of neurotransmitter synthesis and general function [55]. Other mechanisms involve stimulating or sedating CNS activity and regulating or supporting the healthy function of endocrine system [56, 57]. Traditional antipsychotics have been the first step in treating schizophrenia, that is, thorazine (chlorpromazine) is dopamine antagonist, which effectively blocks the action of dopamine and diminishes positive symptoms in approximately 75–80% of people with schizophrenia who take such antipsychotic medication [58]. Traditional antipsychotics have sedative properties which affect patients quickly; such sedation and improvement in psychotic symptoms can take anywhere from 5 days to 6 weeks [59].

A huge scientific literature focusing on psychoactive herbal extracts and their phytochemicals, encompassing hundreds of thousands of scientific papers, has emerged over recent decades. The vast majority of these papers describe *in vitro* investigations of the potential mechanisms of action of putatively psychoactive phytochemicals, whereas a much smaller proportion explores their effects *in vivo* on animals and only a tiny minority investigates their efficacy in humans. Zhang [60] identified extracts and constituents from 85 individual medicinal plants that have demonstrated potential efficacy for treating psychiatric disorders on the basis of animal behavioral models alone.

A study indicated antipsychotic activity along with antianxiety and anticonvulsant from the hydroalcoholic extract of *Euphorbia neriifolia* leaves in mice and rats [61]. The observation of another study indicated that the anticataleptic activity exhibited by ethanolic extract of *Randia dumetorum* Lam fruits does not possess antidopaminergic and antiserotonergic activity. Catalepsy usually associated with catatonic schizophrenia [62].

Methanolic extract of *Aegle marmelos* leaves possessed potential anxiolytic and antidepressant activities in albino mice and also may be served as a potential resource for natural psychotherapeutic agent [63]. In India, *Aegle marmelos* highly reputed ayurvedic medicinal tree and has been used in nervous disorder and as tonic for brain [64, 65]. A survey study conducted by Rahmatullah et al. [66, 67] reported that TMP of Santals tribe in Bangladesh used *Coccinia grandis* for the treatment of mental disorder.

Ocimum americanum possessed relaxant effects [68] and can be considered as beneficial to patients with mental disorders. The seed of *Brassica juncea* and leaves juice of *Ocimum americanum* were mixed with leaves of *Acorus calamus* L. (Acoraceae) for treating mental disorders as well being possessed with evil spirits; such combined formulation was used by the TMP of the Tonchongya tribe of Bangladesh, and whether such beings exist or not is scientifically debatable, any possession by "evil spirits" can be considered as a sort of mental disorder with the status of the patient being in a state of delirium [69]. *A. calamus* is also used to make brahmyadiyoga (an Ayurvedic medicine system) and has been used for the treatment of schizophrenia. An important general issue is the cost of treatment, as Ayurvedic treatments are cheaper and therefore more accessible to poor people than chlorpromazine, let alone the more recent atypical antipsychotics [70, 71].

The effect of acetone soluble fraction of methanolic extract of roots of the *Vitex negundo* (50 and 100 mg/kg, i.p.) was studied on haloperidol-induced catalepsy in mice, amphetamine induced stereotyped behaviour in rats, and dopamine-induced contraction isolated vas deferens preparation of rat. The acetone soluble fraction of methanolic extract of isolated of *V. negundo* significantly potentiated haloperidol induced catalepsy, antagonized dose dependent amphetamine-induced stereotyped behaviour, and also antagonized dopamine induced contractions of rat vas deference. The result suggests that the methanolic extract of *Vitex negundo* possessed antidopaminergic principle [72]. Another study results in mice indicated that roots of *Vitex negundo* have an effective anxiolytic agent [73].

Since the discovery of the endocannabinoid system, a growing body of psychiatric research has emerged focusing on the role of this system in major psychiatric disorders like schizophrenia, bipolar disorder, major depression, and anxiety disorder. A compound found in *Cannabis sativa* can treat schizophrenia as effectively as antipsychotic medications, with far fewer side effects, according to a preliminary clinical trial. Researchers led by Markus Leweke of the University of Cologne in Germany studied 39 people with schizophrenia who were hospitalized for a psychotic episode. Nineteen patients were treated with amisulpride, an antipsychotic medication that is not approved in the U.S. but is comparable to other medications that are antipsychotic. The rest of the patients were given cannabidiol (CBD), a substance found in *C. sativa* that is thought to be responsible for some of its mellowing or anxiety-reducing effects [74]. Unlike the main ingredient in marijuana, THC, which can produce psychotic reactions and may worsen schizophrenia, CBD has antipsychotic effects, according to previous research in both animals and humans. The use of CBD for schizophrenia is becoming more and more common. Studies from around the world are showing great promise [75]. Moreover, fMRI results strongly suggest that the antipsychotic effects of CBD involve the striatum and temporal cortex that have been traditionally associated with psychosis [76].

Antipsychotic-like activity of *Morinda citrifolia* in mice demonstrated the antidopaminergic effect, suggesting that this plant has antipsychotic-like activity which can be utilized in the treatment of psychiatric disorders [77].

No available scientific literature is found regarding antipsychotic effects of six plants which were used by the traditional medical practitioners' of Rangamati Sadar Upazila, Bangladesh, and these six species are *A. augusta* L.f, *L. polyantha* Juss., *P. retrofractum* Vahl., *F. hirta* Vahl., *T. peruviana* (Pers.) K. Schum, and *Datura metel* L. However, it is very much important to conduct proper scientific study for the evaluation of antipsychotic effects of these plants. Bangladesh has a very rich diversity of medicinal plant species which has been used by the traditional healers of several districts for the treatment of different diseases like mental health problems, brain disorders, malaria, cardiovascular disorders, diabetes, tumor, snake bite, and rheumatoid arthritis [78–85]. Thus the body of the existing ethnomedical knowledge has led to great developments in schizophrenia as well as can be the source for the discovery of new antipsychotic drugs.

5. Conclusions

The use of psychoactive plants is practically a universal human phenomenon. Except for a few cultures lacking access to psychoactive plants, humans tend to use them routinely. The psychological and behavioral effects of such plants have been long recognized and information about their uses has been passed down through generations. However, with the advent of modern science we are able to better understand the composition of these plants and how they interact with the nervous system.

The available scientific literature strongly suggests that at least some of the plants used by the traditional medical practitioners of Bangladesh may have strong scientific basis for their use in the treatment of schizophrenia like psychotic episodes. This ethnobotanical data provides an interesting basis for further phytotherapeutical research towards discovery of novel and efficacious antipsychotic drugs, especially concerning uncommonly used species (i.e., *A. augusta* L.f, *L. polyantha* Juss., *P. retrofractum* Vahl., *F. hirta* Vahl., *T. peruviana* (Pers.) K. Schum, and *Datura metel* L.). Although some formulations have drawn attention, in depth clinical trials of each one of the plants presented in the table should be conducted which will be a major tool to prove the benefits for a schizophrenia patient as well as to evaluate more scientific researches for discovering the new antipsychotic drugs with giving less side effects.

Conflict of Interests

The authors declare that there is no conflict of interests regarding the publication of this paper.

Acknowledgments

The authors are grateful to Robin S. Rosenberg and Stephen M. Kosslyn, authors of the book of "Abnormal Psychology," for Chapter 12. The book was very helpful in developing the concept in the field of schizophrenia. Thanks are also due to the traditional medical practitioners of Rangamati for their cooperation and help during the ethnomedicinal survey. All authors edited the paper and read and approved the final paper.

References

[1] S. Hodgins, "Mental disorder, intellectual deficiency, and crime: evidence from a birth cohort," *Archives of General Psychiatry*, vol. 49, no. 6, pp. 476–483, 1992.

[2] S. Hodgins, S. A. Mednick, P. A. Brennan, F. Schulsinger, and M. Engberg, "Mental disorder and crime: evidence from a Danish birth cohort," *Archives of General Psychiatry*, vol. 53, no. 6, pp. 489–496, 1996.

[3] I. I. Gottesman, *Schizophrenia Genesis: The Origin of Madness*, Freeman, New York, NY, USA, 1991.

[4] J. Perälä, J. Suvisaari, S. I. Saarni et al., "Lifetime prevalence of psychotic and bipolar I disorders in a general population," *Archives of General Psychiatry*, vol. 64, no. 1, pp. 19–28, 2007.

[5] C. J. L. Murray and A. D. Lopez, Eds., *The Global Burden of Disease. A Comprehensive Assessment of Mortality and Disability from Diseases, Injuries, and Risk Factors in 1990 and Projected to 2020*, Harvard School of Public Health, Cambridge, Mass, USA, 1996.

[6] E. F. Torrey, *Surviving Schizophrenia: A Manual for Families, Consumers, and Providers*, Quill, New York, NY, USA, 4th edition, 2001.

[7] A. H. M. Firoz, M. E. Karim, M. F. Alam, A. H. M. Rahman, M. N. Zaman, and V. Chandra, "Community based Multicentric Service Oriented Research on mental illness with focus on prevalence, medical care, awareness and attitude towards mental illness in Bangladesh. WHO published data, 2003–2005," *Bangladesh Journal of Psychiatry*, vol. 20, no. 1, pp. 9–32, 2006.

[8] J. Addington and P. Bumett, "Working with families in the early stages of Psychosis," in *Psychological Interventions in Early Psychosis: A Treatment Handbook*, J. F. M. Gleeson and P. D. McGorry, Eds., pp. 99–116, John Wiley & Sons, Chichester, UK, 2004.

[9] Department of Health, *The Policy Implementation Guide for Mental Health*, Her Majesty's Stationery Office (HMSO), London, UK, 2001.

[10] M. A. Mohit, "Diagnosis of patients attending Out Patient Department (OPD) of NIMH," *Bangladesh Journal Psychiatry*, vol. 15, no. 1, pp. 5–12, 2001.

[11] M. Gelder, D. Gath, R. Mayou, and P. Cowen, *Oxford Text Book of Psychiatry*, Oxford University Press, Oxford, UK, 5th edition, 2005.

[12] A. Fahmida, M. A. Wahab, and M. M. Rahman, "Pattern of psychiatric morbidity among the patients admitted in a private psychiatric clinic," *Bangladesh Journal of Medical Science*, vol. 8, no. 1, pp. 1–2, 2009.

[13] H. Freeman, "Schizophrenia and city residence," *British Journal of Psychiatry*, vol. 164, no. 23, pp. 39–50, 1994.

[14] P. B. Mortensen, C. B. Pedersen, T. Westergaard et al., "Effects of family history and place and season of birth on the risk of schizophrenia," *The New England Journal of Medicine*, vol. 340, no. 8, pp. 603–608, 1999.

[15] D. Babić and R. Babić, "Complementary and alternative medicine in the treatment of schizophrenia," *Psychiatria Danubina*, vol. 21, no. 3, pp. 376–381, 2009.

[16] G. Elkins, M. H. Rajab, and J. Marcus, "Complementary and alternative medicine use by psychiatric inpatients," *Psychological Reports*, vol. 96, no. 1, pp. 163–166, 2005.

[17] U. Dhar, R. S. Rawal, S. S. Samant, S. Airi, and J. Upreti, "People's participation in Himalayan biodiversity conservation: a practical approach," *Current Science*, vol. 76, no. 1, pp. 36–40, 1999.

[18] J. M. Balick and P. A. Cox, *Plants, People and Culture: the Science of Ethnobotany*, Scientific American Library, New York, NY, USA, 1996.

[19] A. H. Gilani and A. U. Rahman, "Trends in ethnopharmacology," *Journal of Ethnopharmacology*, vol. 100, no. 1-2, pp. 43–49, 2005.

[20] M. M. Romeiras, M. C. Duarte, B. Indjai, and L. Catarino, "Medicinal plants used to treat neurological disorders in West Africa: a case study with Guinea-Bissau Flora," *American Journal of Plant Sciences*, vol. 3, no. 7, pp. 1028–1036, 2012.

[21] M. A. H. Mollik, M. S. H. Hossan, A. K. Paul, M. Taufiq-Ur-Rahman, R. Jahan, and M. Rahmatullah, "A comparative analysis of medicinal plants used by folk medicinal healers in three districts of Bangladesh and inquiry as to mode of selection of medicinal plants," *Ethnobotany Research and Applications*, vol. 8, pp. 195–218, 2010.

[22] M. Rahmatullah, M. A. H. Mollik, M. N. Ahmed et al., "A survey of medicinal plants used by folk medicinal practitioners in two villages of Tangail district, Bangladesh," *American-Eurasian Journal of Sustainable Agriculture*, vol. 4, no. 3, pp. 357–362, 2010.

[23] M. S. Hossan, A. Hanif, B. Agarwala et al., "Traditional use of medicinal plants in Bangladesh to treat urinary tract infections and sexually transmitted diseases," *Ethnobotany Research and Applications*, vol. 8, pp. 61–74, 2010.

[24] M. Rahmatullah, D. Ferdausi, M. A. H. Mollik, R. Jahan, M. H. Chowdhury, and W. M. Haque, "A survey of medicinal plants used by Kavirajes of Chalna area, Khulna district, Bangladesh," *African Journal of Traditional, Complementary and Alternative Medicines*, vol. 7, no. 2, pp. 91–97, 2010.

[25] F. I. Jahan, M. R. U. Hasan, R. Jahan et al., "A comparison of medicinal plant usage by folk medicinal practitioners of two adjoining villages in Lalmonirhat district, Bangladesh," *American-Eurasian Journal of Sustainable Agriculture*, vol. 5, no. 1, pp. 46–66, 2011.

[26] B. Berlin and E. A. Berlin, "Anthropological issues in medical anthropology," in *Ethnobotany and the Search for New Drugs*, G. Prance, Ed., Ciba Foundation Symposium No. 185, pp. 240–258, John Wiley and Sons, New York, NY, USA, 1994.

[27] C. H. Browner, B. R. Ortiz de Montellano, and A. J. Rubel, "A methodology for cross-cultural ethnomedical research," *Current Anthropology*, vol. 29, pp. 681–702, 1988.

[28] G. J. Martin, *Ethnobotany: A "People and Plants" Conservation Manual*, Chapman and Hall, London, UK, 1995.

[29] M. N. Alexiades, Ed., *Selected Guidelines for Ethno Botanical Research: A Field Manual*, The New York Botanical Garden, New York, NY, USA, 1996.

[30] P. Maundu, "Methodology for collecting and sharing indigenous knowledge: a case study," *Indigenous Knowledge and Development Monitor*, vol. 3, pp. 3–5, 1995.

[31] "The plant list database," http://www.theplantlist.org/.

[32] M. Ayyanar and S. Ignacimuthu, "Traditional knowledge of Kani tribals in Kouthalai of Tirunelveli hills, Tamil Nadu, India," *Journal of Ethnopharmacology*, vol. 102, no. 2, pp. 246–255, 2005.

[33] S. Bhattarai, R. P. Chaudhary, C. L. Quave, and R. S. L. Taylor, "The use of medicinal plants in the trans-himalayan arid zone of Mustang district, Nepal," *Journal of Ethnobiology and Ethnomedicine*, vol. 6, article 14, 2010.

[34] C. A. Ross, R. L. Margolis, S. A. J. Reading, M. Pletnikov, and J. T. Coyle, "Neurobiology of Schizophrenia," *Neuron*, vol. 52, no. 1, pp. 139–153, 2006.

[35] S. E. Arnold, K. Talbot, and C. Hahn, "Neurodevelopment, neuroplasticity, and new genes for schizophrenia," *Progress in Brain Research*, vol. 147, pp. 319–345, 2005.

[36] P. J. Harrison and D. R. Weinberger, "Schizophrenia genes, gene expression, and neuropathology: on the matter of their convergence," *Molecular Psychiatry*, vol. 10, no. 1, pp. 40–68, 2005.

[37] J. L. Rapoport, A. M. Addington, S. Frangou, and M. R. C. Psych, "The neurodevelopmental model of schizophrenia: update 2005," *Molecular Psychiatry*, vol. 10, no. 5, pp. 434–449, 2005.

[38] B. Dean, "Understanding the pathology of schizophrenia: recent advances from the study of the molecular architecture of postmortem CNS tissue," *Postgraduate Medical Journal*, vol. 78, no. 917, pp. 142–148, 2002.

[39] A. B. Goodman and A. B. Pardee, "Meeting report; 'Molecular neurobiological mechanisms in schizophrenia: seeking a synthesis," *Biological Psychiatry*, vol. 48, no. 3, pp. 173–183, 2000.

[40] H. Y. Meltzer, "Biochemical studies in schizophrenia," *Schizophrenia Bulletin*, vol. 2, no. 1, pp. 10–18, 1976.

[41] S. Kapur, "Psychosis as a state of aberrant salience: a framework linking biology, phenomenology, and pharmacology in schizophrenia," *The American Journal of Psychiatry*, vol. 160, no. 1, pp. 13–23, 2003.

[42] M. Huttunen, "The evolution of the serotonin-dopamine antagonist concept," *Journal of Clinical Psychopharmacology*, vol. 15, supplement 1, no. 1, pp. 4S–10S, 1995.

[43] B. P. Riley and P. McGuffin, "Linkage and associated studies of schizophrenia," *The American Journal of Medical Genetics*, vol. 97, pp. 23–44, 2000.

[44] S. I. Deutsch, J. Mastropaolo, B. L. Schwartz, R. B. Rosse, and J. M. Morihisa, "A "glutamatergic hypothesis" of schizophrenia. Rationale for pharmacotherapy with glycine," *Clinical Neuropharmacology*, vol. 12, no. 1, pp. 1–13, 1989.

[45] C. Abbott and J. Bustillo, "What have we learned from proton magnetic resonance spectroscopy about schizophrenia? A critical update," *Current Opinion in Psychiatry*, vol. 19, no. 2, pp. 135–139, 2006.

[46] L. Tebartz van Elst, G. Valerius, M. Büchert et al., "Increased prefrontal and hippocampal glutamate concentration in schizophrenia: evidence from a magnetic resonance spectroscopy study," *Biological Psychiatry*, vol. 58, no. 9, pp. 724–730, 2005.

[47] D. A. Lewis and B. Moghaddam, "Cognitive dysfunction in schizophrenia: convergence of γ-aminobutyric acid and glutamate alterations," *Archives of Neurology*, vol. 63, no. 10, pp. 1372–1376, 2006.

[48] E. F. Walker, C. B. Logan, and D. Walder, "Indicators of neurodevelopmental abnormality in schizotypal personality disorder," *Psychiatric Annals*, vol. 29, no. 3, pp. 132–136, 1999.

[49] E. F. Walker, D. J. Walder, and F. Reynolds, "Developmental changes in cortisol secretion in normal and at-risk youth," *Development & Psychopathology*, vol. 13, no. 3, pp. 721–732, 2001.

[50] X. Y. Zhang, D. F. Zhou, L. Y. Cao, G. Y. Wu, and Y. C. Shen, "Cortisol and cytokines in chronic and treatment-resistant patients with schizophrenia: association with psychopathology and response to antipsychotics," *Neuropsychopharmacology*, vol. 30, no. 8, pp. 1532–1538, 2005.

[51] T. Ohnuma, S. J. Augood, H. Arai, P. J. McKenna, and P. C. Emson, "Measurement of GABAergic parameters in the prefrontal cortex in schizophrenia: focus on GABA content, GABA(A) receptor α-1 subunit messenger RNA and human GABA transporter-1 (hGAT-1) messenger RNA expression," *Neuroscience*, vol. 93, no. 2, pp. 441–448, 1999.

[52] M. M. Huntsman, B. V. Tran, S. G. Potkin, W. E. Bunney Jr., and E. G. Jones, "Altered ratios of alternatively spliced long and short $\gamma 2$ subunit mRNAs of the γ-amino butyrate type A receptor in prefrontal cortex of schizophrenics," *Proceedings of the National Academy of Sciences of the United States of America*, vol. 95, no. 25, pp. 15066–15071, 1998.

[53] D. O. Kennedy and E. L. Wightman, "Herbal extracts and phytochemicals: plant secondary metabolites and the enhancement of human brain function," *Advances in Nutrition*, vol. 2, no. 1, pp. 32–50, 2011.

[54] M. Spinella, *The Psychopharmacology of Herbal Medicine: Plant Drugs that Alter the Mind, Brain and Behavior*, MIT Press, Cambridge, UK, 2011.

[55] J. Sarris, "Herbal medicines in the treatment of psychiatric disorders: a systematic review," *Phytotherapy Research*, vol. 21, no. 8, pp. 703–716, 2007.

[56] V. Kumar, "Potential medicinal plants for CNS disorders: an overview," *Phytotherapy Research*, vol. 20, no. 12, pp. 1023–1035, 2006.

[57] D. S. Avinash, "Herbal medicine and anxiety disorders: an overview," *Journal of Medicinal Plants Studies*, vol. 1, no. 6, pp. 18–23, 2013.

[58] M. F. Green, *Schizophrenia Revealed: From Neurons to Social Interactions*, W.W. Norton, New York, NY, USA, 2001.

[59] B. Rosenbaum, K. Valbak, S. Harder et al., "The Danish National Schizophrenia Project: prospective, comparative longitudinal treatment study of first-episode psychosis," *British Journal of Psychiatry*, vol. 186, pp. 394–399, 2005.

[60] Z. Zhang, "Therapeutic effects of herbal extracts and constituents in animal models of psychiatric disorders," *Life Sciences*, vol. 75, no. 14, pp. 1659–1699, 2004.

[61] P. Bigoniya and A. C. Rana, "Psychopharmacological profile of hydro-alcoholic extract of Euphorbia neriifolia leaves in mice and rats," *Indian Journal of Experimental Biology*, vol. 43, no. 10, pp. 859–862, 2005.

[62] M. M. Ghaisas, P. B. Ninave, G. P. Ganu, V. S. Zope, M. B. Tanwar, and A. D. Deshpande, "Effect of *Randia dumetorum* Lam on clonidine and haloperidol-induced catalepsy in mice," *Pharmacologyonline*, vol. 2, pp. 42–50, 2008.

[63] S. Kothari, M. Minda, and S. D. Tonpay, "Anxiolytic and antidepressant activities of methanol extract of *Aegle marmelos* leaves in mice," *Indian Journal of Physiology and Pharmacology*, vol. 54, no. 4, pp. 318–328, 2010.

[64] K. P. S. Raj and M. R. Patel, "Some medicinal plants of Cambay and its immediate vicinity and their uses in Indian indigenous system of medicine," *Indian Drugs*, vol. 15, pp. 145–152, 1978.

[65] J. K. Maheshwari and J. P. Singh, "Plants used in ethnomedicine by the Kols of Allahabad district Uttar Pradesh," *Bulletin of Medico-Ethno-Botanical Reserch*, vol. 5, pp. 105–121, 1984.

[66] M. Rahmatullah, A. Hasan, and W. Parvin, "Medicinal plants an formulations used by the sore clan of the Santal tribe in Rajshahi District, Bangladesh for treatment of various ailemnts," *African Journal of Traditional, Complementary, and Alternative Medicines*, vol. 9, no. 3, pp. 350–359, 2012.

[67] M. Rahmatullah, Md. A. H. Mollik, A. T. M. A. Azam et al., "Ethnobotanical survey of the Santal tribe residing in Thakurgaon District, Bangladesh," *American-Eurasian Journal of Sustainable Agriculture*, vol. 3, no. 4, pp. 889–898, 2009.

[68] M. H. Boskabady, S. Kiani, and B. Haghiri, "Relaxant effects of *Ocimum basilicum* on guinea pig tracheal chains and its possible mechanism(s)," *DARU*, vol. 13, no. 1, pp. 28–33, 2005.

[69] M. Md. Rashid, F. B. Rafique, N. Debnath et al., "Medicinal plants and formulations of a community of the Tonchongya tribe in Bandarban district of Bangladesh," *The American-Eurasian Journal of Sustainable Agriculture*, vol. 6, no. 4, pp. 292–298, 2012.

[70] N. L. Soh and G. Walter, "Traditional and alternative medicine treatments in child and adolescent mental health," in *IACAPAP e-Textbook of Child and Adolescent Mental Health*, J. M. Rey, Ed., International Association for Child and Adolescent Psychiatry and Allied Professions, Geneva, Switzerland, 2012.

[71] V. Agarwal, A. Abhijnhan, and P. Raviraj, "Ayurvedic medicine for schizophrenia," *Cochrane Database of Systematic Reviews*, vol. 3, Article ID CD006867, 2010.

[72] L. B. Borse, A. K. Muthu, A. Thangatripathi, and S. L. Borse, "Antidopaminergic activity of *vitex negundo* (linn) roots," *Asian Journal of Chemistry*, vol. 24, no. 7, pp. 3171–3173, 2012.

[73] R. S. Adnaik, P. T. Pai, V. D. Sapakal, N. S. Naikwade, and C. S. Magdum, "Anxiolytic activity of *Vitex negundo* linn. in experimental models of anxiety in mice," *International Journal of Green Pharmacy*, vol. 3, no. 3, pp. 243–247, 2009.

[74] F. M. Leweke, D. Piomelli, F. Pahlisch et al., "Cannabidiol enhances anandamide signaling and alleviates psychotic symptoms of schizophrenia," *Translational Psychiatry*, vol. 2, article e94, 2012.

[75] S. Deiana, "Medical use of cannabis. Cannabidiol: a new light for schizophrenia?" *Drug Testing and Analysis*, vol. 5, no. 1, pp. 46–51, 2013.

[76] A. W. Zuardi, J. A. Crippa, J. E. Hallak et al., "A critical review of the antipsychotic effects of cannabidiol: 30 years of a translational investigation," *Current Pharmaceutical Design*, vol. 18, no. 32, pp. 5131–5140, 2012.

[77] P. Vijayapandi, N. Megala, and M. Zahurin, "Antipsychotic-like activity of noni (*Morinda citrifolia* Linn.) in mice," *BMC Complementary and Alternative Medicine*, vol. 12, article 186, 2012.

[78] M. N. K. Azam, M. A. Mannan, and M. N. Ahmed, "Medicinal plants used by traditional medical practitioners of Barendra and Shamatat (Rajshahi Khulna division) region in Bangladesh for treatment of cardiovascular disorders," *Journal of Medicinal Plants Studies*, vol. 2, no. 2, pp. 9–14, 2014.

[79] M. Rahmatullah, S. Hossain, A. Khatun, S. Seraj, and R. Jahan, "Medicinal plants used by various tribes of Bangladesh for treatment of Malaria," *Malaria Research and Treatment*, vol. 2012, Article ID 371798, 5 pages, 2012.

[80] M. A. H. Mollik, "A preliminary study on the efficacy of medicinal plants from the Lawacherra Rain Forest used for all forms of brain disorders," *Alzheimer's & Dementia*, vol. 6, supplement 4, p. S44, 2010.

[81] M. N. Ahmed, M. N. K. Azam, U. S. Zohora, and M. N. Hasan, "Use of medicinal plants against snake venom to treat snake bite by folk medicinal practitioners in Barandra and Shamatat region of Bangladesh," in *Proceedings of the International Conference Updates on Natural Products in Medicine and Healthcare Systems*, Khulna, Bangladesh, July 2013.

[82] M. N. Hasan, M. N. Ahmed, M. Z. A. Bhuiyan, M. M. Rahman, M. N. K. Azam, and M. Rahmatullah, "Medicinal plants used in treatment of tumors: results from a survey of folk medicinal practitioners," in *Proceedings of the International Conference on Green Chemistry for Sustainable Development*, Jessore, Bangladesh, July 2012.

[83] M. Rahmatullah, R. Jahan, A. K. Azad et al., "A randomized survey of medicinal plants used by folk medicinal practitioners in six districts of Bangladesh to treat rheumatoid arthritis," *Advances in Natural and Applied Sciences*, vol. 4, no. 2, pp. 124–127, 2010.

[84] M. Rahmatullah, M. N. K. Azam, Z. Khatun et al., "Medicinal plants used for treatment of diabetes by the Marakh sect of the Garo tribe living in Mymensingh district, Bangladesh," *The African Journal of Traditional, Complementary and Alternative Medicines*, vol. 9, no. 3, pp. 380–385, 2012.

[85] M. A. H. Mollik, "Beideyes in Kurigram district of Bangladesh: their knowledge of common mental health problems and possible role in primary health care," *Alzheimers Dementia*, vol. 6, no. 4, article S337, 2006.

Permissions

All chapters in this book were first published in SCHIZORT, by Hindawi Publishing Corporation; hereby published with permission under the Creative Commons Attribution License or equivalent. Every chapter published in this book has been scrutinized by our experts. Their significance has been extensively debated. The topics covered herein carry significant findings which will fuel the growth of the discipline. They may even be implemented as practical applications or may be referred to as a beginning point for another development.

The contributors of this book come from diverse backgrounds, making this book a truly international effort. This book will bring forth new frontiers with its revolutionizing research information and detailed analysis of the nascent developments around the world.

We would like to thank all the contributing authors for lending their expertise to make the book truly unique. They have played a crucial role in the development of this book. Without their invaluable contributions this book wouldn't have been possible. They have made vital efforts to compile up to date information on the varied aspects of this subject to make this book a valuable addition to the collection of many professionals and students.

This book was conceptualized with the vision of imparting up-to-date information and advanced data in this field. To ensure the same, a matchless editorial board was set up. Every individual on the board went through rigorous rounds of assessment to prove their worth. After which they invested a large part of their time researching and compiling the most relevant data for our readers.

The editorial board has been involved in producing this book since its inception. They have spent rigorous hours researching and exploring the diverse topics which have resulted in the successful publishing of this book. They have passed on their knowledge of decades through this book. To expedite this challenging task, the publisher supported the team at every step. A small team of assistant editors was also appointed to further simplify the editing procedure and attain best results for the readers.

Apart from the editorial board, the designing team has also invested a significant amount of their time in understanding the subject and creating the most relevant covers. They scrutinized every image to scout for the most suitable representation of the subject and create an appropriate cover for the book.

The publishing team has been an ardent support to the editorial, designing and production team. Their endless efforts to recruit the best for this project, has resulted in the accomplishment of this book. They are a veteran in the field of academics and their pool of knowledge is as vast as their experience in printing. Their expertise and guidance has proved useful at every step. Their uncompromising quality standards have made this book an exceptional effort. Their encouragement from time to time has been an inspiration for everyone.

The publisher and the editorial board hope that this book will prove to be a valuable piece of knowledge for researchers, students, practitioners and scholars across the globe.

List of Contributors

Ravi Philip Rajkumar
Department of Psychiatry, Jawaharlal Institute of Postgraduate Medical Education and Research (JIPMER), Dhanvantari Nagar, 605 006 Pondicherry, India

Saeed Shoja Shafti
University of Social Welfare and Rehabilitation Sciences (USWR), Razi Psychiatric Hospital, P.O. Box 18735-569, Tehran, Iran

Mahsa Gilanipoor
Razi Psychiatric Hospital, P.O. Box 18735-569, Tehran, Iran

Jihun Hamm
Department of Computer Science and Engineering, The Ohio State University, Columbus, OH 43210, USA

Amy Pinkham
Southern Methodist University, Dallas, TX 75205, USA

Ruben C. Gur and Christian G. Kohler
Department of Psychiatry, Neuropsychiatry Section, University of Pennsylvania, Philadelphia, PA 19104, USA

Ruben C. Gur
Philadelphia Veterans Administration Medical Center, Philadelphia, PA 19104, USA

Ragini Verma
Department of Radiology, Section of Biomedical Image Analysis, University of Pennsylvania, Philadelphia, PA 19104, USA

David H. Adams, Lu Zhang, Brian A. Millen, Bruce J. Kinon and Juan-Carlos Gomez
Lilly Research Laboratories, Eli Lilly and Company, Lilly Corporate Center, Indianapolis, IN 46285, USA
Brendan P. Murphy
Early in Life Mental Health Service, Southern Health, Melbourne, VIC 3175, Australia
School of Psychology and Psychiatry, Monash University, Melbourne, VIC 3800, Australia

Terence Y. Pang and Anthony J. Hannan
Howard Florey Institute, Florey Neuroscience Institutes, University of Melbourne, Melbourne, VIC 3052, Australia

Tina-Marie Proffitt, Mirabel McConchie, Melissa Kerr, Connie Markulev and Patrick D. McGorry
Orygen Youth Health Research Centre, University of Melbourne, Melbourne, VIC 3052, Australia

Colin O'Donnell
St. Davnet's Hospital, Monaghan, County Monaghan, Ireland

Gregor E. Berger
Department of Child and Adolescent Psychiatry, University of Zurich, 8032 Zurich, Switzerland

Erika Jääskeläinen, Nina Rautio, Tanja Nordström, Ina Rissanen, Emmi Keskinen, Riikka Marttila, Svetlana Filatova, Tiina-Mari Paaso and Jouko Miettunen
Center for Life Course Epidemiology and Systems Medicine, University of Oulu, P.O. Box 5000, 90014 Oulu, Finland

Marianne Haapea, Pauliina Juola, Matti Penttilä, Kristiina Moilanen, Anja Husa, Erika Jääskeläinen, Nina Rautio, Tanja Nordström, Ina Rissanen, Emmi Keskinen, Tiina-Mari Paaso,
Riikka Marttila, Svetlana Filatova and Jouko Miettunen
Medical Research Center Oulu, Oulu University Hospital and University of Oulu, P.O. Box 5000, 90014 Oulu, Finland

Marianne Haapea, Pauliina Juola, Jenni Koivukangas, Matti Penttilä, Matti Isohanni, Kristiina Moilanen, Anja Husa, Erika Jääskeläinen, Ina Rissanen, Emmi Keskinen, Jouko Miettunen,
Riikka Marttila and Svetlana Filatova
Department of Psychiatry, Center for Clinical Neurosciences, University of Oulu, P.O. Box 5000, 90014 Oulu, Finland

Marianne Haapea, Pauliina Juola, Matti Penttilä, Matti Isohanni, Kristiina Moilanen, Anja Husa, Svetlana Filatova and Jouko Miettunen
Department of Psychiatry, Oulu University Hospital, P.O. Box 26, 90029 Oulu, Finland

Nina Rautio
Unit of Primary Health Care, Oulu University Hospital, P.O. Box 10, 90029 Oulu, Finland

Jenni Koivukangas
Aurora Doctoral Programme, Th le Institute, University of Oulu, P.O. Box 7300, Oulu, Finland

Rajeev Krishnadas
Sackler Institute of Psychobiological Research, Southern General Hospital, Room 25, University Corridor, Ground Floor, Neurology Building, Glasgow G51 4TF, UK

Seethalakshmi Ramanathan
Hutchings Psychiatric Center, NYS Office of Mental Health, Syracuse, NY 13210, USA

Eugene Wong
Gartnavel Royal Hospital, Glasgow G12 0XH, UK

Ajita Nayak
Department of Psychiatry, KEM Hospital, Mumbai 400012, India

Brian Moore
Newcastle General Hospital, 1st Floor, Building 15, Westgate Road, Newcastle upon Tyne NE4 6BE, UK

Annika Clamor, A. Malika Warmuth and Tania M. Lincoln
Department of Clinical Psychology and Psychotherapy, University of Hamburg, Von-Melle-Park 5, 20146 Hamburg, Germany
Florent Auger, Patrick Duriez, Françoise Martin-Nizard, Nicolas Durieux, Régis Bordet and Olivier Pétrault
Universite´ Lille Nord de France, 59000 Lille, France

Régis Bordet, Patrick Duriez and Florent Auger
De´partement de Pharmacologie Me´dicale, CHULille, EA 1046, 59000 Lille, France

Florent Auger
Inserm, U837, 59000 Lille, France

Olivier Pétrault, Régis Bordet, Nicolas Durieux, Patrick Duriez and Florent Auger
IMPRT-IFR114, 59000 Lille, France

Françoise Martin-Nizard and Patrick Duriez
Faculte´ de Pharmacie, 59006 Lille, France

Françoise Martin-Nizard
Inserm, U1011, 59000 Lille, France

Françoise Martin-Nizard
Institut Pasteur de Lille, 59019 Lille, France

Olivier Pétrault
UArtois, 62300 Lens, France

Olivier Pétrault
Laboratoire de Pharmacologie Me´dicale, EA 1046, Faculte´ de Me´decine, Universite´ Lille2, Po^le Pecherche, 1 Place de Verdun, 59045 Lille Cedex, France

Esme Fuller-Thomson and Bailey Hollister
Factor-Inwentash Faculty of Social Work, University of Toronto, Toronto, ON, Canada M5S 1V4

Alexandre González-Rodríguez
Barcelona Clinic Schizophrenia Unit (BCSU), Neurosciences Institute, Hospital Clinic of Barcelona, University of Barcelona, 170 Villarroel Street, 08036 Barcelona, Spain

Oriol Molina-Andreu
Department of Mental Health, Hospital Universitari Mu´tua de Terrassa, 5 Doctor Robert Street, 08221 Terrassa, Spain

Marina Garriga
Barcelona Clinic Schizophrenia Unit (BCSU), Bipolar Disorders Unit, Neurosciences Institute, Hospital Clinic of Barcelona, University of Barcelona, 170 Villarroel Street, 08036 Barcelona, Spain

Rafael Penadés, Alexandre Pons, Rosa Catalán and Miguel Bernardo
Barcelona Clinic Schizophrenia Unit (BCSU), Neurosciences Institute, Hospital Clinic of Barcelona, Department of Psychiatry and Clinical Psychobiology, University of Barcelona, 170 Villarroel Street, 08036 Barcelona, Spain
Centro de Investigacio´n Biome´dica en Red en Salud Mental (CIBERSAM), Institut d'Investigacions Biome`diques August Pi i Sunyer (IDIBAPS), 149 Rossello´ Street, 08036
Barcelona, Spain

Alexander M. Rapp, Karin Langohr, Dorothee E. Mutschler and Barbara Wild
Department of Psychiatry, University of Tuebingen, Calwerstraße 14, 72076 Tuebingen, Germany

Ann Blomgren Mannerheim and Eleni Siouta
Karolinska Institute, Division of Nursing, Department of Neurobiology, Care Science and Society, 171 77 Stockholm, Sweden

Ulla Hellström Muhli
Department of Sociology, Uppsala University, Box 624, 751 26 Uppsala, Sweden

Eleni Siouta
Department of Learning, Informatics, Management and Ethics (LIME), Karolinska Institute, 171 77 Stockholm, Sweden
Sophiahemmet University, Box 5605, 114 86 Stockholm, Sweden

Shahram Khademvatan
Health Research Institute, Infectious and Tropical Diseases Research Center, Department of Medical Parasitology, Ahvaz Jundishapur University of Medical Sciences, P.O. Box 613715794, Ahvaz, Iran

Niloufar Khajeddin
Department of Psychiatry, Ahvaz Jundishapur University of Medical Sciences, Ahvaz, Iran

Sakineh Izadi
Department of Psychology, Shahid Chamran University, Ahvaz, Iran

Elham Yousefi
Research Institute for Infectious Disease of Digestive System, Department of Medical Parasitology, Ahvaz Jundishapur University of Medical Sciences, Ahvaz, Iran

Quintino R. Mano, Gregory G. Brown, Heline Mirzakhanian, Khalima Bolden, Kristen S. Cadenhead and Gregory A. Light
San Diego Veterans Affairs Healthcare System, San Diego, CA 92161, USA
VISN-22 Mental Illness, Research, Education and Clinical Center (MIRECC), VA San Diego Healthcare System, San Diego, CA 92161, USA
Department of Psychiatry, University of California, San Diego, School of Medicine, San Diego, CA, USA

Adam Gater, Chloe Tolley, Chris Marshall and Linda Abetz-Webb
Adelphi Mill, Grimshaw Lane, Bollington, Cheshire SK10 5JB, UK

Diana Rofail
Roche Products Ltd., Hexagon Place, 6 Falcon Way, Welwyn Garden City, Hertfordshire AL7 1TW, UK

Steven H. Zarit
305 Health & Human Development East, The Pennsylvania State University, University Park, PA
16802, USA

Carmen Galani Berardo
F. Hoffmann La-Roche Ltd., Grenzacherstrasse 124, 4070 Basel, Switzerland

Anna Dietrich-Muszalska and Justyna Kopka
Department of Biological Psychiatry, The Chair of Experimental and Clinical Physiology, Medical University of Lodz, 6/8 Mazowiecka Street, 92-215 Lodz, Poland

Bogdan Kontek
Department of General Biochemistry, Faculty of Biology and Environmental Protection, University of Lodz, 90-236 Lodz, Poland

Martin Wiesjahn, Esther Jung, Fabian Lamster and Winfried Rief
Department of Psychology, Division of Clinical Psychology and Psychotherapy, Philipps-Universität Marburg, 35032 Marburg, Germany

Tania M. Lincoln
Institute of Psychology, Department of Clinical Psychology and Psychotherapy, Universität
Hamburg, 20146 Hamburg, Germany

Youssef Kouidrat and Jean-Daniel Lalau
Department of Endocrinology, University of Picardie-Jules Verne, CHU d'Amiens, Amiens, France

Youssef Kouidrat
Department of Nutrition, Hôpital maritime, Assistance Publique-Hôpitaux de Paris (AP-HP), 62600 Berck, France

Ali Amad
Psychiatry Department and SCA-lab, PSYchiC team, Université de Lille, 59100 Lille, France

Gwenole Loas
Department of Psychiatry, Erasme Hospital, ULB, 1070 Brussels, Belgium

Hanne Skarsholm
The Psychiatry in the Region of Southern Denmark, Søndre, Sdr. Boulevard 29, 5000 Odense C, Denmark

Henrik Stoevring
Department of Public Health, Aarhus University, 8000 Aarhus C, Denmark

Bent Nielsen
Department of Psychiatry, The Psychiatry in the Region of Southern Denmark, 5000 Odense, Denmark

Md. Nasir Ahmed and Md. Nur Kabidul Azam
Ethnobotany & Ethnomedicine Division, TechB Herbal Solution, Bheramara, Kushtia 7040, Bangladesh